简明妇产科学

Obstetrics and Gynecology: A Short Textbook

（中英文对照）

主　编　温　菁　张　莉

副主编　贾琳钰　路旭宏　王学慧
　　　　魏　巍

编　者　马晓秋　刘　芳　刘　健
　　　　佟春艳　陈艺华

绘　图　王秀敏

科学出版社

北　京

内 容 简 介

本书是根据双语教学课程的需求，参考国家卫健委"十三五"规划教材《妇产科学》（第 9 版）而编写的中英文对照《简明妇产科学》。共分 24 章介绍女性生殖系统解剖、生理、妊娠、产前检查与保健、正常分娩、异常分娩及妇产科疾病。本书以中英文对照、条目的形式编排，帮助读者学习掌握必备的妇产科相关英语知识，并在每一章节末附有重点关键词汇、练习题等以便读者复习。内容精练、实用、易于掌握，适于广大医学院校师生、临床医师参考阅读。

图书在版编目（CIP）数据

简明妇产科学＝Obstetrics and Gynecology：A Short Textbook：汉英对照 /
温菁，张莉主编.—北京：科学出版社，2020.8
ISBN 978-7-03-065718-3

Ⅰ.①简…　Ⅱ.①温…　②张…　Ⅲ.①妇产科学－汉、英　Ⅳ.①R71

中国版本图书馆CIP数据核字（2020）第131853号

责任编辑：马　莉 / 责任校对：郭瑞芝
责任印制：李　彤 / 封面设计：龙　岩

科 学 出 版 社 出版
北京东黄城根北街 16 号
邮政编码：100717
http://www.sciencep.com

北京凌奇印刷有限责任公司 印刷

科学出版社发行　各地新华书店经销
*

2020 年 8 月第　一　版　开本：787×1092　1/16
2020 年 8 月第一次印刷　印张：18 1/2
字数：430 000
POD定价：98.00元
（如有印装质量问题，我社负责调换）

主编简介

温菁，女，大连大学附属中山医院妇产科教研室主任，主任医师，教授，研究生导师，妇产科学课程专业负责人。长期从事妇产科临床、教学、科研工作。社会兼职：大连市医学会妇产科专科分会委员、辽宁省中西医结合学会妇科内分泌及绝经专业委员会常务委员、辽宁省免疫学会妇产科基础与临床免疫专业委员会委员、辽宁省住院医师规范化培训妇产科专业基地评审专家委员会委员。研究方向为妇科内分泌，发表论文50余篇，获得大连市科技进步奖二等奖1项，教学成果奖3项。

张莉，女，大连大学英语学院副院长，副教授，硕士生导师，从事大学英语教学工作20余年，讲授课程主要包括：大学英语、高级英语视听说、雅思写作、英文佳片赏析、教师领导力。主要研究领域：英语教育与教学、专门用途英语、中西文化比较。近年来主持省级以上教改课题2项，主编教材3部，参编、参译图书及教材多部，2020年作为主要参与人获校级教学成果一等奖。

Editors in Chief

Wen Jing, female, is the director of the Department of Obstetrics and Gynecology, Zhongshan Hospital Affiliated to Dalian University, chief physician, professor, postgraduate tutor, and head of obstetrics and gynecology program. She has long been engaged in clinical, teaching and research work in obstetrics and gynecology. Her social part-time jobs include member of the Obstetrics and Gynecology Specialty Branch of Dalian Medical Association, standing member of Gynecological Endocrinology and Menopause Professional Committee of Liaoning Association of Integrative Medicine, member of Basic and Clinical Immunology Committee of Obstetrics and Gynecology of Liaoning Society for Immunology, expert of Liaoning Evaluation of Professional Base of Obstetrics and Gynecology for Standardized Training of Resident Physicians. She focuses on gynecological endocrinology research and has published more than 50 papers. She has won a second prize of Dalian Science and Technology Progress Award and 3 teaching achievement awards.

Zhang Li, female, is the associate dean of English College, Dalian University. As an associate professor and a professional master tutor, she has engaged in college English teaching for more than twenty years and the courses she has taught include College English, Advanced English Listening and Speaking, IELTS Writing, Appreciation of English Movies, Teacher Leadership. Her research interests include English education and teaching, English for special purposes, and comparison of Chinese and Western cultures. In recent years, she has presided over 2 teaching reform projects at the provincial level and above, edited 3 textbooks, and contributed to the writing and translation of several books. In 2020, she won the first prize of the teaching achievements of Dalian University as a major participant.

前 言

国家教育部在加强大学本科教学的多项措施中，要求各高校都要努力创造条件开设双语教学课程。目前，我国没有统一的妇产科学中英文对照双语教材，原版英文教材又不符合我国教学大纲的要求，因此我们编写此教材的目的是为临床医学专业的教师和学生提供一本方便学习、有利于提高专业英语水平的教材，使广大学生及教师通过阅读本教材，掌握妇产科必备的英文专业知识，努力培养与国际接轨的高素质医学生。

本教材应广大学生的要求，采用短语提纲式内容、附有重点词汇、练习题，便于学生复习使用。对于相关概念、单位参考标准值、诊断及治疗标准、用药剂量等问题，以国家卫健委"十三五"规划教材《妇产科学》（第9版）为标准。作为本土化自编中英文教材，着力提高学生学会如何在英语环境中交流和应用妇产科学知识的能力。

在本教材的编写过程中，受诸多方面因素的影响，书中可能存在疏漏和不妥之处，敬请同学及教师批评指正，我们将不断对本教材进行改正和完善。

温 菁

2020年5月

Preface

Among the measures to strengthen undergraduate teaching, the Ministry of Education requires that all colleges and universities make efforts to create conditions to offer bilingual teaching courses. At present, however, there are no uniform bilingual teaching materials for obstetrics and gynecology in China, and the original English teaching materials fail to meet the requirements of our syllabus. Our purpose of writing this textbook, therefore, is to provide both teachers and students of clinical medicine with a reference book, which is convenient to learn and conducive to improving their professional English. Through reading this book, students and teachers may master the necessary English professional knowledge of obstetrics and gynecology, and strive to cultivate or become high-quality medical students with international standards.

At the request of students, this textbook adopts phrase outlines, with key words and exercises, which is convenient for study and review. The standards for relevant concepts, units, diagnosis, treatment and dosage are based on *Obstetrics and Gynecology* (the 9th edition), a textbook of the National Health Commission for the 13th Five-Year Plan. As localized teaching materials in Chinese and English, this textbook aims to improve the students' ability to learn how to communicate and apply the professional knowledge of obstetrics and gynecology in an English environment.

Due to many factors there may be something improper and omissions in this book, and comments and suggestions both from students and teachers are welcome, which will help us continue to make it revised and polished.

Wen Jing
May, 2020

目　录

Contents

第1章　女性生殖系统解剖

CHAPTER 1　Anatomy of female reproductive system

第一节　外生殖器

外生殖器包括：阴阜、大阴唇、小阴唇、阴蒂、阴道前庭、前庭大腺、阴道口、处女膜及会阴（图1-1）。

1.阴阜

含有脂肪组织，外有皮肤遮盖，皮肤上生有阴毛。

2.大阴唇

皮肤皱褶，外层阴唇有色素沉着并有毛发覆盖，内层皮下为结缔组织、脂肪、血管和神经。

Section 1　External genital organs

External genital organs include mons pubis, labium majus, labium minus, clitoris, vestibule, major vestibular gland, vaginal orifice, hymen and perineum（Figure 1-1）.

1.Mons pubis

Composed of fatty tissue and covered by skin and tuft of hairs.

2.Labium majus

Cutaneous folds, with outer layer of the labium pigmented and covered with hair, and inner connective tissue, fat, blood vessels and nerves.

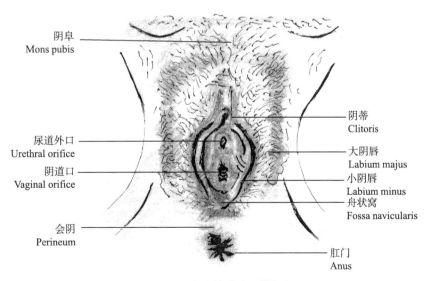

图1-1　正常女性外生殖器解剖

Figure 1-1　Normal anatomy of female external genitalia

1

3.小阴唇

位于大阴唇之内侧，亦是皮肤皱褶。此阴唇无毛囊，但有皮脂腺。

4.阴蒂

位于两侧小阴唇之前端，含有勃起组织。阴蒂含有丰富的神经末梢，所以非常敏感。

5.阴道前庭

在阴道前庭内，前有尿道口，后有阴道口。

6.前庭大腺（又称巴氏腺）

7.阴道口，处女膜及会阴

第二节　内生殖器

内生殖器包括：阴道、子宫、输卵管和卵巢（图1-2）。

1.阴道

（1）阴道为上宽下窄的管道，前壁长7～9cm，后壁长10～12cm，子宫颈与阴道之间的圆周状隐窝，称

3.Labium minus

Cutaneous folds, inside the labium majus. No hair follicles but sebaceous glands.

4.Clitoris

Located between the anterior ends of the labium minus, and composed of erectile tissue. Rich in nerve endings and therefore very sensitive.

5.Vaginal vestibule

The structures found in the vestibule are the external urethral orifice anteriorly and the vaginal orifice posteriorly.

6.Major vestibular gland（Bartholin's gland）

7.Vaginal orifice, hymen and perineum

Section 2　Internal genital organs

Internal genital organs include vagina, uterus, fallopian tubes, and ovaries（Figure 1-2）.

1.Vagina

（1）A channel with wide top and narrow bottom, anterior wall 7 ～ 9cm long, posterior wall 10 ～ 12cm long. The circumferential recess

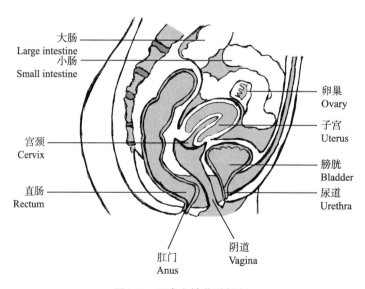

图1-2　正常女性盆腔解剖

Figure 1-2　Normal female pelvic anatomy

阴道穹窿。

（2）阴道黏膜由复层扁平细胞组成，呈坑状。经多次分娩此坑状会逐渐消失，黏膜内无腺体，阴道分泌物由淋巴液和脱落的上皮细胞组成。

（3）阴道为性交器官，亦为月经排出之路及分娩时产道的一部分。

2.子宫

（1）解剖结构
- 子宫底、子宫体、子宫角、子宫颈、子宫腔、子宫峡部、子宫颈管。
- 子宫为倒梨形，壁厚，肌性器官，位于膀胱和直肠之间。
- 重：约50g；长度：7～8cm，宽度：3～5cm；厚度：2～3cm；容量：5ml。子宫体与子宫颈的比例因年龄和卵巢功能而异，青春期前为1∶2，育龄期为2∶1，绝经后为1∶1。
- 子宫峡部：在非孕期长约1cm，在妊娠末期达7～10cm，形成子宫下段。
- 子宫颈管：成年女性长为2.5～3cm。

（2）组织结构
- 子宫内膜：功能层/基底层。
- 子宫肌层：厚约0.8cm，内层环形，中层交叉，外层纵形。
- 浆膜层：直肠子宫陷凹，又称道格拉斯陷凹。

（3）韧带：子宫有4对韧带。

between cervix and vagina is called vaginal fornix.

（2）Vaginal mucosae lined by stratified squamous epithelium and ridged. The ridges obliterated with repeated childbearing. No glands and the vaginal secretion composed of transudation of lymph and cast-off epithelial cells.

（3）The vagina serves as an organ for coitus, the canal for menstrual flow and the passage for childbirth.

2.Uterus

（1）Anatomic structure
- Fundus uteri, corpus uteri, cornua uteri, cervix uteri, uterine cavity, isthmus uteri, and cervical canal.
- A pear-shaped, thick-walled, muscular organ, located between the bladder and rectum.
- Weight: About 50g, length: 7～8cm, width: 3～5cm, thickness: 2～3cm, volume: 5ml. The ratio of uterine corpus to cervix varies with age and ovarian function, with 1∶2 before puberty, 2∶1 for women of childbearing age and 1∶1 after menopause.
- Isthmus uteri: About 1cm long in non-pregnancy, 7～10cm in the third trimester, forming the lower uterine segment.
- Cervical canal: About 2.5～3cm long for adult women.

（2）Histologic structure
- Endometrium: Functional/basal layer.
- Myometrium: About 0.8cm thick, with annular inner layer, crossed middle layer, vertical outer layer.
- Serosal layer: Rectouterine pouch, also called Douglas pouch.

（3）Ligaments: The ligaments of uterus are 4 pairs in number.

■ 圆韧带。

■ 阔韧带（卵巢韧带和骨盆漏斗韧带）。

■ 主韧带。

■ 宫骶韧带。

3.输卵管

■ 输卵管为一对细长而弯曲的肌性管道，为卵子与精子结合的场所及运送受精卵的通道。全长8～14cm。由内向外分为4部分。

■ 间质部。

■ 峡部。

■ 壶腹部。

■ 伞部（漏斗）。

4.卵巢

（1）卵巢为一对性腺器官，是产生卵子并分泌甾体激素的性器官。当性器官完全成熟时，卵泡破裂，释放卵子，变成黄体。随后，黄体被瘢痕组织所取代，形成了一个白体。

（2）卵巢为两个扁椭圆形状的器官，位于子宫两侧，大小为4cm×3cm×1cm。卵巢分为两个部分：皮质（外层）和髓质（内层）。

（3）皮质表面是一层灰白色的生发上皮细胞，皮质内含有原始卵泡和成熟卵泡（赫拉夫卵泡）。髓质含有疏松结缔组织及肌纤维，内含血管、神经与淋巴管。

第三节　血管、淋巴和神经

1.盆腔血管（图1-3）

（1）卵巢动脉：自腹主动脉发

■ Round ligaments.

■ Broad ligaments (ovarian ligament and infundibulopelvic ligament).

■ Cardinal ligaments.

■ Uterosacral ligaments.

3.Fallopian tube (oviduct)

■ A pair of slender and curved muscular tubes, where the ovum and sperm combine, also the channel for transporting the fertilized ovum. Total length: 8 ～ 14cm. Divided into 4 parts from the inside out.

■ Interstitial portion.

■ Isthmic portion.

■ Ampulla portion.

■ Fimbrial portion (infundibulum).

4.Ovary

（1）A pair of gonadal organs, the sexual organs to produce and secrete steroid hormone. When they are fully mature, the follicle bursts, releasing the ovum and becoming corpus luteum. The corpus luteum is replaced by scar tissue afterwards, forming corpus albicans.

（2）Located on either side of the uterus and ellipse-shaped. Size: 4cm×3cm×1cm. An ovary is made up of the cortex (outer layer) and the medulla (inner layer).

（3）The primordial and mature follicles (Graafian follicles) are in the cortex, the covering of which is formed by the grey-colored germinal epithelium. The medulla contains loose connective tissue and muscle fibres, with blood vessels, nerves and lymphatics inside.

Section 3　Vascular, lymphatic and nervous systems

1.Pelvic vasculature (Figure 1-3)

（1）Ovarian artery: Arising from aorta, but

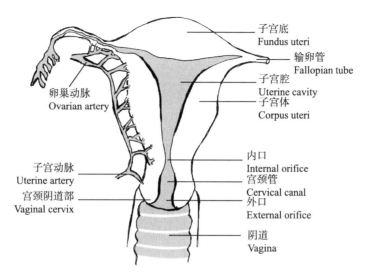

图1-3 子宫的血液供应

Figure 1-3 Blood supply of the uterus

出，但左侧发自左肾动脉。

（2）子宫动脉：自髂内动脉分出。

（3）阴道动脉：为髂内动脉或子宫动脉分支。

（4）阴部内动脉：为髂内动脉的终末分支。

2.淋巴引流

（1）外生殖器淋巴群
- 腹股沟浅淋巴结。
- 腹股沟深淋巴结。

（2）盆腔淋巴群
- 髂淋巴群。
- 骶前淋巴群。
- 腰淋巴群。

3.盆腔神经

（1）外生殖器神经：由骶神经丛的阴部神经支配。

（2）内生殖器神经：由交感神经系统和副交感神经支配。

the left side from left renal artery.

（2）Uterine artery: Arising from internal iliac artery.

（3）Vaginal artery: Arising from internal iliac artery or from the uterine artery.

（4）Internal pudendal artery: The terminal branch of the internal iliac artery.

2.Lymphatic drainage

（1）External genital organ lymph group
- Superficial inguinal lymph nodes.
- Deep inguinal lymph nodes.

（2）Pelvic lymph group
- Iliac lymph group.
- Presacral lymph group.
- Lumbar lymph group.

3.Pelvic innervation

（1）External genital organ: Controlled by pudendal nerve arising from sacral plexus.

（2）Internal genital organ: Controlled by sympathetic nervous system and parasympathetic nervous system.

第四节 骨 盆

Section 4 Pelvis

1.组成

（1）骨骼：骶骨（骶骨岬），尾骨，髋骨（髂骨，坐骨，耻骨）。（图1-4）

（2）关节：耻骨联合，骶髂关节，骶尾关节。（图1-4）

（3）韧带：骶结节韧带，骶棘韧带（图1-5）。

1.Composition

（1）Bone: Sacrum（sacral promontory）, coccyx, coxae（ilium, ischium, pubis）.（Figure 1-4）

（2）Joint: Pubic symphysis, sacroiliac joint, sacrococcygeal joint.（Figure 1-4）

（3）Ligament: Sacrotuberous ligament, sacrospinous ligament（Figure 1-5）.

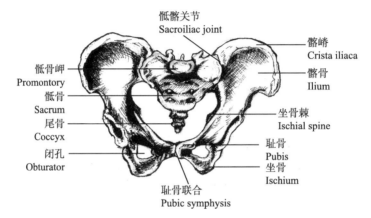

图1-4 女性骨盆正面观

Figure 1-4 Anterior view of maternal pelvis

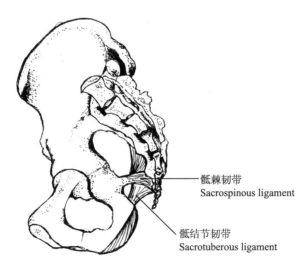

图1-5 骨盆的韧带

Figure 1-5 Ligament of maternal pelvis

2．骨盆的分界

- 骨盆以骶骨岬上缘、髂耻缘及耻骨联合上缘连线为界，将骨盆分为大骨盆（假骨盆）和小骨盆（真骨盆）。

3．骨盆的类型

（1）女型：我国最常见，为女性正常骨盆，占52%～58.9%。

（2）扁平型：较常见，占23.2%～29%。

（3）类人猿型：较少见，占14.2%～18%。

（4）男型：少见，占1%～3.7%。

上述为理论上的归类，临床所见多是混合型骨盆。

第五节 邻近器官

1．尿道

- 长4～5cm，直径约0.6cm。女性尿道短而直，与阴道邻近，容易引起泌尿系统感染。

2．膀胱

- 排空的膀胱位于耻骨联合和子宫之间，膀胱充盈时可凸向盆腔甚至腹腔。

3．输尿管

- 全长约30cm，管壁厚1mm，内径粗细不一，最细部分的内径为3～4mm，最粗为7～8mm，全程周围丰富的血管丛营养输尿管，盆腔手术时要注意保护输尿管血供，避免因缺血形成输尿管瘘。

2.Boundary of pelvis

- Pelvis is divided into the pelvis major (false pelvis) and the pelvis minor (true pelvis) bounded by the upper margin of the sacral promontory, the ilium, and the upper margin of the pubic symphysis.

3.Type of pelvis

（1）Gynecoid type: The most common in China in the female normal pelvis, accounting for 52%～58.9%.

（2）Platypelloid type: Relatively common, accounting for 23.2%～29%.

（3）Anthropoid type: Less common, accounting for 14.2%～18%.

（4）Android type: Rare, accounting for 1%～3.7%.

The above is a classification in theory, but the most clinical findings are mixed pelvis.

Section 5　Neighbouring organs

1.Urethra

- 4～5cm long and 0.6cm in diameter. Female urethra is short and straight, near the vagina, and vulnerable to urinary tract infection.

2.Bladder

- The emptied bladder is located between the pubic symphysis and the uterus. When the bladder fills, it protrudes into the pelvic cavity and even the abdominal cavity.

3.Ureter

- The total length is about 30cm, the tube wall thickness is 1mm, and the internal meridian thickness varies, ranging from 3～4mm to 7～8mm. The abundant vascular plexus around provide nutrition for ureter. In pelvic surgery attention should be paid to the ureteral blood supply to avoid ureteral

4.直肠

■ 全长15～20cm。

5.阑尾

重点专业词汇

1.阴道

2.子宫

3.输卵管

4.卵巢

5.圆韧带

6.阔韧带

7.主韧带

8.宫骶韧带

9.骨盆漏斗韧带

10.间质部

11.峡部

12.壶腹部

13.伞部（漏斗）

14.生发上皮

15.卵泡

16.髓质

17.皮质

18.白体

19.黄体

练习题

1.维持子宫前倾的主要韧带是：（A）

A.圆韧带

B.阔韧带

C.宫骶韧带

D.主韧带

E.骨盆漏斗韧带

2.关于子宫解剖，下列哪项错误？（E）

A.大小约7cm×5cm×3cm

B.容积5ml

C.重量50g

D.成人宫颈与宫体比例1∶2

E.子宫峡部非妊娠状态2～3cm

fistula due to ischemia.

4.Rectum

■ The total length is about 15～20cm.

5.Appendix

Key words

1.Vagina

2.Uterus

3.Fallopian tube（oviduct）

4.Ovary

5.Round ligament

6.Broad ligament

7.Cardinal ligament

8.Uterosacral ligament

9.Infundibulopelvic ligament

10.Interstitial portion

11.Isthmic portion

12.Ampulla portion

13.Fimbrial portion（infundibulum）

14. Germinal epithelium

15.Follicle

16.Medulla

17.Cortex

18.Corpus albicans

19.Corpus luteum

Exercises

1.The main ligament to maintain anteversion position is:（A）

A.Round ligament

B.Broad ligament

C.Uterosacral ligament

D.Cardinal ligament

E.Infundibulopelvic ligament

2.Which of the following is not correct about the uterine anatomy？（E）

A.Size: About 7cm×5cm×3cm

B.Volume: 5ml

C.Weight: About 50g

D.Adult women cervical corpus ratio is 1∶2

E.The uteri isthmus in nonpregnant status is

3.关于卵巢的解剖，下列哪项错误？（B）

A.大小约 4cm×3cm×1cm

B.外层是髓质

C.卵巢表面覆盖生发上皮

D.皮质内含有大量卵泡

E.髓质内含有血管、神经和淋巴管

（温　菁）

2～3cm

3.Which of the following is not correct about the ovary anatomy?（B）

A.Size: About 4cm×3cm×1cm

B.The outer layer is medulla

C.The covering of the ovary is germinal epithelium

D.The cortex contains numerous follicles

E.The medulla contains blood vessels, nerves and lymphatics

第2章 女性生殖系统生理

CHAPTER 2　Physiology of female reproductive system

第一节　女性一生不同时期的生理特点

1. 胎儿期
- 胚胎、胎儿。

2. 新生儿期
- 出生后4周内，此阶段有乳房增大、泌乳、阴道出血。

3. 儿童期
- 从出生后4周到12岁左右。

4. 青春期
- 月经初潮——性成熟，10～19岁。

（1）乳房萌发：约经过3.5年发育成熟。

（2）肾上腺功能初现：阴毛先发育，约2年后发育腋毛。

（3）生长加速：每年长9cm，初潮后减缓。

（4）月经初潮：晚乳房发育2.5年，青春期重要标志，卵巢成熟，月经调节机制建立。

5. 性成熟期
- 始于18岁，历时约30年。

6. 绝经过渡期
- 围绝经期：开始于40岁，持续1～2年或10～20年〔绝经前、绝经（最后一次月经）、绝经后〕。

7. 绝经后期
- 60岁后又称老年期。

Section 1　The changes of female in different periods

1.Fetal period
- Embryo, fetus.

2.Neonatal period
- ≤ 4 weeks, breast enlargement, lactation, vaginal bleeding.

3.Childhood
- From 4 weeks after birth to the age of 12.

4.Puberty or adolesence
- Menarche—sexual maturity, at the age of 10 ～ 19.

（1）Thelarche: It takes about 3.5 years to reach maturity.

（2）Adrenal adrenarche: Pubic hair development, about 2 years later armpit hair begins to develop.

（3）Growth spurt: 9 cm per year, slowing down after menarche.

（4）Menarche: 2.5 years later than breast development, the important signs of puberty, ovarian maturing, menstrual mediation mechanism established.

5.Sexual maturity
- From the age of 18, for about 30 years.

6.Menopause transition period
- Peri-menopausal period: From the age of 40, for 1 ～ 2 years or 10 ～ 20 years 〔pre-menopause, menopause（last time of menorrhea）, and post-menopause〕.

7.Post-menopausal period
- Senility: From the age of 60.

第二节 月 经

- 月经初潮：女性第一次月经来潮称月经初潮，大约在青春期始动后2年出现，即发生在13～15岁，最初2年无周期性排卵。
- 出血的第1日为月经周期的第1日。
- 正常月经周期是21～35日，平均28日。
- 每次月经持续时间为2～8日。
- 正常月经量为20～60ml（＜80ml），月经血呈暗红色，不凝状。

第三节 卵巢功能

1.卵巢具有生殖和内分泌双重功能

（1）生殖功能：产生卵母细胞和排卵。

（2）内分泌功能：产生女性激素。

2.生殖周期分为三个阶段

（1）月经期：月经第1～4日。

（2）卵泡期：月经第5～14日。

- 一定数量的卵泡发育。
- 只有一个成熟卵泡。
- 其他卵泡闭锁。
- 排卵：月经第14日，排出卵子。

（3）黄体期：如果没有妊娠发生，黄体期为月经第15～28日。

Section 2 Menstruation

- Menarche: The first menses of the female occurs about two years after the onset of puberty, between 13 and 15 years old, anovulatory in the first two years.

- The first menstrual bleeding day is the first day of the menstrual cycle.

- The normal length of menstrual cycle is 21～35 days, with an average of 28 days.

- The duration of the cycle is 2～8 days.

- The normal volume of menstrual blood is 20～60ml（＜80ml）, dark red and non-clotting.

Section 3 The function of ovary

1.The ovary has reproductive and endocrine functions

（1）Reproductive function: Producing oocytes and ovulating.

（2）Endocrine function: Producing female hormone.

2.Reproductive cycle is devided into 3 phases

（1）Menstruation: From the first day to the 4th day of menses.

（2）Follicular phase: From the 5th day to the 14th day of menses.

- With a certain number of follicles developing.
- Only one mature follicle.
- Others becoming atretic.
- Ovulation: Releasing oocyte on the 14th day of menses.

（3）Luteal phase: From the 15th day to 28th day of menses, unless pregnancy occurs.

3.卵巢的发育

（1）从青春期开始到绝经前，卵巢在形态上和功能上发生周期性变化称为卵巢周期。

（2）卵巢周期分为几个阶段：

■ 卵泡的发育过程：始基卵泡→初级卵泡→次级卵泡→卵泡闭锁/卵泡发育→成熟卵泡→排卵→黄体→白体。

4.黄体形成及退化

■ 排卵后卵泡壁塌陷，颗粒细胞和卵泡膜细胞包裹共同形成黄体。若卵子未受精，黄体在排卵后9～10日开始退化，逐渐被结缔组织所替代，外观白色，称白体。

5.卵巢类固醇激素

（1）雌激素

■ 产生于颗粒细胞和卵泡膜细胞。

■ 月经的第7日血浆雌激素水平开始升高，在排卵前达最高峰，排卵后7～8日形成又一个高峰。

■ 对促卵泡素产生负反馈。

■ 对黄体生成素产生正反馈。

（2）孕激素

■ 产生于黄体。

■ 排卵后7～8日达最高峰，并维持11日。

■ 对促卵泡素和黄体生成素产生负反馈。

6.卵巢激素的生理作用（表2-1）

3.Development of ovary

（1）From puberty to pre-menopause, ovarian changes in morphology and function are called ovarian cycle.

（2）Ovarian cycle is divided into the following phases：

■ Development of follicles: Primordial follicles→primary follicles→secondary follicles→follicular atresia/developing follicles→maturity follicles→ovulation→corpus luteum→corpus albicans.

4.Corpus luteum formation and degeneration

■ After ovulation, the follicular wall collapses, and granulosa cells and theca cells encapsulate together to form corpus luteum. If the ovum is not fertilized, the corpus luteum begins to degenerate on the 9th or 10th day after ovulation, and it is gradually replaced by the connective tissue and appears white, called corpus albicans.

5.Ovarian steroid hormones

（1）Estrogen

■ From granulosa cells and theca cells.

■ Rising in plasma on the 7th day of menstrual cycle, reaching its peak before ovulation, and another peak occurring on the 7th or 8th day after ovulation.

■ Negative feedback to FSH.

■ Positve feedback to LH.

（2）Progesterone

■ From corpus luteum.

■ Maximal production occurring on the 7th or 8th day after ovulation and lasting for 11 days.

■ Negative feedback to FSH and LH.

6.Physiological functions of ovarian hormones（Table 2-1）

表2-1 卵巢激素的生理作用

Table 2-1 Physiological functions of ovarian hormones

名称	雌激素 Estrogen	孕激素 Progesterone
子宫肌层 Uterine muscle	促进作用 Promotion	抑制作用 Inhibition
子宫内膜 Endometrium	增生 Proliferation	分泌 Secretion
宫颈 Cervix	闭合 Closed	扩张 Expansion
输卵管 Fallopian tube	促进 Promotion	抑制 Inhibition
阴道上皮 Vaginal epithelium	增生 Hyperplasia	脱落 Falling off
乳房 Breast	腺管增生 Ductal hyperplasia	腺泡发育 Gland bubble growth
下丘脑、垂体 Hypothalamus, pituitary	正负反馈 Positive and negative feedback	负反馈 Negative feedback
代谢 Metabolism	水钠潴留 Water-sodium retention	水钠排泄 Water-sodium excretion
体温 Body temperature		升高 0.3~0.5 ℃ Rising 0.3~0.5 ℃

第四节 激素周期性改变的临床表现

1.子宫内膜

（1）子宫内膜从形态学上可分为功能层和基底层，功能层受卵巢激素的影响发生周期性变化并脱落，基底层在功能层脱落后修复子宫内膜重新形成功能层。

（2）子宫内膜从基底层开始发生周期性改变（图2-1）。

■ 增生期：月经周期的第5～14日（间质增厚，腺体扩

Section 4　Clinical manifestations of hormone changes in menstruation

1.Endometrium

（1）Endometrium can be morphologically divided into a functional layer and a basal layer. The functional layer changes periodically under the influence of ovarian hormones, then falls off. The basal layer repairs the endometrium and the functional layer reforms.

（2）Endometrium changes periodically from the basal layer in the menstruation cycle（Figure 2-1）.

■ Proliferative phase: From the 5th day to the 14th day of the menstrual cycle（stroma

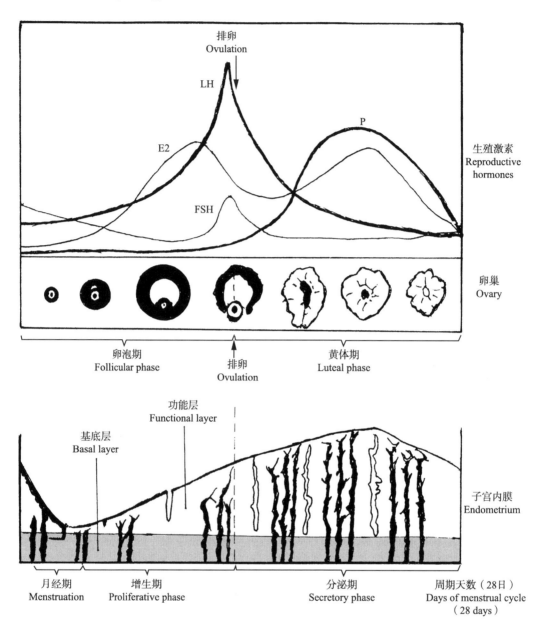

图2-1 卵巢及子宫内膜周期性变化和激素水平关系

Figure 2-1   Relationship between ovarian and endometrial changes and hormone levels

大）。在卵泡期，排卵时子宫内膜厚度最大。

- 分泌期：月经周期的第15～28日（在黄体期，间质疏松、水肿、血管扭曲、腺体弯曲）。

thickened, and gland elongated）. In the follicular phase, the thickness is greatest when ovulation occurs.

- Secretory phase: 15th ～ 28th day of the menstrual cycle（stroma loose, edematous, vessel twisted, gland tortuous in the corpus luteum phase）.

- 月经期：月经周期的第 1 ～ 4 日。子宫内膜自基底层开始脱落并出血。

2.子宫颈内膜

（1）子宫颈也受激素的影响发生周期性改变。

（2）子宫颈腺体在卵泡期分泌稀薄、透明、水样黏液，排卵前达高峰，在黄体期黏液变黏稠、浑浊、拉丝度差。

3.阴道

- 卵泡期受雌激素的影响，阴道上皮细胞成熟增生，黄体期阴道上皮细胞分泌性改变并脱落。采集阴道脱落细胞，可了解雌激素水平和有无排卵。

4.乳房

- 雌激素促进乳腺管增生，而孕激素则促进乳腺小叶及腺泡生长。

第五节　下丘脑-垂体-卵巢轴（H-P-O轴）

月经周期主要受下丘脑-垂体-卵巢轴的神经内分泌反馈调节（图2-2）。

1.下丘脑

- 下丘脑弓状核神经细胞分泌的 GnRH（下丘脑促性腺激素释放激素），直接通过垂体门脉系统输送到腺垂体，调节垂体的性腺激素的合成和分泌。
  - 脉冲式分泌方式。
  - 分泌特征为周期性脉冲式释放。

- Menstrual phase: From the 1st day to the 4th day of the menstrual cycle. Endometrium sloughed from the basal layer and bleeding.

2.Endocervix

（1）Cervix also changes in response to the reproductive cycle.

（2）Cervical glands secrete thin, clear and watery mucus in the follicular phase, reaching a peak before ovulation. Mucus becomes thick, opaque, tenacious in the corpus luteum phase.

3.Vagina

- Epithelial cells mature and proliferate in the follicular phase due to estrogen, and undergo secretory changes of vaginal epithelium in the corpus luteum phase. Vaginal exfoliated cells are collected to know the estrogen level and ovulation.

4.Breast

- Estrogen promotes proliferation of mammary ducts, whereas progesterone causes growth of lobules and alveoli.

Section 5　Hypothalamic-pituitary-ovarian axis（H-P-O axis）

The cycle of menstruation is based on the feedback loop of H-P-O axis（Figure 2-2）.

1.Hypothalamus

- GnRH（hypothalamic gonadotropin releasing hormone）, secreted by hypothalamic arcuate nerve cells, is directly transported to the pituitary gland through the pituitary portal system to regulate the synthesis and secretion of the pituitary gonadal hormone.
  - Pulsed secretion.
  - Characterized by periodic pulsed release.

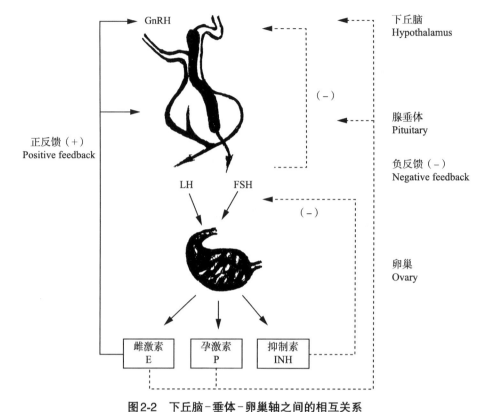

图2-2 下丘脑-垂体-卵巢轴之间的相互关系

Figure 2-2 Relationship between hypothalamic-pituitary-ovarian axis

- 受性激素和神经递质的影响。

2.垂体

■ 主要产生促性腺激素
- 卵泡刺激素（FSH）。
- 黄体生成素（LH）。
  ①由垂体前叶腺体分泌的蛋白类激素。
  ②脉冲式分泌方式。
  ③受雌激素、孕激素和其他因素的影响。

3.卵巢

（1）卵巢性激素是类固醇类激素，主要为雌二醇（E2）和孕酮（P）。

（2）卵巢分泌的雌激素和孕激素对下丘脑和垂体具有反馈调节作用。

- Influenced by gonadal hormone and neurotransmitters.

2.Pituitary

■ Producing gonadotropins
- Follicle-stimulating hormone（FSH）.
- Luteinizing hormone（LH）.
  ①Protein hormones secreted by the anterior pituitary gland.
  ②Pulsed secretion.
  ③Influenced by estrogen, progesterone and other factors.

3.Ovary

（1）Ovarian sex hormones are steroid hormones, mainly estradiol（E2）and progesterone（P）.

（2）Estrogen and progesterone have feedback regulation effect on hypothalamus and pituitary.

（3）雌激素对性腺轴产生正负反馈作用，一定水平的雌激素负反馈作用于下丘脑，卵泡接近成熟时雌激素分泌达到≥200pg/ml，并持续48小时以上，即可发挥正反馈作用。

（4）孕激素对性腺轴主要产生负反馈作用。

4.性腺轴的反馈作用
- 反馈的概念
  - GnRH、FSH、LH的分泌量和频率受雌激素和孕激素的影响。
  - 负反馈：导致GnRH、FSH、LH的分泌量降低。
  - 正反馈：导致LH分泌量的增加，并促发排卵。

重点专业词汇

1.生殖周期

2.月经

3.卵巢周期

4.下丘脑-垂体-卵巢轴

5.反馈

6.雌激素

7.孕激素

8.卵泡

9.排卵

10.黄体

11.白体

12.增生期（又称卵泡期）

13.分泌期（又称黄体期）

练习题

1.下列哪项激素可以致子宫内膜增生期改变？（C）

A.孕激素

B.雄激素

C.雌激素

D.人绒毛膜促性腺激素

（3）Estrogen has positive and negative feedback effects on the gonadal axis, and a certain level of estrogen has negative feedback effect on the hypothalamus. When follicles are approaching maturity, estrogen secretion reaches ≥200pg/ml and lasts for more than 48 hours, then positive feedback role can be played.

（4）Progesterone mainly has negative feedback effect on the gonadal axis.

4.Feedback of H-P-O axis
- The concept of feedback
  - The magnitude and the rate of GnRH, FSH, LH are determined by estrogen, progesterone.
  - Negative feedback: Resulting in a decrease in secretion of GnRH, FSH and LH.
  - Positive feedback: Resulting in an increase in LH secretion and ovulation.

Key words

1.Reproductive cycle

2.Menstruation

3.Ovarian cycle

4.H-P-O axis

5.Feedback

6.Estrogen

7.Progesterone

8.Follicles

9.Ovulation

10.Corpus luteum

11.Corpus albicans

12.Proliferative phase（Follicular phase）

13.Secretory phase（Luteal phase）

Exercises

1.Which of the following hormones can make endometrial proliferative phase change？（C）

A.Progesterone

B.Androgen

C.Estrogen

D.Human chorionic gonadotropin

E.泌乳素

2.雌激素、孕激素对下丘脑和腺垂体的反馈作用是：（D）

A.雌激素负反馈，孕激素正反馈

B.雌激素正反馈，孕激素负反馈

C.雌激素负反馈，孕激素负反馈

D.雌激素正反馈和负反馈，孕激素负反馈

E.雌激素负反馈，孕激素正反馈和负反馈

3.关于月经周期排卵后的改变，下列哪项是正确的？（D）

A.90%阴道角化层细胞脱落

B.基础体温单相型

C.月经前3天宫颈黏液呈现典型的羊齿状结晶

D.内膜分泌期改变

E.宫颈黏液稀薄

4.月经期后内膜再生起源于：（C）

A.肌层

B.致密层

C.基底层

D.海绵层

E.功能层

（温 菁）

E.Prolactin

2.The feedback effects of estrogen and progesterone hormones on hypothalamus and pituitary are：（D）

A.Estrogen—negative feedback, progesterone—positive feedback

B.Estrogen—positive feedback, progesterone—negative feedback

C.Estrogen—negative feedback, progesterone—negative feedback

D.Estrogen—positive and negative feedback, progesterone—negative feedback

E.Estrogen—negative feedback, progesterone—positive and negative feedback

3.Which of the following is true about changes after ovulation in the menstrual cycle？（D）

A.90% exfoliated cells of the keratinized layer of vagina

B.The basal body temperature of single-phase type

C.3 days before menstruation, cervical mucus typically shows ferning

D.Endometrial secretion phase change

E.Thin cervical mucus

4.After menstruation endometrial regeneration occurs in：（C）

A.Myometrium

B.Dense layer

C.Basal layer

D.Sponge layer

E.Functional layer

第 3 章 妊 娠 生 理

CHAPTER 3   Physiology of pregnancy

妊娠：胚胎或胎儿在母体内发育成长的过程是从受精卵受精开始的，胎儿及其附属物自母体排出则是妊娠的终止。

人胚的概念：从受精后8周内妊娠称为胚胎；妊娠11周后至分娩称为胎儿。

Pregnancy: The condition of being with child or gravid, is the process of embryo and fetus growing and developing in the uterus. It begins with fertilization and the expelling of the fetus with placenta and membranes is the termination of pregnancy.

Human embryo: Pregnancy within 8 weeks after fertilization is termed embryo; the period from 11 weeks of pregnancy to delivery is termed fetus.

第一节 受精，受精卵发育、输送与着床

Section 1   Fertilization, development, transport and implantation of fertilized ovum

1.受精

- 获能的精子与次级卵母细胞相遇于输卵管，结合形成受精卵的过程称为受精（图3-1）。

2.着床

（1）受精卵→分裂球→桑葚胚→早期胚囊→进入宫腔→晚期胚囊→着床，包括定位、黏附、侵入。

（2）着床必须具备的条件

- 透明带消失。
- 合体滋养细胞出现。
- 囊胚与子宫内膜发育同步。

- 足够量的孕酮。

1.Fertilization

- The capacitated sperm and the secondary oocytes meet in the fallopian tube, and combine to form the fertilized ovum. The process is called fertilization (Figure 3-1).

2.Implantation

（1）Fertilized ovum (zygote)→blastomere→morula→early blastocyst→into uterine cavity→late blastocyst→implantation, including positioning, adhesion and invasion.

（2）The necessity factors

- Disappearance of zone pellucida.
- Appearance of syncytiotrophoblastic cells.
- Synchronistical development of blastosphere and endometrium.
- Sufficient progesterone.

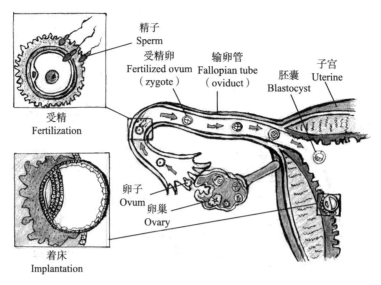

图3-1 受精及受精卵发育、输送与着床

Figure 3-1 Fertilization and development, transport and implantation of fertilized ovum

3.蜕膜反应

- 子宫内膜增厚，血管增加，间质水肿。

3.Decidua formation

- Thicker, more vascular and edematous endometrium.

第二节 胚胎、胎儿的发育特征

（1）胚胎：妊娠10周之内（受精后8周）称胚胎。

（2）胎儿：妊娠11周后（受精后9周）称胎儿。

（3）胎儿长度：妊娠20周内，月份的平方；妊娠20周后，月份乘5。

Section 2 Developmental characteristics of embryo and fetus

（1）Embryo: The first 10 weeks of pregnancy（8 weeks after fertilization）termed embryo.

（2）Fetus: After 11 weeks of pregnancy（9 weeks after fertilization）.

（3）Fetal length: < 20 weeks, m^2; > 20 weeks, $m \times 5$.

第三节 胎盘、胎膜、脐带和羊水

1.胎盘（图3-2）

（1）胎盘的组成：羊膜、叶状绒毛膜、底蜕膜。

（2）胎盘的大小和重量：重

Section 3 Placenta, fetal membrane, umbilical cord and amniotic fluid

1.Placenta（Figure 3-2）

（1）Structure of placenta: Amniotic membrane, chorion frondosum, and basal decidua.

（2）Size and weight of placenta: Weight

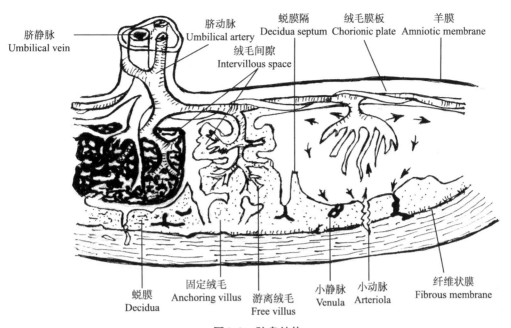

图3-2 胎盘结构

Figure 3-2 Structure of placenta

450 ～ 650g, 直径16 ～ 20cm, 厚度1 ～ 3cm。

（3）胎盘的功能：从母体输送胎儿氧气和营养，相反，二氧化碳和其他代谢废物则从胎儿排泄到母体。

（4）交换方式：简单扩散、易化扩散、主动运输。

■ 气体交换。

■ 营养供应。

■ 排泄胎儿代谢产物。

■ 防御功能。

■ 合成功能：人绒毛膜促性腺激素（hCG）、人胎盘生乳素（HPL）、雌激素、孕激素、缩宫素酶，耐热性碱性磷酸酶（HSAP）。

2.胎膜，脐带，羊水

（1）胎膜：绒毛膜和羊膜。

（2）脐带：连接胎儿与胎盘表

450 ～ 650g, diameter 16 ～ 20cm, thickness 1 ～ 3cm.

（3）Function of placenta: Oxygen and nutrients are transferred from mother to fetus, while carbon dioxide and other metabolic wastes are excreted from fetus into mother.

（4）Method of transfer: Simple diffusion, facilitated diffusion and active transport.

■ Gas exchange.

■ Nutrients transfer.

■ Excretion of fetal metabolites.

■ Defense function.

■ Synthesis function: Human chorionic gonadotropin（hCG）, human placental lactogen（HPL）, estrogen, progesterone, oxytocinase, heat stable alkaline phosphatase（HSAP）.

2.Fetal membrane, umbilical cord, and amniotic fluid

（1）Fetal membrane: Chorion and amnion.

（2）Umbilical cord: The cord-like tissue that

面的索条状组织。长度：30～100cm（55cm）；直径：0.8～2.0cm。

（3）羊水：12周前羊水50ml，中期妊娠400ml，足月达1000ml。

- 羊水来源：妊娠早期羊水来自母体血清透析液，20周后为胎儿尿液。

- 羊水功能：有助于缓冲胎儿，使其肌肉骨骼发育，保护胎儿免受创伤；保持温度和最低限度的营养供给；促进胎儿肺和胃肠道的正常生长和发育。

第四节 妊娠期母体的变化

1. 生殖系统的变化

（1）子宫

- 子宫大小：增大（7cm×5cm×3cm至35cm×25cm×22cm），容量（5～5000ml），重量（50～1100g），妊娠早期、中期和晚期的厚度（1cm→2.0～2.5cm→0.5～1.0cm）；不同部位增大的速度不同（宫底强，宫颈弱），因此从底部到子宫颈的收缩性逐渐减弱，有助于胎儿娩出。

- 子宫血流：随着妊娠周数增加，子宫肌细胞更加肥大，血供更丰富（450～650ml/min）。

- 子宫内膜：受精卵着床后，子宫内膜称为蜕膜，分为

connects the fetus to the surface of the placenta. Length: 30 ～ 100cm（55cm）, diameter: 0.8 ～ 2.0cm.

（3）Amniotic fluid: 50ml before 12 weeks, 400ml at mid pregnancy, 1000ml at term.

- Source of amniotic fluid: Ultrafiltrate of maternal plasma in early pregnancy, and fetal urine after 20 weeks.

- Function of amnionic fluid: To cushion the fetus, allow for musculoskeletal development and protect it from trauma; to maintain temperature and minimum nutrient supply; to promote the normal growth and development of the lungs and gastrointestinal tract.

Section 4　Changes during pregnancy

1.Changes of reproductive tract

（1）Uterus

- Size: Increase in size（from 7cm×5cm×3cm to 35cm×25cm×22cm）, capacity（5 ～ 5000ml）, weight（50 ～ 1100g）, thickness in the first, second and third trimesters（1cm→2.0 ～ 2.5cm→0.5 ～ 1.0cm）; the rate of the hypertrophy of different parts varies（fundus→inferior portion→cervix）and the contractility decreases from fundus to cervix, which helps the delivery of fetus.

- Uterine blood flow: Hypertrophy of the uterine muscular cells with the increase of pregnant weeks, and more vascular（450 ～ 650ml/min）.

- Endometrium: After implantation, endometrium is called decidua, which is

底蜕膜、包蜕膜、真蜕膜（图3-3）。

■ 峡部：柔软变长（1cm至7～10cm），形成子宫下段。

■ 宫颈：血流丰富，宫颈水肿，宫颈腺体增生。

（2）卵巢：增大，新生卵泡和排卵停止。妊娠7周黄体产生雌激素和孕激素，妊娠10周后开始萎缩，取而代之的是胎盘功能。

（3）输卵管：伸长但不增厚。

（4）阴道：紫蓝色（Chadwick征），脱落的阴道上皮细胞糖原水平增加，乳酸含量增多。

（5）外阴：色素沉着。

子宫收缩：Braxton Hicks收缩，无痛宫缩，稀发，不规律，不对称。子宫内的压力：5～25mmHg，持续时间＜30秒。

2.乳房

■ 随着乳腺腺泡增生，导致乳腺增大并出现结节，乳头增大变黑，易勃起。乳晕颜色

divided into basal decidua, capsular decidua and true decidua（Figure 3-3）.

■ Isthmus: Soft and longer（from 1cm to 7～10cm）, forming lower uterine segment.

■ Cervix: Increased vascularity, edema of the entire cervix, and hyperplasia of cervical glands.

（2）Ovary: Enlarged, and no ovulation and new follicle. Corpus luteum produces E and P from week 7 of pregnancy, but starts to atrophy after week 10 of pregnancy. The function is replaced by placenta.

（3）Fallopian tube: Prolonged without hypertrophy.

（4）Vagina: Bluish coloration（Chadwick's sign）; desquamation of epithelium with more glycogen→acidity increased.

（5）Vulva: Pigmentation.

Uterine contraction: Braxton Hicks contraction, contraction without pain, rare, irregular, and asymmetric. Intrauterine pressure: 5 ～ 25mmHg, duration＜30 seconds.

2.Breast

■ With the increase in size and nodular sensation, due to the hypertrophy of the mammary alveoli, the nipples soon become

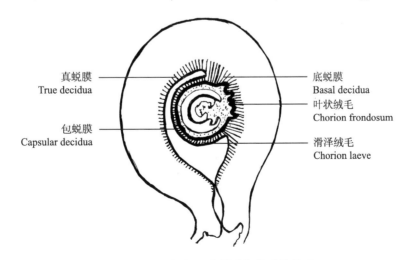

图3-3 早期妊娠子宫蜕膜与绒毛的关系

Figure 3-3 Relationship between decidua and villi in early pregnancy

加深，其外围的皮脂腺肥大形成散在的结节状隆起，称为蒙氏结节。

3.循环系统

（1）心脏：妊娠期增大的子宫使膈肌升高，心脏由此向左前上方移位发生一定程度的扭转。血容量增加10%，心率每分钟增加10～15次。

（2）心排血量：从妊娠10周开始增加，妊娠32～34周达高峰。

（3）血压：有少许的改变。

（4）下肢静脉压力：静脉压增加，妊娠后期明显增加，可导致妊娠期间脚踝水肿、腿部及外阴静脉曲张。

仰卧位低血压综合征：长时间仰卧位→下腔静脉受压→心脏回流减少→心排血量减少→血压下降→低血压。

4.血液系统

（1）血容量：妊娠6～8周开始增加，妊娠32～34周达高峰，平均增加约1450ml（血浆增加1000ml，红细胞增加450ml→血液稀释）。

（2）血液成分：红细胞$3.6×10^{12}$/L，血红蛋白110g/L，白细胞（10～12）$×10^9$/L，妊娠期血液处于高凝状态→由于血液稀释血浆蛋白略有减少。

5.泌尿系统

（1）肾血浆流量（RPF）和肾小球滤过率（GFR），分别增加35%和50%，由此造成孕妇和胎儿的代

larger, deeply pigmented and erectile. Scattered around the areola are some roundish nodules called Montgomery's tubercles, which result from hypertrophy of the sebaceous glands.

3.Circulatory system

（1）Heart: The growing uterus pushes the diaphragm upward, thus shifting the heart to the left, upward and somewhat in the direction of the anterior chest wall, with a certain degree of torsion. The capacity increases by 10%, and the heart rate increases by 10～15 bpm.

（2）Cardiac output: Increasing from week 10 of pregnancy, at peak in week 32～34 of pregnancy.

（3）Blood pressure: Few changes if any.

（4）Venous pressure: Increased venous pressure, on the legs demonstrable in later months of pregnancy, which contributes to the ankle edema, varicose veins in the legs and vulva during gestation.

Supine hypotensive syndrome: Supine position for a long time→inferior vena cava compressed→decreased venous return→decreased cardiac output→decreased blood pressure（Bp）→hypotension.

4.Blood system

（1）Volume: Increasing from week 6～8 of pregnancy, at peak in week 32～34 of pregnancy, average increase about 1450ml（1000ml of plasma, 450ml of erythrocytes→hemodilution）.

（2）Composition: RBC $3.6×10^{12}$/L, hemoglobin 110g/L, WBC（10～12）$×10^9$/L, coagulating factors→most increasing→hypercoagulation, plasmal protein decreases mildly due to hemodilution.

5.Urinary system

（1）RPF and GFR increase by about 35% and 50% respectively, resulting in increased excretion of metabolites in the gravida and fetus.

谢产物排泄增多。

（2）在孕激素的影响下，不仅子宫，而且输尿管、肠管和胆管的平滑肌张力降低→输尿管扩张和肾盂积水→造成急性肾盂肾炎，尤其发生在右侧。

6. 呼吸系统

■ 总体上讲，通气量增加，免疫能力下降。

7. 消化系统

■ 受雌激素影响→齿龈肥厚，在孕激素影响下→胃肠道平滑肌张力降低、松弛→胃烧灼感、呕吐、便秘。

8. 皮肤

（1）在乳晕、腹白线、外阴等处偶尔会出现色素沉着，形成不规则、大小不同的褐色斑块，出现在面部和颈部时，称黄褐斑或妊娠斑，通常在分娩后就会消失。

（2）妊娠后期，腹部的皮肤出现淡红色，略凹陷的条纹称为妊娠纹，有时也可出现在胸部和大腿。约1/2的孕妇有妊娠纹。

9. 内分泌变化

（1）脑下垂体：腺垂体（垂体前叶）稍增生。

高水平的雌激素和孕激素→抑制促性腺激素（Gn）释放。

（2）泌乳素：妊娠7周开始增加，分娩前达高峰。

（3）肾上腺皮质素：皮质醇和醛固酮水平分别增加3～4倍。

（4）甲状腺：正常妊娠甲状腺呈中度增大，由于腺体组织增生，血液供应增加并形成新的毛囊。但

（2）Under the influence of progesterone, the condition of atonia not only in uterus, but also on the ureters, the enlarged bowel and bile ducts→dilatation of ureters and renal pelvis associated with stasis of urine→ acute nephropyelitis particularly on the right side.

6. Respiratory system

■ The ventilation volume increases; the immunologic competence declines.

7. Digestive system

■ Estrogen→gingiva hypertrophy, due to progesterone→atonia of stomach and bowel→stomach burn, vomit, and constipation.

8. Skin

（1）The pigmentation of the areola, linea alba, and vulva, occasionally irregular shaped, brownish patches of varying size appear on the face and neck, called chloasma or cyasma, which fortunately disappear after delivery.

（2）During late months of pregnancy, reddish, slightly depressed streaks often appear on the skin of abdomen, sometimes covering the breasts and the thighs. These striae gravidarum occur in 1/2 of all pregnancies.

9. Endocrine changes

（1）Pituitary gland: Hyperplasia of the adenohypophysis（anterior lobe）.

High level of estrogen and progesterone→inhibiting gonadotropin（Gn）release.

（2）PRL:It increases at week 7 of pregnancy and reaches its peak before delivery.

（3）Adrenocortical hormone: The levels of cortisol and aldosterone increase by 3～4 times respectively.

（4）Thyroid gland: The enlargement concomitant with normal pregnancy due to hypertrophy of adenomatous tissue, with the

大多数甲状腺素与甲状腺结合球蛋白结合，所以孕妇无甲状腺功能亢进表现。

10. 新陈代谢的变化

（1）基础代谢率：略有上升。

（2）体重：从妊娠13周开始每周增加350g，整个妊娠期间约增加12.5kg。

（3）碳水化合物代谢。

- 由于高胰岛素分泌，空腹血糖降低。

- 胰岛素抵抗因素。

（4）脂肪代谢：母体脂肪积存多，能量消耗增多时，使血中酮体增加，易发生酮血症。

（5）蛋白质代谢：呈正氮平衡。

（6）水代谢：妊娠期水潴留约7L。

（7）矿物质代谢：在妊娠后期要及时补充钙和铁，避免钙和铁缺乏。

11. 骨、关节和韧带

（1）骨质：通常无变化。

（2）关节和韧带：松弛素→关节和韧带松弛→产道扩大。

重点专业词汇

1. 妊娠

2. 胚胎

3. 胎儿

4. 受精

5. 受精卵

6. 着床

7. 胎盘

8. 胎膜

9. 脐带

10. 羊水

11. 人绒毛膜促性腺激素（hCG）

increase blood supply to set formation of new follicles. But most thyroxin connected with thyroxin binding globulin, and no hyperthyroidism occurs.

10. Metabolic changes

（1）BMR: Mild increase.

（2）Weight: From week 13 of pregnancy increased by 350g per week, and about 12.5kg during the entire pregnancy.

（3）Metabolism of carbohydrate.

- Lower fasting blood glucose due to higher insulin secretion.

- Insulin-resistant factors.

（4）Fat metabolism: Deposit of maternal fat and energy consumption increasing, characterized by increased ketone bodies and tendency to ketosis.

（5）Protein metabolism: Positive nitrogen balance.

（6）Water metabolism: Water retention during pregnancy is about 7L.

（7）Mineral metabolism: In the late months of gestation, calcium and iron supplements are necessary to avoid their deficiency.

11. Bone, joint and ligament

（1）Bone: No changes normally.

（2）Joint and ligament: Relaxin→loose joints and ligaments→birth canal widened.

Key words

1. Pregnancy

2. Embryo

3. Fetus

4. Fertilization

5. Fertilized ovum

6. Implantation

7. Placenta

8. Fetal membrane

9. Umbilical cord

10. Amniotic fluid

11. Human chorionic gonadotropin（hCG）

12.底蜕膜

13.包蜕膜

14.真蜕膜

练习题

1.hCG分泌于：（B）

A.滋养细胞

B.合体滋养细胞

C.颗粒细胞

D.蜕膜细胞

E.卵泡膜细胞

2.关于受精卵的描述下列哪项是错误的？（A）

A.受精4日后受精卵进入宫腔，5日开始植入

B.获能的精子与次级卵母细胞结合形成受精卵

C.受精3日后受精卵形成桑葚胚

D.植入有定位、黏附和侵入3个阶段

E.受精发生于排卵后12小时内

3.正常妊娠，受精卵在什么条件下植入？（A）

A.受精后6～8日，子宫内膜呈分泌期

B.子宫内膜蜕膜反应

C.排卵后2～3日的子宫内膜

D.受精时透明带仍然存在

E.受精卵在桑葚胚期植入

4.植入发生在受精后：（D）

A.2～3日

B.3～4日

C.5～6日

D.6～7日

12.Basal decidua

13.Capsular decidua

14.True decidua

Exercises

1.Human chorionic gonadotropin secretion occurs in:（B）

A.Trophoblast cells

B.Syncytiotrophoblastic cells

C.Granulosa cells

D.Decidual cells

E.Theca cells

2.Which of the following descriptions of the fertilized ovum is wrong?（A）

A.4 days after fertilization, the fertilized ovum enters the uterine cavity, and 5 days later begins the implantation

B.The viable sperm binds to the secondary oocyte to form a fertilized ovum

C.The fertilized ovum forms morula in 3 days after fertilization

D.Three stages of implantation include positioning, adhesion and invasion

E.Fertilization occurs within 12 hours after ovulation

3.Under what condition is the fertilized ovum implanted in normal pregnancy?（A）

A.6 ～ 8 days after fertilization, endometrial secretion stage

B.Endometrial decidual response

C.Endometrium of 2 ～ 3 days after ovulation

D.The zona pellucida still existing while fertilization

E.Fertilized ovum implantation in the morula period

4.Implantation after fertilization:（D）

A.2 ～ 3 days

B.3 ～ 4 days

C.5 ～ 6 days

D.6 ～ 7 days

E.7～8日

5.妊娠8～10周后孕激素主要来源于:(E)

A.绒毛膜

B.胎膜

C.血管合体膜

D.底蜕膜

E.胎盘合体滋养细胞

（温　菁）

E.7～8 days

5．The main source of progesterone after 8～10 weeks of gestation:（E）

A.Chorion

B.Fetal membranes

C.Vasculo-syncytial membrane

D.Basal decidua

E.Placenta syncytiotrophoblastic cells

第4章 妊娠诊断

CHAPTER 4　Diagnosis of pregnancy

第一节　早期妊娠的诊断

1.病史和症状

（1）停经
- 是最早出现、最重要的症状。

- 情绪紧张，慢性疾病和某些药物均可导致月经延期。

- 哺乳期，宫内节育器存在和内分泌紊乱也可能妊娠。

（2）早孕反应
- 疲劳感，头晕，恶心和呕吐（第6周开始出现，第12周消失）。
- 妊娠剧吐：长期呕吐需要住院治疗。
  - 原因：hCG，孕酮升高使胃排空延长。

（3）泌尿症状
- 膀胱易惹综合征，尿频和夜尿症。
  - 原因：雌激素、孕激素升高致使盆腔血流循环增加，增大的子宫压迫。
  - 必须排除尿路感染。

（4）乳房胀痛
- 雌激素升高使乳腺管发育，孕激素升高使腺泡发育。

Section 1　Diagnosis of early pregnancy

1.Medical history and symptoms

（1）Amenorrhea
- The earliest and the most important symptom.

- Emotional stress, chronic diseases and certain medications can lead to delayed menses.

- During lactation, intrauterine devices, or in endocrine disorders, pregnancy may also occur.

（2）Morning sickness
- Fatigue, dizziness, nausea and vomiting（appear in week 6, disappear in week 12）.

- Hyperemesis gravidarum: Prolonged vomiting requires hospitalization.
  - Causes: hCG, elevated progesterone prolongs gastric emptying.

（3）Urinary symptoms
- Bladder irritability, urinary frequency and nocturia.
  - Causes: Enlargement of the uterus and increased circulation in pelvis due to elevated estrogen and progesterone.
  - Urinary infection must be ruled out.

（4）Mastodynia
- The development of mammary ducts（elevated estrogen）and of alveoli（elevated

■ 循环增加致使乳房增大。

2.体征

（1）生殖器官的改变

■ 阴道：紫蓝着色（盆腔血管充血导致）。雌激素、孕激素升高可使阴道分泌物增加。

■ 宫颈：变软及紫蓝着色。宫颈黏液，黏稠状。

■ 黑加征：妊娠6～8周时，双合诊检查子宫峡部极软，感觉宫颈与子宫体之间似不相连，称为黑加征。

■ 腹部增大：子宫增大（妊娠12周后感觉到）。

（2）乳房变化

■ 妊娠6～8周乳房增大，血管充盈。

■ 蒙氏结节：因妊娠6～8周雌激素和孕激素升高，乳晕周围出现的小结节。

■ 妊娠16周可出现初乳分泌或副乳。

3.辅助检查

（1）妊娠试验

■ 尿hCG试验。

■ 血清hCG试验＞5.0U/L。

（2）超声

■ 子宫增大。

■ 妊娠5周可见妊娠囊。

■ 妊娠6周可见胎芽或胎心搏动。

（3）其他

■ 孕激素试验。

■ 宫颈黏液检查。

progesterone）.

■ Increased circulation results in enlargement of breasts.

2.Signs

（1）The changes of genital organs

■ Vagina: Bluish discoloration（congested pelvic vasculature）. Increased vaginal discharge（elevated estrogen and progesterone）.

■ Cervix: Softer and bluish discoloration. The cervical mucus is viscous.

■ Hegar's sign: When gestation 6 ～ 8 weeks, uterine isthmus is extremely soft by bimanual examination, and the uterocervical junction seems not to be connected. It is known as Hegar's sign.

■ Abdominal enlargement: Enlargement of uterus（after 12 weeks of pregnancy）.

（2）Breast changes

■ Breast enlargement and vascular engorgement（week 6 ～ 8 of pregnancy）.

■ Montgomery's tubercles: Small nodules around the areola（week 6 ～ 8 of pregnancy, elevated estrogen and progesterone）.

■ Colostrum secretion or accessory breast（week 16 of pregnancy）.

3.Auxiliary examination

（1）Pregnancy test

■ Urine hCG test.

■ Serum hCG＞5.0U/L.

（2）Ultrasound

■ Enlargement of uterus.

■ Gestational sac（week 5 of pregnancy）.

■ Embryo or fetal heart beat（week 6 of pregnancy）.

（3）Other tests

■ Progesterone test.

■ Cervical mucus examination.

- 基础体温测定（BBT）：双相体温，高温相持续超过3周，诊断妊娠可能性大。

- Basal body temperature（BBT）: Biphasic pattern, which lasts for more than 3 weeks, which is likely to be diagnosed as pregnancy.

第二节 妊娠中、晚期的诊断

Section 2 Diagnosis of mid or late pregnancy

1.症状与体征

预产期（EDC）：月份加9或减3，日加7。

（1）子宫增大（图4-1）

- 妊娠12周：耻骨联合上2指。

- 妊娠16周：耻骨联合与脐之间中点。

- 妊娠20～22周：平脐。

（2）胎动（FM）

- 初次感到：在妊娠18～20周。

- 可以诊断妊娠，推测妊娠周数，判断胎儿的安危。

1.Symptoms and signs

Expected date of confinement（EDC）: m + 9 or m-3, d+7.

（1）Enlargement of uterus（Figure 4-1）

- 12th week: 2 fingers wide above the pubic symphysis.

- 16th week: Midway between the pubic symphysis and the umbilicus.

- 20th ～ 22nd week: At the umbilicus.

（2）Fetal movement（FM）

- The first perception: In week 18 ～ 20.

- Diagnosis of pregnancy, duration of pregnancy, and the safety of fetus.

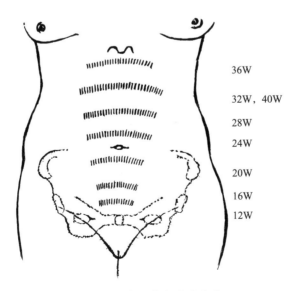

图4-1 妊娠周数与宫底高度

Figure 4-1 Abdominal measurement of uterine height and gestation weeks

（3）胎动计数：每日3次，每次1小时。次数×4=FM/12小时。正常：≥30次/12小时。

（4）胎儿心搏

■ 妊娠18～20周可经听诊器闻及。

■ 正常胎心110～160次/分。

■ 需要与脐带杂音相鉴别。

■ 胎体。

（5）触诊：妊娠20周可触及胎儿轮廓。

2.辅助检查

（1）超声

■ 胎儿数目。

■ 胎产式。

■ 胎先露。

■ 胎方位。

■ 胎儿是否存活。

■ 胎盘与脐带（脐血流）。

■ 胎儿大小。

（2）胎儿心电图（FECG）

第三节　胎姿势、胎产式、胎先露、胎方位（表4-1）

1.胎姿势

■ 指胎儿在子宫内的姿势。

2.胎产式

■ 指胎儿的长轴与母体长轴之间的关系

　● 纵产式：胎儿的长轴与母体平行。

　● 横产式：胎儿的长轴与母体垂直交叉。

3.胎先露

（1）头先露：枕先露（95%），面先露。

（3）Fetal movement counting: 3 times per day, and 1 hour per time. sum×4=FM/12 hours. Normal: ≥30/12 hours.

（4）Fetal heart tones

■ Heard: In week 18～20 with stethoscope.

■ Normal rate: 110～160bpm.

■ Differentiation: Umbilical souffle.

■ Fetal body.

（5）Palpation: Outline of the fetus（the 20th week）.

2.Auxiliary examination

（1）Ultrasound

■ The number of fetus.

■ Fetal lie.

■ Fetal presentation.

■ Fetal position.

■ Fetal death or not.

■ Placenta and cord（velocity of flow）

■ Size of fetus.

（2）Fetal electrocardiography（FECG）

Section 3　Fetal attitude, fetal lie, fetal presentation, and fetal position（Table 4-1）

1.Fetal attitude

■ The position of fetus in the uterus.

2.Fetal lie

■ The relationship of the long axis of the fetus and the long axis of the mother

　● Longitudinal lie: The long axis of the fetus is parallel to the mother's.

　● Transverse lie: The long axis of the fetus crosses the mother's vertically.

3.Fetal presentation

（1）Head presentation: Occiput presentation（95%）, and face presentation.

表4-1 胎产式、胎先露和胎方位的关系和种类

Table 4-1 Relationship and types of fetal lie, fetal presentation and fetal position

产式 Fetal lie	胎先露 Fetal presentation		胎位 Fetal position
纵产式 Longitudinal lie 99.75%	头先露 Head presentation 95.75%～97.55%	枕先露 Occiput presentation 95.55%～97.55%	枕左前、枕左横、枕左后 LOA, LOT, LOP 枕右前、枕右横、枕右后 ROA, ROT, ROP
		面先露 Face presentation 0.2%	颏左前、颏左横、颏左后 LMA, LMT, LMP 颏右前、颏右横、颏右后 RMA, RMT, RMP
	臀先露 Breech presentation 2%～4%		骶左前、骶左横、骶左后 LSA, LST, LSP 骶右前、骶右横、骶右后 RSA, RST, RSP
横产式 Transverse lie 0.25%	肩先露 Shoulder presentation		肩左前、肩左后 LSCA, LSCP 肩右前、肩右后 RSCA, RSCP

（2）臀先露
- 完全臀先露。
- 混合臀先露。
- 不全臀先露：足先露。

4.胎方位
- 胎儿先露部的指示点与母体骨盆的4个象限关系或与母体骨盆横径的关系。

  - 枕先露：枕骨部,O表示。LOA，LOT，LOP。
  - 面先露：下颏，M表示。LMA，LMT，LMP。
  - 臀先露：骶骨，S表示。LSA，LST，LSP。

重点专业词汇
1.停经
2.早孕反应
3.超声

（2）Breech presentation
- Complete breech presentation.
- Frank breech presentation.
- Incomplete breech presentation: Footling presentation.

4.Fetal position
- The relationship of the point of direction of the presenting part to the 4 quadrants of the pelvis or to the transverse diameter of the maternal pelvis.

  - Occiput presentation: The occiput, represented by O. LOA, LOT, LOP.
  - Face presentation: The chin, represented by M. LMA, LMT, LMP.
  - Breech presentation: The sacrum, represented by S. LSA, LST, LSP.

Key words
1.Amenorrhea
2.Morning sickness
3.Ultrasound

4.妊娠囊

5.预产期（EDC）

6.胎姿势

7.胎产式

8.胎先露

9.胎方位

10.枕先露

11.面先露

12.臀先露

练习题

1.早期妊娠诊断方法是：（A）

A.超声

B.尿妊娠试验

C.孕激素试验

D.基础体温测定

E.妇科检查

2.下列哪项确诊早孕？（C）

A.尿频

B.宫颈紫蓝着色

C.宫内妊娠囊

D.尿妊娠试验阳性

E.停经并早孕反应

3.孕妇最早出现胎动感觉是：（C）

A.妊娠14～16周

B.妊娠16～18周

C.妊娠18～20周

D.妊娠20～24周

E.妊娠24周以上

4.每小时正常胎动的次数是：（A）

A.3～5次

B.6～8次

C.9～10次

D.12～14次

E.15～17次

（温 菁）

4.Gestational sac

5.Expected date of confinement（EDC）

6.Fetal attitude

7.Fetal lie

8.Fetal presentation

9.Fetal position

10.Occiput presentation

11.Face presentation

12.Breech presentation

Exercises

1.Early pregnancy diagnosis method is：（A）

A.Ultrasound

B.Urine pregnancy test

C.Progestin trial

D.Basal body temperature measurement

E.Pelvic examination

2.Which of the following can be accurate in the diagnosis of early pregnancy？（C）

A.Frequent urination

B.Cervical bluish discoloration

C.Gestational sac

D.Urine pregnancy test: Positive

E.Menopause with morning sickness

3.Pregnant women first time feel fetal movement in：（C）

A.14～16 weeks

B.16～18 weeks

C.18～20 weeks

D.20～24 weeks

E.More than 24 weeks

4.Normal fetal movement per hour should be：（A）

A.3～5 times

B.6～8 times

C.9～10 times

D.12～14 times

E.15～17 times

第5章 异常妊娠

CHAPTER 5　Abnormal pregnancy

第一节　自 然 流 产

Section 1　Spontaneous abortion

1.定义

- 妊娠不足28周、胎儿体重不足1000g而终止者，称为流产。

1.Definition

- Abortion is termination of pregnancy before 28 weeks of gestation and the fetal weight is less than 1000g.

2.分类

（1）根据孕周

- 早期流产：发生在妊娠12周前。

- 晚期流产：发生在妊娠12周后。

（2）根据临床类型

- 先兆流产：阴道少量出血伴或不伴腹痛，宫颈口未开，胎膜完整（图5-1）。

- 难免流产：在先兆流产基础上，阴道出血增多，腹痛加重，宫口扩张，有时胚胎组织或胎囊堵塞于宫内口（图5-2）。

- 不全流产：难免流产继续发展，部分妊娠组织或胎盘残留于宫腔或宫颈内口。发生大量阴道出血甚至休克（图5-3）。

- 完全流产：妊娠物已全部排出，阴道出血停止，腹痛消失，宫内口关闭（图5-4）。

2.Classification

（1）Gestational age

- Early abortion: Before 12 weeks.

- Late abortion: After 12 weeks.

（2）Clinical classification

- Threatened abortion: Slight vaginal bleeding with or without abdominal pain. The cervical os is closed and the membrane is intact（Figure 5-1）.

- Inevitable abortion: On the basis of threatened abortion, vaginal bleeding has been often severe, and the cervical os becomes dilated in response to the painful intermittent uterine contractions. Sometimes the tissue of embryo or gestation sac may block the cervical os（Figure 5-2）.

- Incomplete abortion: Developed from inevitable abortion, parts of the tissue of embryo or placenta are retained in the uterus or cervical os. Vaginal bleeding may be so severe as to cause shock（Figure 5-3）.

- Complete abortion: The tissue of embryo is expelled intact, bleeding stops, pain ceases, and the os is closed（Figure 5-4）.

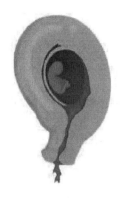 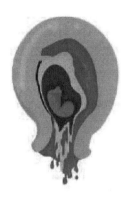 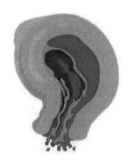 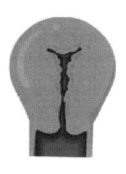

图5-1 先兆流产　　图5-2 难免流产　　图5-3 不全流产　　图5-4 完全流产

Figure 5-1 Threatened　Figure 5-2 Inevitable　Figure 5-3 Incomplete　Figure 5-4 Complete
abortion　　　　　　 abortion　　　　　　 abortion　　　　　　 abortion

- 稽留流产：胚胎已死，滞留于宫腔内未能及时排出。
- 复发性流产（RSA）：与同一性伴侣连续发生2次或2次以上的自然流产。
- 流产合并感染：通常与不全流产或非法堕胎有关。

3.病因

（1）胚胎因素：染色体异常是早期自发流产最常见的原因，占50%～60%。

（2）母体因素

- 全身性疾病：如严重感染、严重贫血或心力衰竭、血栓性疾病、慢性肝脏疾病或高血压等。
- 内分泌异常：黄体功能不全、高催乳素血症、多囊卵巢综合征、甲状腺功能减退、糖尿病血糖控制不良等。
- 生殖器疾病：先天畸形（如单角子宫、双角子宫或纵隔子宫）改变或减小宫腔面积；既往宫腔手术操作的瘢痕，如刮宫、肌瘤切除术或

- Missed abortion: The fetus dies and is retained in uterus.
- Recurrent spontaneous abortion（RSA）: A woman has two or more consecutive spontaneous abortions with the same sexual mate.
- Septic abortion: Usually associated with incomplete or illegal abortion.

3.Etiology

（1）Embryo factors: Chromosome abnormality is responsible for a large percentage of early spontaneous abortions, which accounts for at least 50%～60% of these losses.

（2）Maternal factors

- General diseases: Severe infection, severe anemia or cardiac failure, thrombotic diseases, chronic hepatic diseases or hypertension and so on.
- Endocrine disorders: Corpus luteum insufficiency, hyperprolactinemia, polycystic ovary syndrome, hypothyroidism, poorly controlled diabetes mellitus and so on.
- Genital diseases: Congenital anomalies that distort or reduce the size of the uterine cavity, such as unicornuate, bicornuate, or septate uterus; previous scarring of the uterine cavity following dilatation and

宫颈解剖学的异常或宫颈功能不全。

■ 强烈应激与不良习惯：躯体或心理的创伤，过量吸烟、酗酒或饮咖啡。

■ 免疫功能异常：自身免疫功能异常（抗磷脂综合征、系统性红斑狼疮）和同种免疫功能异常。

（3）父亲因素：精子染色体异常。

（4）环境因素：放射线和砷、铅等化学物质。

4. 诊断

（1）病史

■ 停经史，反复流产史。

■ 腹痛程度，阴道出血情况。

■ 是否有妊娠物排出。

（2）体格检查

■ 全身检查：体温，脉搏，呼吸，血压。

■ 妇科检查

● 子宫大小：与停经周数是否相符且有无压痛。

● 宫颈口：是否扩张。

（3）辅助检查

■ 超声

● 鉴别流产类型。

● 妊娠囊的形态和位置、有无胎心搏动。

■ 妊娠试验。

■ 孕激素测定。

5. 治疗

（1）先兆流产

■ 卧床休息，禁止性生活。

■ 药物治疗。

● 黄体功能不全或孕酮低

curettage, and myomectomy; anatomic abnormalities or functional incompetence of the uterine cervix.

■ Severe stress and bad habits: Severe stress (physical and psychological) and excess smoking, insobriety and excess coffee.

■ Immunologic dysfunction: Abnormal autoimmune diseases (antiphospholipid syndrome, systemic lupus erythematosus) and abnormal alloimmune diseases.

（3）Paternal factors: Chromosome abnormality of sperm.

（4）Environmental factors: Radioactive rays and chemical substances, such as arsenic or lead.

4. Diagnosis

（1）Medical history

■ Amenorrhea, recurrent abortion.

■ The degree of abdominal pain, vaginal bleeding.

■ The products of gestation expelled or not.

（2）Physical examination

■ General examination: Temperature, pulse, respiration, blood pressure.

■ Pelvic examination

● Uterine size: Compared to the expected date of pregnancy, uterine tenderness.

● Cervical os: Open or close.

（3）Auxiliary examination

■ Ultrasound

● Differentiation of varieties of abortion.

● Gestation sac status and position, whether there is fetal heartbeat.

■ Pregnancy test.

■ Progesterone measurement.

5. Treatment

（1）Threatened abortion

■ Bed rest, forbid sexual intercourse.

■ Medical treatment.

● For those with corpus luteum insufficiency

者，黄体酮肌内注射。

● 口服维生素 E。

（2）难免流产与不全流产

■ 一旦确诊应及时行清宫术。

■ 使用抗生素预防感染。

■ 刮出组织并送病理检查。

（3）完全流产：证实宫腔内无残留物，不需特殊处理。

（4）稽留流产

■ 一旦确诊，需要尽快清宫。

■ 因为胎儿死亡，胎盘释放凝血酶原激酶进入血液循环，导致弥散性血管内凝血（DIC）。

● 清宫前，应检查血常规、凝血功能，并做好输血准备。

● 提高子宫肌对缩宫素的敏感性。

● 炔雌醇1mg每日2次口服，连服5日。

（5）复发性流产：首先要检查发生习惯性流产的原因，针对原因进行治疗。

（6）流产合并感染：控制感染的同时尽快清除宫内残留物。

重点专业词汇

1.先兆流产

2.难免流产

3.不全流产

4.完全流产

5.稽留流产

6.复发性流产

7.流产合并感染

练习题

1.自然流产最常见的原因可能

or low progestin, progesterone by intramuscular injection.

● Vitamin E, take orally.

（2）Inevitable and incomplete abortion

■ Once diagnosed, dilatation & curettage（D&C）.

■ Antibiotics used for preventive infection.

■ Tissue sent for pathological examination.

（3）Complete abortion: If the uterus empty, no need for further interference.

（4）Missed abortion

■ Dilation & curettage（D&C）is necessary as soon as possible after diagnosis.

■ Placenta releases thrombokinase into blood circulation due to the death of the fetus, leading to disseminated intravascular coagulation（DIC）.

● Check the blood routine examination and coagulation function before curettage and prepare for blood transfusion.

● Improve myometrium sensitivity to the oxytocin.

● Ethinyloestradiol 1mg, bid, po, for 5d.

（5）Recurrent spontaneous abortion: Find out the causes of habitual abortion and give treatment.

（6）Septic abortion: Control infection and remove remnants as soon as possible.

Key words

1.Threatened abortion

2.Inevitable abortion

3.Incomplete abortion

4.Complete abortion

5.Missed abortion

6.Recurrent spontaneous abortion

7.Septic abortion

Exercises

1.The most common reason of spontaneous

是：（E）

　　A.孕妇患甲状腺功能低下

　　B.孕妇接触放射性物质

　　C.孕妇细胞免疫调节失调

　　D.母儿血型不合

　　E.遗传基因异常

　　2.关于流产的治疗原则，以下哪项是错误的？（D）

　　A.先兆流产于妊娠早期可肌内注射黄体酮

　　B.难免流产可选用适宜方式清除子宫内容物

　　C.不全流产应尽快行刮宫术

　　D.流产感染出血不多时，抗感染和刮宫治疗可同时进行

　　E.子宫内口松弛症应在妊娠14～18周行宫颈环扎术

　　3.患者30岁，停经17周，1个月来间断少量阴道出血，腹部无明显压痛、反跳痛，子宫颈口未开，子宫增大如孕8周，最可能的诊断为：（E）

　　A.先兆流产

　　B.难免流产

　　C.不全流产

　　D.完全流产

　　E.稽留流产

第二节　异位妊娠

1.定义

　　（1）受精卵在子宫体腔以外着床称为异位妊娠，习称宫外孕。

abortion is:（E）

　　A.Hypothyroidism

　　B.Radiations

　　C.Cell immunologic disorders

　　D.Blood group incompatibility

　　E.Genetic abnormalities

　　2.Which of the following is wrong about the treatment principle of abortion?（D）

　　A.For threatened abortion, supplement progesterone by intramuscular injection at first trimester

　　B.For inevitable abortion, evacuate the uterus by appropriate methods

　　C.Curettage should be promptly performed to incomplete abortion

　　D.If septic abortion is less bleeding, antibiotic therapy and curettage should be done at the same time

　　E.If cervical incompetence, a cervical cerclage should be done between 14 and 18 weeks' gestation

　　3.A 30-year-old patient had menopause for 17 weeks. In recent 1 month, she had intermittent less vaginal bleeding. No obvious tenderness and rebound tenderness were found by abdominal palpation. Her cervical os was close, and the size of uterus was about 8 weeks of pregnancy. The most possible diagnosis is:（E）

　　A.Threatened abortion

　　B.Inevitable abortion

　　C.Incomplete abortion

　　D.Complete abortion

　　E.Missed abortion

Section 2　Ectopic pregnancy

1.Definition

　　（1）The fertilized ovum embeds outside the uterine cavity, and the condition is called ectopic or extrauterine pregnancy.

（2）最常见的是输卵管妊娠（占异位妊娠95%左右），但亦可着床在卵巢、腹腔、阔韧带、宫颈。所以我们主要介绍输卵管妊娠（图5-5）。

2.病因

（1）输卵管炎症：主要病因。

（2）输卵管妊娠史或手术史。

（3）输卵管发育不良或功能异常。

（4）辅助生殖技术。

（5）避孕失败。

3.临床表现

（1）症状

■ 停经：多数有6～8周停经史。有20%～30%异位妊娠女性在每个月来月经时间会有少量阴道出血而误认为月经而没有意识到妊娠。

■ 腹痛：最主要的症状，可以是单侧的，也可以双侧的，可以是局部的，也可以是全身的，取决于腹腔内出血量。

■ 阴道出血，可有蜕膜管型。

　　● 晕厥与休克：取决于出血量及出血速度，与阴道出

（2）The commonest site is in the fallopian tube（95%）, but the pregnancy may occasionally be embedded in the ovary, the abdomen, the broad ligament or in the cervix uteri. So we introduce the tubal pregnancy mainly herewith（Figure 5-5）.

2.Etiology

（1）Tubal inflammatory disease: The main cause.

（2）The history of tubal pregnancy or tubal surgery.

（3）Tubal dysplasia or dysfunction.

（4）Assisted reproductive techniques.

（5）Contraceptive failure.

3.Clinical manifestations

（1）Symptoms

■ Amenorrhea: Mostly the history of amenorrhea 6 ～ 8 weeks, 20% ～ 30% women with ectopic pregnancies have spotting at the time of their expected menses, and thus do not realize they are pregnant.

■ Abdominal pain: The main symptom that pain can be unilateral or bilateral, localized or generalized, depending on the amount of intra-abdominal bleeding.

■ Bleeding and decidual cast

　　● Syncope and shock: Depending on the amount of blood and the speed of

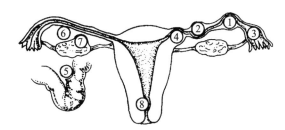

图5-5　异位妊娠的发生部位

Figure 5-5　Location of ectopic pregnancy

①输卵管壶腹部妊娠　Ampulla portion pregnancy；②输卵管峡部妊娠　Isthmic portion pregnancy；③输卵管伞部妊娠　Fimbrial portion pregnancy；④输卵管间质部妊娠　Interstitial portion pregnancy；⑤腹腔妊娠　Abdominal pregnancy；⑥阔韧带妊娠　Broad ligament pregnancy；⑦卵巢妊娠　Ovarian pregnancy；⑧宫颈妊娠　Cervical pregnancy

血量不成正比。

● 腹部包块。

（2）体征

■ 一般情况：腹腔内出血较多时生命体征不平稳。

■ 腹部检查：压痛、反跳痛，有时可触及包块。

■ 盆腔检查：附件压痛和（或）宫颈举摆痛，附件包块，子宫变软，略大。

bleeding, not proportional to the amount of vaginal bleeding.

● Abdominal mass.

（2）Signs

■ General condition: Intra-abdominal hemorrhage is severe and the vital signs are unstable.

■ Abdominal examination: Tenderness, rebound tenderness, sometimes palpable mass.

■ Pelvic examination: Adnexal tenderness and/or cervical motion tenderness, adnexal mass, uterus softening and a slight increase in size.

4.诊断

（1）症状＋体征。

（2）辅助诊断方法

■ hCG：尿或血 hCG。

■ 孕酮测定：＜5ng/ml，应考虑宫内妊娠流产或异位妊娠。

■ 超声图像：宫腔内无孕囊，附件区有包块，腹腔有游离液体。

■ 腹腔镜检查：诊断的金标准，诊断的同时手术治疗。

■ 后穹窿穿刺术：可靠的诊断方法，抽出不凝血（图5-6）。

4.Diagnosis

（1）Symptoms ＋ signs.

（2）Auxiliary diagnostic techniques

■ hCG: Urinary and serum hCG.

■ Progestin assay: ＜ 5ng/ml, considering abortion or ectopic pregnancy.

■ Ultrasound imaging: Empty uterus, adnexal mass, free peritoneal fluid.

■ Laparoscopy: The golden criterion for diagnosis and accompanied by surgical management.

■ Culdocentesis: A reliable diagnostic method, drawing out the blood non-congealable（Figure 5-6）.

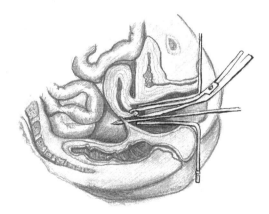

图5-6 后穹窿穿刺术

Figure 5-6 Schematic diagram of culdocentesis

■ 诊断性刮宫：很少应用。

5.处理

（1）药物治疗：甲氨蝶呤。

- 适应证
  - 没有禁忌证。
  - 输卵管妊娠未发生破裂。
  - 妊娠囊直径≤4cm。
  - 血清hCG＜2000U/L。
  - 无明显内出血。

（2）手术治疗：分保守手术和根治手术。

- 适应证
  - 生命体征不平稳或有腹腔内出血征象。
  - 持续性异位妊娠者。
  - 异位妊娠有进展者。
  - 随诊不可靠者。
  - 药物治疗禁忌证或无效者。

重点专业词汇

1.异位妊娠

2.输卵管妊娠

3.停经

4.晕厥

5.后穹窿穿刺术

6.腹腔镜

7.甲氨蝶呤

练习题

1.以下哪一项不是输卵管妊娠的原因？（B）

A.慢性输卵管炎

B.子宫颈炎

C.输卵管手术史

D.宫内节育器（IUD）

E.辅助生殖技术（ART）

2.以下哪项不是异位妊娠手术治疗的指征？（E）

A.生命体征不平稳

B.腹腔内出血

C.血hCG＞3000U/L

■ Diagnostic curettage: Rarely used.

5.Management

（1）Medical treatment: Methotrexate.

- Indications
  - No contraindication.
  - Tubal pregnancy without rupture.
  - The diameter of gestation sac ≤4cm.
  - Serum hCG＜2000U/L.
  - No internal hemorrhage.

（2）Surgical treatment: Conservative surgery and radical surgery.

- Indications
  - Unstable vital signs or internal hemorrhage.
  - Persistent ectopic pregnancy.
  - Ectopic pregnancy aggravating.
  - Follow-up unreliable.
  - Medical treatment contraindication or invalid.

Key words

1.Ectopic pregnancy

2.Tubal pregnancy

3.Amenorrhea

4.Syncope

5.Culdocentesis

6.Laparoscopy

7.Methotrexate

Exercises

1.Which of the following is not related to tubal pregnancy?（B）

A.Chronic salpingitis

B.Cervicitis

C.Prior tubal surgery

D.Intrauterine device（IUD）

E.Assisted reproductive techniques（ART）

2.Which of the following is not the indication of surgical management of ectopic pregnancy?（E）

A.Unstable vital signs

B.Intraperitoneal hemorrhage

C.Serum hCG＞3000U/L

D.发现胎心搏动

E.患者有停经史及阴道出血

第三节 早 产

1.定义

妊娠满28周至不足37周间分娩者。

2.分类

（1）自发性早产。

（2）未足月胎膜早破早产（PPROM）。

（3）治疗性早产。

3.预测

（1）阴道超声检查宫颈长度：＜25mm。

（2）阴道后穹窿分泌物胎儿纤连蛋白检测：阳性。阴性预测价值更高。

4.临床表现及诊断

（1）临床表现：子宫收缩伴少许阴道出血或血性分泌物。

（2）早产临产诊断

■ 出现规则宫缩（20分钟≥4次，或60分钟≥8次），伴有宫颈的进行性改变。

■ 宫颈扩张1cm以上。

■ 宫颈展平≥80%。

5.治疗

治疗原则：若胎膜完整，在母胎情况允许时尽量保胎至34周。

（1）卧床休息。

（2）糖皮质激素：地塞米松6mg肌内注射，每12小时1次，共4次。

D.Fetal heart beat

E.The patient had amenorrhea and vaginal bleeding

Section 3　Preterm birth

1.Definition

Labor occurring after 28 weeks' but before 37 weeks' gestation.

2.Classification

（1）Spontaneous preterm labor.

（2）Preterm premature rupture of membranes（PPROM）.

（3）Preterm birth for medical and obstetrical indications.

3.Prediction

（1）Vaginal ultrasound examination for cervical length: ＜25mm.

（2）Fetal fibronectin from vaginal posterior fornix secretion: Positive. The higher negative predictive value.

4.Clinical manifestation and diagnosis

（1）Clinical manifestation: Uterine contractions with a little vaginal bleeding or bloody excretion.

（2）Diagnosis of preterm labor

■ Regular uterine contractions（20min≥4 times, or 60min≥8 times）with the cervical gradual change.

■ Cervical dilation of at least 1cm.

■ Cervical effacement≥80%.

5.Treatment

Principle: If the membrane is intact, no contraindications for mother and fetus, expectant management is usually recommended till 34 weeks' gestation.

（1）Bed rest.

（2）Corticosteroids: Dexamethasone 6mg intramuscular every 12 hours for a total of 4 doses.

（3）抑制宫缩治疗

■ β-肾上腺素能受体激动剂。

■ 硫酸镁：不作为宫缩抑制剂，建议＜32周使用，有保护胎儿脑神经作用。

■ 阿托西班。

■ 钙通道阻滞剂。

■ 前列腺素合成酶抑制剂。

（4）控制感染：尤其B族链球菌培养。

（5）终止早产指征

■ 宫缩进行性增强，经过治疗无法控制者。

■ 有宫内感染者。

■ 衡量母胎利弊，继续妊娠对母胎的危害大于胎肺成熟对胎儿的好处时。

■ 孕周已达34周，顺其自然，不必干预。

（6）分娩期处理：临产后慎用吗啡、哌替啶等抑制新生儿呼吸中枢的药物。

重点专业词汇

1.早产

2.早产临产

3.皮质类固醇

4.宫缩抑制剂

练习题

1.以下哪项符合早产的定义？（C）

A.妊娠满20周至不足37周间分娩者

B.妊娠满24周至不足37周间分娩者

C.妊娠满28周至不足37周间分娩者

D.妊娠满20周至不足28周间

（3）Tocolysis therapy

■ β-adrenergic receptor agonists.

■ Magnesium sulfate: Not as tocolysis but to protect fetal cranial nerve before 32 weeks' gestation.

■ Atosiban.

■ Calcium-channel blockers.

■ Prostaglandin synthetase inhibitors.

（4）Antibiotics: Especially Group B streptococcal culture.

（5）Indications for termination of pregnancy

■ The uterine contractions are more frequent and intense, and tocolytic therapy fails.

■ Intrauterine infection.

■ During the period of the pregnancy, corticosteroids have not been shown to be beneficial to fetus and mother, on the contrary, maybe dangerous for them.

■ Once a pregancy has continued beyond 34 weeks' gestation, expectant management is usually recommended.

（6）The management of delivery: Drug use should be careful such as morphine and pethidine, which may restrain neonatal respiratory center.

Key words

1.Preterm birth

2.Preterm labor

3.Corticosteroids

4.Tocolysis

Exercises

1.Which of the following is the definition of preterm birth?（C）

A.Labor between 20 weeks and less than 37 weeks of gestation.

B.Labor between 24 weeks and less than 37 weeks of gestation.

C.Labor between 28 weeks and less than 37 weeks of gestation.

D.Labor between 20 weeks and less than 28

分娩者

E.妊娠满28周至不足35周间分娩者

2.以下哪项不属于治疗性早产？（D）

A.子痫前期

B.胎盘早剥

C.前置胎盘出血

D.细菌性阴道病

E.血型不合溶血

3.以下哪项与早产临产诊断无关？（E）

A.出现规则宫缩（20分钟≥4次，或60分钟≥8次）

B.宫颈逐渐缩短

C.宫颈扩张1cm以上

D.宫颈展平≥80%

E.胎膜破裂

第四节 过 期 妊 娠

1.定义

■ 平时月经周期规则，妊娠达到或超过42周尚未分娩者。

2.对母儿影响

（1）围生儿风险：胎儿窘迫、胎粪吸入综合征、新生儿窒息及巨大儿。

（2）母体风险：产程延长和难产率、手术产率增高。

3.诊断

（1）核对孕周：早孕试验，孕早期超声，临床参数（例如：末次月经，胎动时间，早孕反应）。

（2）判断胎儿安危状况。

weeks of gestation.

E.Labor between 28 weeks and less than 35 weeks of gestation.

2.Which of the following is not belonged to the preterm birth for medical and obstetrical indications?（D）

A.Preeclampsia

B.Placental abruption

C.Placenta previa bleeding

D.Bacterial vaginosis

E.Hemolytic disease caused by blood group incompatibility

3.Which of the following is not related to the diagnosis of preterm labor?（E）

A.Regular uterine contractions（20min≥4 times, or 60min≥8 times）

B.The cervix gradually shortening

C.Cervical dilation of ＞1 cm

D.Cervical effacement ≥80%

E.Rupture of membrane

Section 4　Postterm pregnancy

1.Definition

■ Menstrual cycle regular, confirmation of gestational age: 42 weeks or beyond.

2.Effects on gravida and fetus

（1）Perinatal infant risks: Fetal distress, meconium aspiration syndrome, neonatal asphyxia and macrosomia.

（2）Maternal risks: Prolonged stage of labor and increase in the rate of dystocia and operative delivery.

3.Diagnosis

（1）Confirming accurate gestational age: Early pregnancy test, ultrasound examination and clinical parameters（such as LMP, quickening, and morning sickness）.

（2）To adequately assess the risk of fetal

4.处理

（1）妊娠41周以后，应考虑终止妊娠，避免过期妊娠。

（2）促宫颈成熟：宫颈Bishop评分＜7分。

（3）引产术：缩宫素，酌情人工破膜。

（4）产程处理：连续胎心监测。

（5）剖宫产术：适当放宽指征。

重点专业词汇

1.过期妊娠

2.月经周期

3.胎儿窘迫

4.巨大儿

5.难产

练习题

过期妊娠可能带来的母儿不良影响不包括哪一项？（E）

A.胎儿窘迫

B.巨大儿

C.产程延长

D.手术产率增高

E.羊水栓塞

（刘　芳）

compromise.

4.Management

（1）Terminate the pregnancy at 41 weeks avoiding a gestation to progress beyond 42 weeks.

（2）Cervical ripening: Cervical Bishop score ＜7.

（3）Induction of labor: Oxytocin, amniotomy in necessity.

（4）Management of the stage of labor: Consecutive monitoring of fetal heart rate.

（5）Cesarean section: Do it appropriately.

Key words

1.Postterm pregnancy

2.Menstrual cycle

3.Fetal distress

4.Macrosomia

5.Dystocia

Exercises

Which of the following is not the harmful effect of postterm pregnancy for the mother and fetus？（E）

A.Fetal distress

B.Macrosomia

C.Prolonged stage of labor

D.Increase in the rate of operative delivery

E.Amniotic fluid embolism

第6章 产前检查与保健

CHAPTER 6 Prenatal examination and care

第一节 概 述

1.产前保健的目的

（1）产前保健包括对孕妇进行规范的产前检查、健康教育与指导、胎儿健康的监护与评估、孕期营养及体重管理和用药指导等。

（2）降低孕产妇和围生儿并发症的发生率及死亡率、减少出生缺陷。

2.围生期的定义

- 世界卫生组织对围生期的定义提出4种可能：
  - 从妊娠满28周至产后1周。
  - 从妊娠满20周至产后4周。
  - 从妊娠满28周至产后4周。
  - 从胚胎形成至产后1周。

目前，我国采取第一种定义。

第二节 产前检查

1.检查时间与次数

（1）首次产前检查的时间应从确诊妊娠早期开始，一般在妊娠6～8周。

Section 1 Introduction

1.Purpose of prenatal care

（1）Prenatal care includes normative prenatal examination, health education and guidance for pregnant women, monitoring and evaluating fetal health, nutrition and weight management during pregnancy, and medication guidance and so on.

（2）Reduce the incidence and mortality of maternal and perinatal complications, and birth defects as well.

2.Definition of perinatal period

- There are 4 possible definitions given by the World Health Organization（WHO）:
  - From the 28th week of pregnancy to the first week of postpartum.
  - From the 20th week of pregnancy to the 4th week of postpartum.
  - From the 28th week of pregnancy to the 4th week of postpartum.
  - From the formation of embryo to the first week of postpartum.

The first definition is adopted by our country at present.

Section 2 Prenatal examination

1.Time and frequency

（1）The first prenatal examination should begin from the early stage of confirmed pregnancy, generally 6～8 weeks of gestation.

（2）妊娠20～36周为每4周检查1次。

（3）妊娠37周以后每周检查1次。

（4）共行产前检查9～11次，高危孕妇酌情增加检查次数。

2.首次产前检查

（1）问病史

- 年龄、职业。
- 本次妊娠经过。
- 推算预产期：按末次月经第1日算起，月份减3或加9，日数加7。
- 月经史和孕产史。
- 既往史和手术史。
- 家族史。
- 婚姻状况。

（2）全身检查：发育、营养、身高、体重指数、血压、乳房与乳头、脊柱及下肢是否畸形，妇科检查，辅助检查等。

（3）健康教育。

3.妊娠中晚期产前检查

（1）询问孕妇：有无异常症状、体征出现。

（2）全身检查：血压、体重、水肿，血常规、尿常规。

（3）产科检查

- 腹部检查：孕妇排空膀胱后仰卧在舒适的检查床上

  - 视诊：腹部的形状和大小。
  - 触诊：测量宫高、腹围，然后进行四步触诊法。

站在孕妇右侧，前三步检查者面向孕妇面部，第四步时面向孕妇

（2）Once every 4 weeks between 20 and 36 weeks' gestation.

（3）Once a week after the 37th week of gestation.

（4）Total prenatal examinations should be 9～11 times, and pregnant women at high risk should have more.

2.First antenatal visit

（1）History

- Age and occupation.
- History of present pregnancy.
- Calculate the expected date of confinement: Based on the first day of the last menstrual period: m−3, or m＋9, d＋7.
- Menstrual history and obstetric history.
- Previous medical and surgical histories.
- Family history.
- Marital status.

（2）General examination: Development, nutrient, height, body mass index, blood pressure, breast and nipple, whether malformation on spine and lower limbs, gynecological examination, auxiliary examination and so on.

（3）Health education.

3.Second and third trimester antenatal visit

（1）Consulting with the pregnant woman: Abnormal symptoms and signs.

（2）General examination: Blood pressure, weight, edema, blood routine and urine routine examination.

（3）Obstetric examination

- Abdominal examination: The woman should lie comfortably on the couch after emptying the urinary bladder.

  - Inspection: Abdominal shape and size.
  - Palpation: Measure the length of uterus and abdomen circumference, then do four maneuvers of Leopold.

Standing by the pregnant woman's right side, the last maneuver requires that the health

足端（图6-1）。

第一步：检查者两手指腹触诊宫底，判断宫底的胎儿部分，若为胎头则硬而圆，若为胎臀则柔软、宽且形态不规则。

第二步：检查者的双手手掌置于腹部两侧，轻轻深按进行检查。通常胎背平坦饱满，另一侧则为胎儿肢体，感觉不规则或有小突起，有时可感觉到肢体活动。

第三步：检查者右手置于耻骨联合上方握住胎先露部，进一步确认胎先露，左右推动先露部，若不能移动表示已经衔接。

care provider face the woman's feet, while other maneuvers face the woman's face（Figure 6-1）.

First step: The health care provider uses finger pulps to palpate the fundus of uterus, to judge the portion of fetus. The fetal head is hard and round while the breech is soft, wide and irregular.

Second step: The health care provider uses palms of both hands along side of the abdomen and palpates the abdomen gently and deeply. Usually the fetal back is flat and full, and on the other side are limbs of fetus that feel like small irregular bumps and sometimes the movement of limbs.

Third step: The health care provider puts his right hand above the pubic symphysis and holds the presenting part to identify the presentation first, then moves it back and forth. If the presenting part can not be moved, the presentation is actively engaged.

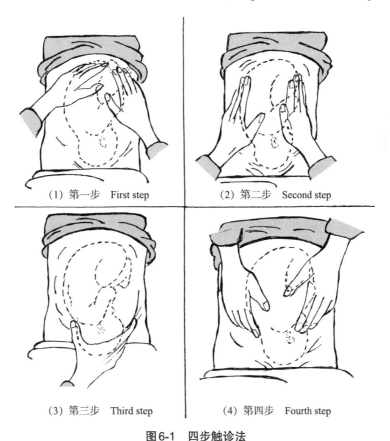

(1) 第一步　First step　　　(2) 第二步　Second step

(3) 第三步　Third step　　　(4) 第四步　Fourth step

图6-1　四步触诊法

Figure 6-1　Four maneuvers of Leopold

第四步：检查者双手分别置于胎先露的两侧，再次确认胎先露部分，沿骨盆入口向下深按，判断入盆程度。

- 听诊：胎心在靠近胎背处听得最清楚。
- 骨盆测量（图6-2至图6-5）
  - 骨盆外测量
    · 髂棘间径：23～26cm。

Fourth step: The health care provider puts both hands on both sides of the presenting part to confirm again and then move gently down the side toward the pubis inlet to judge the extent of engagement.

- Auscultation: Fetal heart sounds are best heard over the fetal back.
- Pelvimetry（Figure 6-2 to Figure 6-5）
  - External pelvimetry
    · Interspinal diameter: 23～26cm.

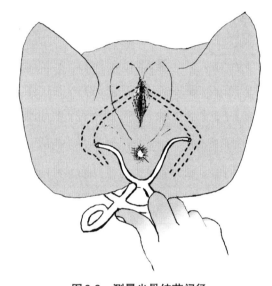

图6-2　测量坐骨结节间径
Figure 6-2　Measurement of intertuberal diameter

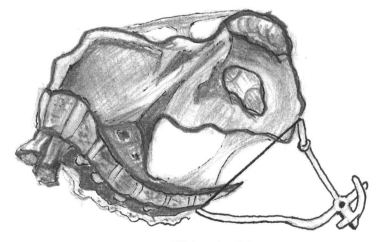

图6-3　测量出口后矢状径
Figure 6-3　Measurement of posterior sagittal diameter of outlet
出口后矢状径：8～9cm　Posterior sagittal diameter of outlet: 8～9cm

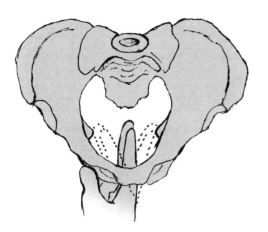

图6-4 测量坐骨棘间径

Figure 6-4 Measurement of bi-ischial diameter

坐骨棘间径：10cm   Bi-ischial diameter: 10cm

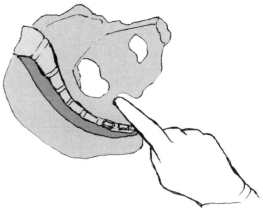

图6-5 测量坐骨切迹宽度

Figure 6-5 Measurement of incisura ischiadica diameter

坐骨切迹（骶棘韧带）宽度：5.5～6.0cm（3横指）

Incisura ischiadica/diameter of sacrospinal ligament: 5.5～6.0cm（3 transverse fingers）

- 髂嵴间径：25～28cm。
- 骶耻外径：18～20cm。
- 坐骨结节间径/出口横径：8.5～9.5cm。
- 如果坐骨结节间径＜8cm（图6-2），应加测出口后矢状径（图6-3），若出口后矢状径＋坐骨结节间径＞15cm，表示骨盆出口狭窄不明显。
  - 骨盆内测量
    - 对角径：耻骨联合下缘至骶岬上缘中点的距离，正常值12.5～13cm（图6-6，图6-7）。

- 阴道检查：在妊娠早期初诊时进行。
- 肛门指诊检查。

（4）胎儿情况：胎产式、胎方位、胎心率、胎儿大小、胎动及羊水量。

（5）辅助检查

- Intercristal diameter: 25～28cm.
- External conjugate: 18～20cm.
- Intertuberal diameter/transverse outlet: 8.5～9.5cm.
- If the intertuberal diameter below 8cm, we should measure the posterior sagittal diameter of outlet, if the two values＞15cm, the pelvic outlet contraction is not obvious.

- Internal pelvimetry
  - Diagonal conjugate: The distance from the inferior border of pubic symphysis to the superior border's middle point of sacral promontory. The normal value is 12.5～13cm(Figure 6-6, Figure 6-7).

- Vaginal examination: This should be made at the first visit.
- Rectal examination.

（4）Fetal conditions: Fetal lie, fetal position, fetal heart rate, fetal size, fetal movement, and amniotic fluid volume.

（5）Auxiliary examination

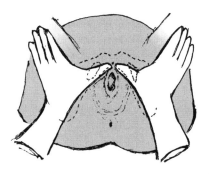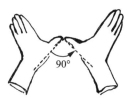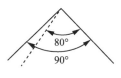

图6-6　测量耻骨弓角度

Figure 6-6　Measurement of angle of subpubic arch

耻骨弓角度＞90°　Angle of subpubic arch ＞ 90°

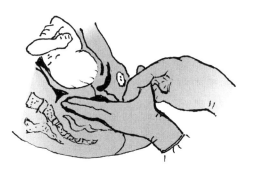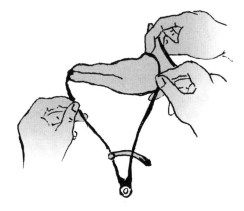

图6-7　测量对角径

Figure 6-7　Measurement of diagonal conjugate

- 实验室检查：血常规、肝功能、病毒等。
- 超声检查。
- 羊水检查。
- 胎儿遗传染色体疾病检查。
- 胎盘功能检查。

第三节　胎儿健康状况评估

1.胎儿宫内监护

（1）确定是否为高危儿

- 孕龄＜37周或≥42周。
- 出生体重＜2500g。
- 巨大儿（≥4000g）。

- Laboratory examination: Blood routine test, liver function, virus and so on.
- Ultrasound examination.
- Amniotic fluid analysis.
- Examination of fetal genetic diseases.
- Examination of placental function.

Section 3　Assessment of fetal health condition

1.Fetal intrauterine monitoring

（1）High risk infant

- Gestational age ＜37 weeks or ≥42 weeks.
- Birth weight ＜2500g.
- Macrosomia （≥4000g）.

- 出生后1分钟Apgar评分≤4分。
- 产时感染。
- 高危孕产妇的胎儿。
- 手术产儿。
- 新生儿的兄姐有新生儿期死亡。
- 双胎或多胎儿。

（2）胎儿宫内监护的内容

- 妊娠早期：确定孕周。
- 妊娠中期：胎儿发育的筛查，胎儿染色体的筛查。
- 妊娠晚期：定期产检，胎动计数，电子胎儿监护。

（3）电子胎儿监护

- 监测胎心率
  - 胎心率基线：指在无胎动和无子宫收缩影响时，10分钟以上的胎心率平均值。正常胎心率为110～160次/分。
    · 心动过速：胎心率＞160次/分，历时10分钟以上。
    · 心动过缓：胎心率＜110次/分，历时10分钟以上。
  - 一过性胎心率变化
    · 加速：指宫缩或胎动时，胎心率增加15次/分，持续15秒以上。

    · 减速
    ① 早期减速（ED）（图6-8）：当子宫收缩时胎心开始下降，胎心最低点与宫缩高峰相一致。为宫缩时胎头受压引起。
    ② 变异减速（VD）（图6-9）：脐带受压所致。

- 1 minute after birth Apgar score ≤ 4.
- Intrapartum infection.
- High risk pregnancy.
- Operative delivery.
- Perinatal death of neonate's brother or sister.
- Twin pregnancy or multiple pregnancy.

（2）Items of fetal intrauterine monitoring

- First trimester: Gestational age.
- Second trimester: The screening of the fetal development and fetal chromosome.
- Third trimester: Periodic prenatal care, fetal movement count, electronic fetal monitoring.

（3）Electronic fetal monitoring

- Monitoring fetal heart rate
  - Fetal heart rate baseline: Mean fetal heart rate over a 10-minute period without fetal movement and uterine contraction. Normal fetal heart rate（FHR）is 110 ～ 160bpm.
    · Tachycardia: FHR ＞ 160bpm, for above 10 minutes.
    · Bradycardia: FHR ＜ 110bpm, for above 10 minutes.
  - Transient fetal heart rate change
    · Acceleration: When the uterus contracts or the fetus moves, the fetal heart rate rises over the baseline 15bpm for above 15 seconds.
    · Deceleration
    ① Early deceleration（ED）（Figure 6-8）: The fetal heart rate begins to fall when the uterus contracts, and the fetal heart rate arrives to the nadir when the contraction arrives to the peak. The reason is the fetal head compressed.
    ② Variable deceleration（VD）（Figure 6-9）: Umbilical cord compressed.

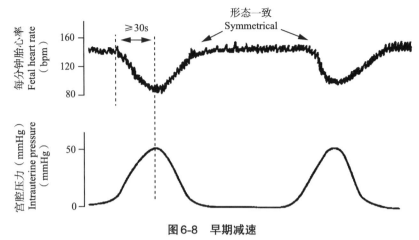

图6-8　早期减速

Figure 6-8　Early deceleration

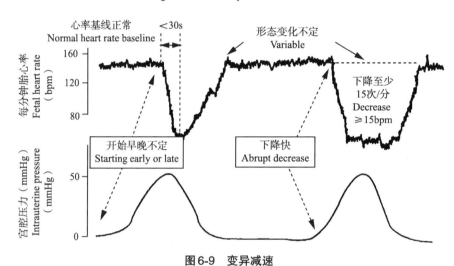

图6-9　变异减速

Figure 6-9　Variable deceleration

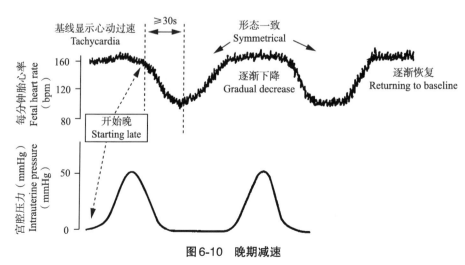

图6-10　晚期减速

Figure 6-10　Late deceleration

③晚期减速（LD）（图 6-10）：晚期减速多在宫缩高峰后开始出现，并在宫缩结束后恢复。一般认为是胎儿缺氧、胎盘功能不良的表现。

■ 预测胎儿宫内储备能力

● 无应激试验（NST）
● 反应型NST的评价标准：
①基线位于110～160次/分。
②基线变异波动于6～25次/分。
③20分钟内≥2次加速，＞15次/分，持续15秒以上。

④无减速或偶发减速，持续时间＜30秒。

● 缩宫素激惹试验（OCT），又称宫缩应激试验（CST）
· 诱发宫缩，了解宫缩时胎心率的变化，测定胎儿的储备能力。

● 胎儿生物物理评分（BPP）

①Manning评分的5个项目：无应激试验、胎儿呼吸运动、胎动、肌张力、羊水量。
②8～10分无急慢性缺氧；6～8分可能有急性或慢性缺氧；4～6分有急性或慢性缺氧；2～4分有急性缺氧伴慢性缺氧；0分有急性缺氧。

③Late deceleration（LD）（Figure 6-10）: The onset and recovery of late deceleration occur, respectively, after the peak and end of the contraction. It is related to fetal hypoxia or placental dysfunction.

■ Assessment of intrauterine fetal reserve capacity
● Non-stress test（NST）
● The criteria for the reaction type NST:
①Baseline between 110 and 160 bpm.

②The variability of baseline between 6 and 25 bpm.
③The presence of periodic accelerations（above two accelerations in 20 minutes）of fetal heart rate of 15bpm over baseline for 15 seconds.
④The absence or little of decelerations of the fetal heart rate, continuous time below 30 seconds.
● Oxytocin challenge test（OCT）/ Contraction stress test（CST）
· Induce contractions to know the relationship between fetal heart rate and contractions, to measure the fetal reserve capacity.

● Biophysiological profile（BPP）（Manning score）
①The criteria of Manning score has 5 items: NST, fetal breath, fetal movement, muscle tension, amniotic fluid.
②Score 8～10 normal; score 6～8 probably acute or chronic hypoxia; score 4～6 acute or chronic hypoxia; 2～4 acute hypoxia with chronic hypoxia; score 0 acute hypoxia.

2.胎盘功能检查

（1）胎动计数：≥6次/2小时为正常。

（2）孕妇尿雌三醇值：＞15mg/24小时为正常值；10～15mg/24小时为警戒值；＜10mg/24小时为危险值。

（3）孕妇血清人胎盘生乳素（hPL）：妊娠足月＜4mg/L或突然下降50%提示胎盘功能低下。

3.胎儿成熟度检查

（1）正确推算预产期。

（2）宫高、腹围预测胎儿大小：胎儿体重（g）=宫高（cm）×腹围（cm）+200。

（3）超声测量：双顶径（BPD）＞8.5cm。

（4）羊水卵磷脂/鞘磷脂比值：＞2，胎儿肺成熟。

（5）羊水泡沫试验。

重点专业词汇

1.围生医学

2.末次月经

3.预产期

4.四步触诊法

5.加速

6.早期减速

7.变异减速

8.晚期减速

9.无应激试验（NST）

10.缩宫素激惹试验（OCT）

11.宫缩应激试验（CST）

练习题

1.我国围生期的定义：（A）

A.从妊娠满28周至产后1周

B.从妊娠满20周至产后4周

2.Placental function examination

（1）Fetal movement counting ≥ 6 times/2 hours.

（2）Estriol in maternal urine: Normal value ＞15mg/24h; warning value 10～15mg/24h; risk value ＜10mg/24h.

（3）Human placental lactogen in maternal serum（hPL）: Term pregnancy ＜4mg/L or suddenly drop 50%, hypofunction of placenta.

3.Fetal maturity tests

（1）Confirm the expected date of confinement.

（2）Measure the weight by the height of uterus and abdomen circumference: fetal weight（g）=uterine height（cm）×abdomen circumference（cm）+200.

（3）Ultrasound: Biparietal diameter（BPD）＞8.5cm.

（4）Lecithin/sphingomyelin ratio in amniotic fluid: ＞2, fetal lung maturity.

（5）Foam stability test.

Key words

1.Perinatology

2.Last menstrual period

3.Expected date of confinement

4.Four maneuvers of Leopold

5.Acceleration

6.Early deceleration

7.Variable deceleration

8.Late deceleration

9.Non-stress test（NST）

10.Oxytocin challenge test（OCT）

11.Contraction stress test（CST）

Exercises

1.The definition of perinatal period in our country:（A）

A.From the 28th week of pregnancy to the first week of postpartum

B.From the 20th week of pregnancy to the 4th

C.从妊娠满28周至产后4周

D.从胚胎形成至产后1周

E.从妊娠满20周至产后1周

2.产前检查至少应该进行多少次？（B）

A.10次

B.9次

C.8次

D.11次

E.12次

3.关于骨盆测量以下哪项在正常范围？（B）

A.坐骨切迹宽度可容纳2横指

B.耻骨弓角度90°

C.骶耻外径17cm

D.坐骨结节间径7cm

E.对角径11cm

4.关于电子胎心监护，哪一项提示脐带受压？（D）

A.无应激试验阴性

B.加速

C.早期减速

D.变异减速

E.晚期减速

5.一位孕妇，30岁，平素月经规律，末次月经2018年3月27日，她的预产期是：（D）

A.2018年12月30日

B.2018年12月3日

C.2018年12月27日

D.2019年1月3日

E.2019年1月5日

（刘 芳）

week of postpartum

C.From the 28th week of pregnancy to the 4th week of postpartum

D.From the formation of embryo to the first week of postpartum

E.From the 20th week of pregnancy to the first week of postpartum

2.How many times should be done for prenatal examination at least?（B）

A.10 times

B.9 times

C.8 times

D.11times

E.12 times

3.Which of the following is the normal range about pelvimetry?（B）

A.Incisura ischiadica width can accommodate 2 horizontal fingers

B.Angle of pubic arch is 90 degree

C.External conjugate is 17cm

D.Intertuberous diameter is 7cm

E.Diagonal conjugate is 11cm

4.Which one prompts the compression of the umbilical cord about electronic fetal heart monitoring?（D）

A.NST negative

B.Acceleration

C.Early deceleration

D.Variable deceleration

E.Late deceleration

5.A 30-year-old pregnant woman has regular menstruation, her last menstrual period is Mar. 27th, 2018, what's her expected date of confinement?（D）

A.Dec. 30th, 2018

B.Dec. 3rd, 2018

C.Dec. 27th, 2018

D.Jan. 3rd, 2019

E.Jan. 5th, 2019

第7章 正常分娩

CHAPTER 7 Normal labor

第一节 概 述

1.分娩定义

（1）妊娠满28周（196天）及以上，胎儿及其附属物从临产开始到全部从母体娩出的过程称为分娩。

（2）分娩是生理过程，在此期间妊娠的产物（即胎儿、胎膜、脐带和胎盘）被排出子宫外。

2.分类

（1）早产：28周～＜37周。

（2）足月产：37周～＜42周。

（3）过期产：≥42周。

第二节 分娩动因

（1）分娩发动是炎症细胞因子、机械性刺激等多因素综合作用的结果。

（2）宫颈成熟是分娩发动的必备条件。

（3）缩宫素与前列腺素是促进宫缩的最直接因素。

第三节 影响分娩的因素

（1）子宫收缩力是临产后的主要产力。

Section 1 Introduction

1.Definition of labor

（1）The procedure of the fetus and its appendages from the beginning of the birth to the full delivery of the mother at the end of 28 weeks（196 days）and above is called childbirth.

（2）Labor is physiologic process during which the products of conception（i.e., the fetus, membranes, umbilical cord, and placenta）are expelled outside of the uterus.

2.Classification

（1）Premature delivery: 28 weeks ～＜37 weeks.

（2）Term delivery: 37 weeks ～＜42 weeks.

（3）Postterm delivery: ≥42 weeks.

Section 2 Labor motivation

（1）The onset of labor is the result from multiple factors such as inflammatory cytokines and mechanical stimulation.

（2）One of the key factors of delivery is cervix maturation.

（3）Oxytocin and prostaglandins are the most direct factors to promote uterine contraction.

Section 3 Key factors for labor

（1）Uterine contractions is the main forces of labor during childbirth.

（2）腹肌和膈肌收缩力是第二产程胎儿娩出的重要辅助力量（产力）。

（3）肛提肌收缩力是协助胎儿内旋转及胎头仰伸所必需的力量（产力）。

（4）骨盆三个平面的大小与形状、子宫下段形成、宫颈管消失与宫口扩张、会阴体伸展直接影响胎儿通过产道（产道）。

（5）胎儿大小及胎方位也是分娩难易的影响因素（胎儿）。

（6）精神鼓励和心理安慰有助于产妇顺利分娩（精神）。

1.产力

定义：将胎儿及其附属物从宫腔内逼出的力量。产力包括：子宫收缩力、腹壁肌及膈肌收缩力、肛提肌收缩力。

（1）子宫收缩力：临产后的主要产力，贯穿于分娩全过程，特点为：

- 节律性。
- 对称性。
- 极性。
- 缩复作用。

（2）腹壁肌及膈肌收缩力：是第二产程胎儿娩出的重要辅助力量。

（3）肛提肌收缩力：协助胎先露在盆腔进行内旋转，第二产程协助胎头仰伸及娩出，第三产程协助胎盘娩出。

2.产道

产道是胎儿娩出的通道，分为骨产道和软产道。

（2）The abdominal muscles and diaphragm contractions（abdominal pressure）are important auxiliary force at the second stage（forces of labor）.

（3）Anal levator contractions are necessary force to assist the fetus for the internal rotation and extension of fetal head（forces of labor）.

（4）The size and shape of the three planes of the pelvis, lower segment of uterus, effacement of cervix, dilatation of cervix, and extension of the perineum body directly affect the fetal passage through the birth canal（birth canal）.

（5）Fetal size and fetal position are also the factors affecting the difficulty of delivery（fetus）.

（6）Emotional support and psychological comfort are conducive to the smooth delivery of pregnant women（psychological factors）.

1.Forces of labor

Definition: The force to expel the fetus and its appendages from the intrauterine, including: uterine contractions, the abdominal muscles and diaphragm contractions, and anal levator contractions.

（1）Uterine contractions: The main force of labor after childbirth throughout the entire process, characterized by:

- Rhythmic.
- Symmetry.
- Polarity.
- Retraction.

（2）The abdominal muscles and diaphragm contractions: Necessary force to assist in the second stage of labor.

（3）Anal levator contractions: Help the fetus with internal rotation in the pelvis. In the second stage of labor, assist in the extension and delivery of fetal head, and in the third stage of labor, assist in the placenta delivery.

2.Birth canal

Fetus birth canal is a channel divided into bony canal and soft birth canal.

（1）骨产道（真骨盆）

- 骨盆的大小、形状与分娩是否顺利关系密切。
- 骨盆腔分为3个假想平面。

■ 骨盆入口平面

- 真结合径：耻骨联合上缘中点至骶岬上缘正中点的距离，正常值平均为11cm。

■ 中骨盆平面：骨盆最小平面，骨盆腔最狭窄部分。

- 中骨盆横径（坐骨棘间径）。
- 两坐骨棘间的距离，正常值平均为10cm。

■ 骨盆出口平面：由两个不在同一平面的三角形组成。

- 出口横径（坐骨结节间径）。
- 两坐骨结节末端内缘的距离，正常值平均为9cm。

■ 骨盆轴与骨盆倾斜度

- 骨盆轴：连接骨盆各平面中点的假想曲线。此轴上段向下向后，中段向下，下段向下向前。分娩时，胎儿沿此轴完成一系列分娩机制。

- 骨盆倾斜度：女性站立时，骨盆入口平面与地平面所形成的角度，一般为60°。

（2）软产道：是由子宫下段、宫颈、阴道及盆底软组织构成的弯曲通道。

■ 子宫下段形成：由非孕时

（1）Bony canal（true pelvis）

- The size and the shape of pelvis is directly related to the delivery process.
- The pelvic cavity is divided into three imaginary planes.

■ Pelvic inlet plane

- Conjugation vera: The normal average distance is 11cm, the midpoint of the upper border of the pubic symphysis to the sacral promontory from the upper border of the middle point.

■ Mid-plane of pelvis: The smallest plane of the pelvis and the narrowest part of the pelvic cavity.

- Interspinous diameter.
- The distance between the two ischial spines is 10cm on average.

■ Pelvic outlet plane: It consists of two triangles that are not in the same plane.

- Outlet diameter（biischial diameter）.
- Two ends of the inner edge of the sciatic tuberosities, the normal average distance is 9cm.

■ Pelvic axis and inclination of pelvis

- Pelvic axis: Imaginary line connecting the midpoint of each curve of the pelvis. The upper section of the axis is back and down, the middle down, and the lower downward and forward. Along this axis the fetus completes a series of delivery mechanism.

- Inclination of pelvis: The angle formed by the pelvic inlet plane and the ground plane in a standing women, is generally 60°.

（2）Soft birth canal: It is a curved passage of soft tissue in the lower uterus, cervix, vagina and pelvic floor.

■ Lower segment of uterus: Formed by the

长约1cm的子宫峡部伸展形成。
- 生理缩复环。
- 宫颈的变化
  - 宫颈管消失。
  - 宫口扩张。
- 骨盆底组织、阴道及会阴的变化

3.胎儿
- 胎儿大小
  - 胎头颅骨构成：由两块顶骨、额骨、颞骨及一块枕骨构成。
  - 胎头径线
    ①双顶径。
    ②枕额径。
    ③枕下前囟径。
    ④枕颏径。
- 胎位
  - 纵产式——头位、臀位。
  - 横产式——横位。
  - 头先露时，矢状缝和囟门是确定胎位的重要标志。
- 胎儿畸形。

4.精神心理因素
（1）分娩是生理现象。

（2）产妇的精神心理因素，能影响机体的内部平衡、适应力和健康。

（3）机体产生一系列变化。

（4）耐心安慰，鼓励产妇进食。

（5）必要的呼吸技术和躯体放松技术、家庭式产房、开展导乐分娩。

extension of the isthmus of the uterus about 1cm during non-pregnancy.
- Physiological retraction ring.
- Changes of cervix
  - Effacement of cervix.
  - Dilatation of cervix.
- Changes of pelvic floor tissue, vagina and perineum

3.Fetus
- Fetal size
  - Fetal skull: Composed by two parietal, frontal, temporal bones and an occipital bone.
  - Head diameter
    ①Biparietal diameter.
    ②Occipito-frontal diameter.
    ③Suboccipitobregmatic diameter.
    ④Occipitomental diameter.
- Fetal position
  - Longitudinal lie—head presentation, breech presentation.
  - Transverse lie—shoulder presentation.
  - Sagittal suture and fontanelle are important indicators to determine fetal position in head presentation.
- Fetal malformation.

4.Psychological factors
（1）Childbirth is a physiological phenomenon.

（2）Maternal mental and psychological factors affect the internal balance, adaptability and health of the body.

（3）The body produces a series of changes.

（4）Patiently comfort pregnant women and encourage them to eat.

（5）Necessary breathing techniques and body relaxation techniques, home-like delivery room, and doula delivery.

第四节　枕先露的分娩机制

Section 4　Mechanism of labor: Occiput presentation

胎儿通过一连串适应性转动，以其最小径线通过产道（图7-1）。

The infantile head has to conform to the various pelvic sections during delivery after a series of adaptive rotation（Figure 7-1）.

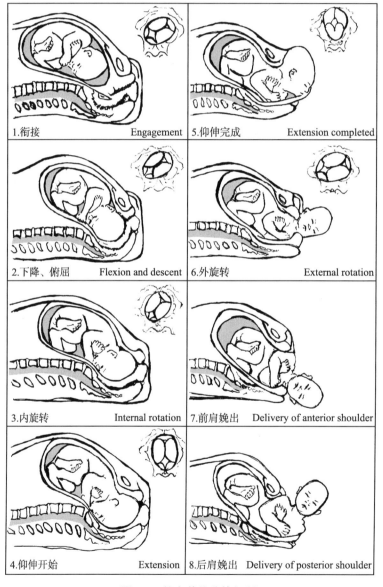

1.衔接　Engagement	5.仰伸完成　Extension completed
2.下降、俯屈　Flexion and descent	6.外旋转　External rotation
3.内旋转　Internal rotation	7.前肩娩出　Delivery of anterior shoulder
4.仰伸开始　Extension	8.后肩娩出　Delivery of posterior shoulder

图7-1　枕左前位分娩机制

Figure 7-1　Schematic diagram of LOA delivery mechanism

下降贯穿分娩全程，是胎儿娩出的首要条件。

（1）衔接：胎头双顶径进入骨盆入口平面，胎头颅骨最低点接近或达到坐骨棘水平。

（2）下降：胎头沿骨盆轴前进的动作称为下降。

■ 胎头下降程度是作为判断产程进展的重要标志。

（3）俯屈：以枕下前囟径取代较大的枕额径。

（4）内旋转：胎头围绕骨盆纵轴向前旋转，使其矢状缝与中骨盆及骨盆出口前后径相一致。

（5）仰伸：宫缩和肛提肌的合力使胎头下降方向转向前。

（6）复位及外旋转：胎头向左旋转45°，而后继续向左旋转45°，保持胎头与胎肩的正常关系。

（7）胎肩及胎儿娩出。

第五节　先兆临产、临产与产程

1.先兆临产
（1）假临产。
（2）胎儿下降感。
（3）见红。
2.临产的诊断
（1）规律且逐渐增强的子宫

Descent is throughout the entire process of childbirth, and it is prerequisite for the successful delivery.

（1）Engagement: Descent of biparietal diameter（BPD）of the fetal head below the plane of the pelvic inlet, the lowest point of fetal skull close to or approaching the level of the ischial spine.

（2）Descent: Fetal head along the axis of the pelvis forward movement throughout the entire process of childbirth.

■ The degree of fetal head descent is an important indicator for judging the progress of labor.

（3）Flexion: Suboccipitobregmatic diameter instead of occipito-frontal diameter.

（4）Internal rotation: The fetal head rotates forward around the longitudinal axis of the pelvis to make the sagittal suture consistent with the anteroposterior diameter of the middle pelvis and the outlet of the pelvis.

（5）Extension: The forces of uterine and levator muscle contraction help to make the fetal head face forward.

（6）Restitution and external rotation: Fetal head rotates 45° to the left, and continues to rotate left 45°, to maintain normal relationship between the shoulder and the fetal head.

（7）Delivery of shoulder and fetus.

Section 5　Threatened labor, labor and stage of labor

1.Threatened labor
（1）False labor.
（2）Lightening.
（3）Show.
2.Diagnosis of labor
（1）Regular and gradually intense uterine

收缩，持续约30秒或以上，间歇5~6分钟。同时伴随进行性宫颈管消失、宫口扩张和胎先露下降。

（2）用强镇静药物不能抑制宫缩。

3. 总产程及产程分期

（1）总产程即分娩全过程，从开始出现规律宫缩直到胎儿、胎盘娩出的全过程。

（2）分娩过程分三个产程

- 第一产程：宫颈扩张期。
- 第二产程：胎儿娩出期。
- 第三产程：胎盘娩出期。

第六节　第一产程的临床经过

必须连续定时观察并记录宫缩与胎心。

产程图显示的宫口扩张曲线与胎头下降曲线能指导产程的处理。

通过阴道检查或肛查判断胎方位、胎先露高低及产道有无异常（图7-2）。

1. 临床表现

- 规律宫缩、宫口扩张、先露下降、胎膜破裂。

2. 产程、母体观察及处理

可采用产程图观察产程。

（1）产程观察及处理

- 子宫收缩。
- 胎心。

contractions for 30 seconds or more, with intervals of 5 ~ 6 minutes, accompanied by progressive cervical effacement, cervical dilation and descent of fetal presentation.

（2）Strong sedatives can not inhibit contractions.

3. Total stage of labor and stage of labor

（1）Total stage of labor: The whole process of delivery, from the beginning of regular contractions to the delivery of fetus and placenta.

（2）Three stages of labor

- The first stage of labor: Dilation of cervix.
- The second stage of labor: Delivery of fetus.
- The third stage of labor: Delivery of placenta.

Section 6　Clinical course of the first stage

The uterine contractions and fetal heart rate must be continuously observed and recorded.

Cervical dilation curve and fetal head decline curve shown in partogram may instruct the treatment of the labor process.

Vaginal examination and anal examination are used to determine the fetal position, the fetal presentation and the abnormality of the birth canal（Figure 7-2）.

1. Clinical manifestations

- Regular contraction, dilation of cervix, descending of presentation, and rupture of membrane.

2. Observation and treatment of labor process and the woman

The partogram can be used to observe the labor process.

（1）The items observed and treatment

- Uterine contractions.
- Fetal heart rate.

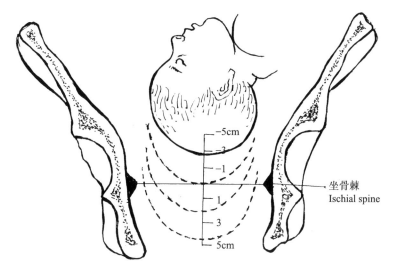

图7-2 阴道检查判断胎头高低

Figure 7-2　Schematic diagram of vaginal examination to determine fetal station

- 宫口扩张及胎头下降：是产程图中两项重要指标，并指导产程处理。
  - 宫口扩张曲线：第一产程分为潜伏期和活跃期。

    ①潜伏期指从临产出现规律宫缩至宫口扩张4～6cm。
    ②活跃期是指宫口扩张4～6cm至10cm。
  - 胎头下降曲线：胎头颅骨最低点与坐骨棘平面的关系。
- 胎膜破裂：一旦发现胎膜破裂，应立即听胎心，并观察羊水的性状，并记录破膜时间。
- 阴道检查。
- 肛门检查。

（2）母体观察及处理
- 精神安慰。
- 血压。

- Cervical dilation and fetal head decline: Two important indexes in partogram used to instruct the treatment of labor process.
  - Cervical dilation curve: The first stage of labor is divided into latent phase and active phase.

    ①Latent phase: The regular contraction appears to cervical dilation 4～6cm.

    ②Active phase: Cervical dilation from 4～6cm to 10cm.
  - Fetal head decline curve: The relationship between the lowest point of fetal skull and the plane of ischial spine.
- Rupture of membranes: Listen to fetal heart immediately, observe amniotic fluid characteristics, and record rupture time simultaneously.
- Vaginal examination.
- Anal examination.

（2）Observation and treatment of the woman
- Spiritual comfort.
- Blood pressure.

■ 饮食与活动。

■ 排尿与排便。

■ 其他。

第七节 第二产程的临床经过

（1）指导产妇正确使用腹压是缩短第二产程的关键。

（2）密切观察宫缩、胎心、先露下降，适时接产。

（3）临床表现

■ 若仍未破膜，应行人工破膜。

■ 产妇有排便感，不自主向下屏气。

■ 胎头拨露。

■ 胎头着冠。

■ 胎儿娩出。

第八节 第三产程的临床经过

（1）新生儿娩出后应准确处理，并立即进行阿普加评分（表7-1）。

（2）胎盘娩出后应仔细检查是否完整。

（3）分娩结束后应检查软产道有无损伤。积极预防产后出血。

1.临床表现

■ 胎盘剥离征象

● 宫体变硬呈球形，宫底升高达脐上。

● 阴道口外露的脐带自行延长。

■ Diet and activity.

■ Urination and defecation.

■ Others.

Section 7　Clinical course of the second stage

（1）To instruct the women to use abdominal pressure correctly is the key to shorten the second stage of labor.

（2）Close observation of contractions, fetal heart rate, presentation decline, timely delivery.

（3）Clinical manifestations

■ Artificial rupture.

■ The woman has defecation feeling, with involuntary downward breath holding.

■ Head visible on vulval gapping.

■ Crowning of head.

■ Fetus delivered.

Section 8　Clinical course of the third stage

（1）The newborn should be treated accurately after delivery, and neonatal Apgar score should be carried out immediately（Table 7-1）.

（2）The placenta should be carefully checked for completeness after delivery.

（3）The soft birth canal should be checked for any damage after delivery. Actively prevent postpartum hemorrhage.

1.Clinical manifestations

■ Signs of placental separation

● Uterus becomes hard and spherical, and rises above umbilicus.

● The umbilical cord exposed in the vaginal margin extends on its own.

表 7-1 新生儿阿普加评分法

Table 7-1 Neonatal Apgar score

体征 Sign	0	1	2
心率 Heart rate	0 Absent	＜100次/分 ＜100 bpm	≥100次/分 ≥100 bpm
呼吸 Breath	无呼吸 Absent	浅慢，不规则 Shallow, irregular	佳，哭声响亮 Good, cry
肌张力 Muscle tone	松弛 Flaccid	四肢稍屈曲 Extremities flexed	四肢屈曲，活动好 Flexed limbs and moving
喉反射 Laryngeal reflexes	无反射 No response	有些动作 Grimace	咳嗽，恶心 Coughs, nausea
皮肤颜色 Skin color	全身苍白 Pale	身体红，四肢发绀 Pink（body），cyanotic（the extremities）	全身粉红 Fully pink

- 阴道少量出血，接产者用手掌尺侧在产妇耻骨联合上方轻压子宫下段时，宫体上升而外露的脐带不再回缩。

- Small amount of vaginal bleeding. When the lower uterine segment is gently pressed above the pubic symphysis with the ulnar side of the palm, the uterus rises and the exposed umbilical cord no longer retracts.

2.处理

（1）新生儿处理

- 清理呼吸道。
- 处理脐带。
- 新生儿阿普加评分。
- 处理新生儿。

（2）协助胎盘娩出。

（3）检查胎盘、胎膜。

（4）检查软产道。

（5）预防产后出血。

2.Management

（1）Newborn treatment

- Respiratory tract cleaning.
- Umbilical cord treatment.
- Neonatal Apgar score.
- Treatment of the newborn.

（2）Assist in the delivery of the placenta.

（3）Examination of placenta and fetal membranes.

（4）Soft birth canal check.

（5）Prevention of postpartum hemorrhage.

重点专业词汇

1.产力

2.子宫收缩力

3.产道

4.缩复作用

5.生理缩复环

6.先兆临产

Key words

1.Forces of labor

2.Uterine contractions

3.Birth canal

4.Retraction

5.Physiological retraction ring

6.Threatened labor

7.胎膜破裂

8.胎头拨露

9.胎头着冠

10.新生儿阿普加评分

练习题

1.哪一项不属于临产后正常宫缩特点？（B）

A.节律性

B.规律性

C.对称性

D.极性

E.缩复作用

2.初产妇，足月巨大儿可能经阴道分娩的是：（A）

A.枕右前位

B.肩左后位

C.肩右后位

D.骶左后位

E.骶右后位

3.正常足月分娩时，哪一条是胎头俯屈后通过产道的胎头径线？（E）

A.双颞径

B.枕额径

C.枕颏径

D.双顶径

E.枕下前囟径

4.胎头于临产后迟迟不入盆，骨盆测量径线最有价值的是哪一个？（C）

A.髂棘间径

B.髂嵴间径

C.骶耻外径

D.坐骨棘间径

E.对角径

5.胎头跨耻征阳性，下列哪项不可能出现？（D）

A.强直性子宫收缩

B.病理性缩复环

7.Rupture of membrane

8.Head visible on vulval gapping

9.Crowning of head

10.Neonatal Apgar score

Exercises

1.Which is not the characteristic of normal contractions during labor?（B）

A.Rhythm

B. Regularity

C. Symmetry

D. Polarity

E. Retraction

2.Primipara, full-term giant baby may be delivered through the vagina with:（A）

A.ROA

B.LSCP

C.RSCP

D.LSP

E.RSP

3.Which is the fetal head diameter line that passes through the birth canal after the fetal head is flexed during normal term delivery?（E）

A.Bitemporal diameter

B.Occipito-frontal diameter

C.Occipitomental diameter

D.Biparietal diameter

E.Suboccipitobregmatic diameter

4.Which is the most valuable of the pelvis measuring diameters when the fetal head is delayed in the pelvis during labor?（C）

A.Interspinous diameter

B. Intercristal diameter

C. External conjugate

D.Interspinous diameter

E. Diagonal conjugate

5.Which of the following is not likely to occur in the positive span-pubis sign?（D）

A.Tetanic contraction of uterine

B. Pathological retraction ring

C.头盆不称

D.胎头衔接

E.子宫收缩乏力

（刘　健）

C.Cephalopelvic disproportion

D. Engagement of fetal head

E. Uterine inertia

第8章 妊娠特有疾病

CHAPTER 8   Pregnancy-specific diseases

第一节　妊娠期高血压疾病

Section 1   Hypertensive disorder of pregnancy

1.分类

（1）妊娠期高血压。

（2）子痫前期。

（3）子痫。

（4）慢性高血压并发子痫前期。

（5）妊娠合并慢性高血压。

2.子痫前期病因及发病机制

（1）尚未完全阐明。

（2）是一种多因素、多机制、多通路致病的疾病。

■ 子宫螺旋小动脉重铸不足。

■ 炎症免疫过度激活。

■ 血管内皮细胞受损。

■ 遗传因素。

■ 营养缺乏。

3.子痫前期病理变化

（1）全身小血管痉挛。

（2）内皮损伤。

（3）局部缺血。

4.子痫前期的诊断

（1）病史。

（2）高血压。

（3）尿蛋白。

（4）辅助检查。

■ 妊娠20周后出现高血压，收

1.Classification

（1）Gestational hypertension.

（2）Preeclampsia.

（3）Eclampsia.

（4）Chronic hypertension with superimposed preeclampsia.

（5）Pregnancy with chronic hypertension.

2.Etiology and pathogenesis of preeclampsia

（1）Not fully yet elucidated.

（2）A multi-factor, multi-mechanism and multi-pathway disease.

■ Inadequate remodeling of uterine spiral arterioles.

■ Overactivation of inflammatory immunity.

■ Damage of vascular endothelial cells.

■ Hereditary factors.

■ Nutrition deficiency.

3.Pathological changes of preeclampsia

（1）Systemic vasospasm.

（2）Endothelial injury.

（3）Regional ischemia.

4.Preeclampsia diagnosis

（1）Medical history.

（2）Hypertension.

（3）Urine protein.

（4）Auxiliary examination

■ Hypertension occurs after 20 weeks of

缩压≥140mmHg和（或）舒张压≥90mmHg。

■ 尿蛋白≥300mg/24h或随机尿蛋白（＋）。

■ 血小板减少。

■ 肝功能损害：血清转氨酶超过正常值2倍。

■ 肾功能损害：血肌酐＞1.1mg/dl或为正常值2倍以上。

■ 肺水肿。

■ 新发生的中枢神经系统异常或视觉障碍。

（5）鉴别诊断：慢性肾炎合并妊娠。

5.子痫前期预测与预防

（1）子痫前期预测

■ 首次产前检查：风险评估。

■ 主张：联合多项指标综合评估预测。

（2）高危因素

■ 孕妇年龄：≥40岁。

■ 子痫前期病史。

■ 抗磷脂抗体阳性。

■ 高血压、慢性肾炎、糖尿病。

■ 初次产检：体重指数（BMI）≥35kg/m^2。

■ 子痫前期家族史（母亲或姐妹）。

■ 本次妊娠：多胎妊娠、首次怀孕、妊娠间隔时间≥10年。

■ 孕早期收缩压≥130mmHg或舒张压≥80mmHg。

（3）生化指标

■ 可溶性酪氨酸激酶-1。

■ 胎盘生长因子。

■ 胎盘蛋白-13。

pregnancy, systolic blood pressure ≥140mmHg and/or diastolic blood pressure ≥90mmHg.

■ Urine protein ≥300mg/24h or random urine protein（＋）.

■ Thrombocytopenia.

■ Liver function damage: Serum transaminase level is more than 2 times of the normal value.

■ Renal dysfunction: Serum creatinine is greater than 1.1mg/dl or is more than 2 times of the normal value.

■ Pulmonary edema.

■ New central nervous system abnormalities or visual disorders.

（5）Differential diagnosis: Chronic nephritis with pregnancy.

5.Prediction and prevention of preeclampsia

（1）Preeclampsia prediction

■ First antenatal examination: Risk assessment.

■ Proposition: Joint evaluation and prediction of multiple indicators.

（2）High risk factors

■ Age of pregnant women: ≥40 years old.

■ History of preeclampsia.

■ Antiphospholipid antibody positive.

■ Hypertension, chronic nephritis and diabetes.

■ Initial antenatal examination: BMI ≥35kg/m^2.

■ Family history of preeclampsia（mother or sister）.

■ This pregnancy: Multiple pregnancy, first pregnancy, pregnancy interval of more than 10 years.

■ Early pregnancy systolic blood pressure ≥130mmHg or diastolic blood pressure ≥80mmHg.

（3）Biochemical indicators

■ Soluble tyrosine kinase-1.

■ Placental growth factor.

■ Placental protein-13.

■ 可溶性内皮因子。

（4）物理指标：子宫动脉血流
搏动指数

（5）联合预测

■ 分子标志物间联合。

■ 分子标志物联合子宫动脉多
普勒血流检测。

（6）子痫前期预防

■ 对低危人群目前尚无有效的
预防方法。

■ 对高危人群可能有效的预防
措施：

- 适度锻炼。
- 合理饮食。
- 补钙。
- 阿司匹林抗凝治疗。

6.子痫前期治疗

■ 治疗基本原则

- 降压、解痉、镇静等。
- 密切监测母儿情况。
- 最有效的治疗措施：终止
  妊娠。

（1）一般处理

■ 妊娠期高血压和子痫前期：
门诊治疗。

■ 重度子痫前期：住院治疗。

■ 适当休息。

■ 保证充足的蛋白质和热量。

■ 不建议：限制食盐摄入。

■ 保证充足睡眠。

■ 地西泮2.5～5mg，必要时
可睡前口服。

（2）降压

■ 降压原则（表8-1）

- 妊娠前已用降压药治疗：
  继续降压。

■ 降压目标

- 无并发脏器功能损伤

■ Soluble endothelial factor.

（4）Physical indicators: Uterine artery blood
flow pulsation index

（5）Joint prediction

■ Combination of molecular markers.

■ Molecular markers combined with uterine
artery Doppler blood flow detection.

（6）Preeclampsia prevention

■ No effective prevention method for low-
risk population at present.

■ Possible effective preventive measures for
high-risk groups:

- Moderate exercise.
- Reasonable diet.
- Calcium supplement.
- Aspirin anticoagulation therapy.

6.Preeclampsia treatment

■ Basic principles of treatment

- Hypotension, spasmolysis, sedation, etc.
- Close monitoring of gravida and fetus.
- The most effective treatment: Termination
  of pregnancy.

（1）General treatment

■ Hypertension in pregnancy and preeclampsia: Outpatient treatment.

■ Severe preeclampsia: Hospitalization.

■ Adequate rest.

■ Adequate protein and calories.

■ Limiting salt intake in not recommended.

■ Adequate sleep.

■ Diazepam 2.5～5 mg, orally before bedtime
if necessary.

（2）Lowering blood pressure

■ Antihypertensive principle（Table 8-1）

- Treatment with antihypertensive drugs
  before pregnancy: Continue to reduce
  blood pressure.

■ Antihypertensive target

- No complications of organ dysfunction

表 8-1　降压原则

Table 8-1　Antihypertensive principle

收缩压和（或）舒张压 Systolic and/or diastolic blood pressure	高血压 Hypertension	降压治疗 Treatment of hypertension
收缩压≥160mmHg 和（或）舒张压≥110mmHg Systolic blood pressure ≥160 mmHg and/or diastolic blood pressure ≥110 mmHg	严重高血压 Severe hypertension	必须降压 Necessary
收缩压≥150mmHg 和（或）舒张压≥100mmHg Systolic blood pressure ≥150 mmHg and/or diastolic blood pressure ≥100 mmHg	非严重高血压 Non-severe hypertension	建议降压治疗 Suggested
收缩压140～150mmHg 和（或）舒张压90～100mmHg Systolic blood pressure 140 ～ 150mmHg and/or diastolic blood pressure 90 ～ 100mmHg		不建议降压治疗 Not recommended

- · 收缩压控制在130～155mmHg。
- · 舒张压应控制在80～105mmHg。
- 并发脏器功能损伤
  - · 收缩压应控制在130～139mmHg，舒张压应控制在80～89mmHg。
  - · 降压过程：力求下降平稳，不可波动过大。
  - · 为保证子宫胎盘血流灌注，血压不建议低于130/80mmHg。

（3）常用的口服降压药物

- 拉贝洛尔：硝苯地平短效或缓释片。
- 肼屈嗪：口服药物不理想，选静脉用药。

（4）解痉

- 硫酸镁是防治子痫的一线药物。
- 用药指征

- · Systolic blood pressure should be controlled at 130 ～ 155mmHg.
- · Diastolic blood pressure should be controlled at 80 ～ 105mmHg.
- Complicated with organ dysfunction
  - · Systolic blood pressure should be controlled at 130 ～ 139mmHg and diastolic blood pressure should be controlled at 80 ～ 89mmHg.
  - · Lowering blood pressure process: Strive to descend smoothly and not undulate too much.
  - · In order to ensure the blood perfusion of uterus and placenta, blood pressure should not be lower than 130/80 mmHg.

（3）Commonly used oral antihypertensive drugs

- Labetalol: Nifedipine（short-acting or sustained-release tablets）
- Hydralazine: Intravenous medication should be chosen if oral medication is not as expected.

（4）Spasmolysis

- Magnesium sulfate is the first-line drug for the prevention and treatment of eclampsia.
- Indications of medication

- 控制子痫抽搐及防止再抽搐。
- 预防重度子痫前期发展成为子痫。
- 重度子痫前期患者临产前用药，预防产时子痫或产后子痫。
- 用药原则
  - 预防和治疗子痫的硫酸镁用药方案：相同。
  - 分娩前未使用硫酸镁：分娩过程可使用硫酸镁，并持续至产后至少24～48小时。
  - 注意：保持硫酸镁血药浓度的稳定性。
- 用药方案
  - 静脉用药：负荷剂量硫酸镁4～6g。
  - 注意事项及使用硫酸镁必备条件
    · 膝腱反射存在。
    · 呼吸≥16次/分。
    · 尿量≥17ml/h或≥400ml/24h。
    · 备有10%葡萄糖酸钙。

7.分娩时机和方式

（1）终止妊娠是唯一有效的治疗措施。

（2）终止妊娠时机

- 妊娠期高血压、子痫前期患者：期待治疗至妊娠37周终止妊娠。
- 重度子痫前期：妊娠＜24周经治疗病情不稳定，建议终止妊娠。
- 孕24～28周根据母胎情况及当地母儿诊治能力决定是

- Control of eclampsia convulsions and prevention of re-convulsions.
- Prevention of the development of severe preeclampsia into eclampsia.
- Prenatal medication for severe preeclampsia to prevent intrapartum or postpartum eclampsia.
- Principles of medication
  - Magnesium sulfate for the prevention and treatment of eclampsia: The same.
  - Magnesium sulfate not used before delivery: Magnesium sulfate can be used during delivery and for at least 24～48 hours after delivery.
  - Attention: Maintain the stability of magnesium sulfate blood concentration.
- Medication regimen
  - Intravenous : Loading dose of magnesium sulfate 4～6g.
  - Notes and requirements for the use of magnesium sulfate
    · Presence of knee tendon reflex.
    · Breath ≥16 times per minute.
    · Urine volume ≥17ml/h or ≥400ml/24h.
    · 10% calcium gluconate available.

7.Timing and mode of delivery

（1）Termination of pregnancy is the only effective treatment.

（2）Timing of termination of pregnancy

- Pregnancy hypertension and preeclampsia patients: Expectant treatment to terminate pregnancy at 37 weeks.
- Severe preeclampsia: If pregnancy is less than 24 weeks and the condition is unstable after treatment, termination of pregnancy is recommended.
- Expectant treatment depends on the maternal condition and local ability of

否期待治疗。

- 孕28～34周
  - 病情不稳定
    - 经积极治疗24～48小时病情仍加重，促胎肺成熟后终止妊娠。

  - 病情稳定
    - 继续期待治疗并建议提前转至早产儿救治能力较强的医疗机构。

  - 妊娠≥34周：应考虑终止妊娠。

8.早发型重度子痫前期的处理

（1）建议住院治疗。

（2）促胎肺成熟、解痉、降压治疗。

（3）严密监测母儿情况。

（4）充分评估病情以明确有无严重的脏器损害，从而决定是否终止妊娠。

（5）当出现以下情况时建议终止妊娠：

- 患者出现持续不适症状或严重高血压。
- 子痫、肺水肿、HELLP综合征。
- 肾功能不全或凝血功能障碍。
- 胎盘早剥。
- 不能存活的胎儿。
- 胎儿窘迫。

9.子痫的治疗

- 处理原则
  - 控制抽搐。
  - 纠正缺氧和酸中毒。

diagnosis and treatment during 24 ～ 28 weeks of pregnancy.

- 28 ～ 34 weeks of pregnancy
  - Unstable condition
    - After active treatment for 24 ～ 48 hours, the condition still aggravates, and the pregnancy should be terminated after the fetal lung matures.
  - Stable condition
    - Continue treatment and recommend that premature infants should be transported to a medical institution with strong ability to treat in advance.
  - Pregnancy ≥ 34 weeks: Termination of pregnancy should be considered.

8.Management of early onset severe preeclampsia

（1）Recommend hospitalization.

（2）Promote fetal lung maturation, relieve spasmolysis and reduce hypertension.

（3）Closely monitor gravida and fetus.

（4）Fully assess the condition to determine whether there is serious organ damage and decide whether to terminate pregnancy.

（5）Termination of pregnancy is recommended when the patient has the following condition:

- Persistent discomfort or severe hypertension.
- Eclampsia, pulmonary edema and HELLP syndrome.
- Renal insufficiency or coagulation dysfunction.
- Placental abruption.
- Unviable fetus.
- Fetal distress.

9.Treatment of eclampsia

- Treatment principles
  - Control convulsions.
  - Correct hypoxia and acidosis.

- 控制血压。
- 抽搐控制后终止妊娠。

（1）一般急诊处理
■ 处理方法
  - 保持气道通畅。
  - 避免声、光等刺激。
（2）控制抽搐
  - 首选药物：硫酸镁。
  - 产后需继续应用硫酸镁24～48小时。
（3）降低颅压
  - 20%甘露醇250ml快速静脉滴注。
（4）控制血压
  - 当收缩压持续≥160mmHg，舒张压≥110mmHg时要积极降压。
（5）纠正缺氧和酸中毒。
  - 面罩和气囊吸氧。
  - 4%碳酸氢钠。
（6）适时终止妊娠：一般抽搐控制后可考虑终止妊娠。

10. 其他类型高血压的治疗

（1）慢性高血压的治疗
■ 降压。
■ 早期识别并发的子痫前期。
（2）产后高血压的治疗
■ 产后同样可以首次发生有严重表现的子痫前期和子痫。

■ 晚期产后高血压
  - 晚期产后高血压的发病机制尚不明确。
  - 可能同妊娠期高血压一样是将来发生慢性高血压疾病的一种预测指标。
  - 血压持续超过150/100

- Control blood pressure.
- Terminate pregnancy after convulsion controlled.

（1）General emergency management
■ Management
  - Keep the airway clear.
  - Avoid stimuli such as sound and light.
（2）Control convulsion
  - Preferred drug: Magnesium sulfate.
  - Magnesium sulfate should be continuously used for 24 ～ 48 hours after delivery.
（3）Reduce intracranial pressure
  - Rapid intravenous drip: 20% mannitol 250ml.
（4）Control blood pressure
  - Lower blood pressure actively: Systolic blood pressure is ≥160mmHg and diastolic blood pressure is ≥110mmHg.
（5）Correct hypoxia and acidosis.
  - Masks and airbags for oxygen inhalation.
  - 4% sodium bicarbonate.
（6）Termination of pregnancy at the right time: Termination of pregnancy can be considered after control of convulsion.

10. Treatment of other types of hypertension

（1）Chronic hypertension
■ Lowering blood pressure.
■ Early identification of preeclampsia.
（2）Treatment of postpartum hypertension
■ Preeclampsia and eclampsia with severe manifestations can also occur for the first time after delivery.

■ Late postpartum hypertension
  - The pathogenesis of late postpartum hypertension is still unclear.
  - It might be a predictor of chronic hypertension in the future, as is pregnancy hypertension.
  - Blood pressure continues to exceed

mmHg。
- 建议降压治疗。
- 先兆子痫症状：建议使用硫酸镁。

第二节 妊娠合并糖尿病

1.分类
（1）孕前糖尿病（PGDM）。

（2）妊娠期糖尿病（GDM）。

2.妊娠期糖代谢的特点

（1）妊娠早中期：空腹血糖约降低10%。

（2）妊娠中晚期
- 孕妇体内拮抗胰岛素样物质增加，胰岛素需求量相应增加。
- 孕妇胰岛素分泌受限。

3.妊娠与糖尿病的相互影响

（1）妊娠对糖尿病的影响
- 原有糖尿病加重。
- 低血糖。

（2）糖尿病对妊娠的影响
- 对孕妇的影响
  - 胚胎发育异常或胚亡。

  - 妊娠期高血压疾病。
  - 感染。
  - 羊水过多。
  - 难产、产道损伤、手术产概率增高。
  - 产后出血。
  - 糖尿病酮症酸中毒。
- 对胎儿的影响
  - 巨大胎儿。

150/100 mmHg.
- Antihypertensive treatment is recommended.
- Preeclampsia symptoms: Magnesium sulfate is recommended.

Section 2　Pregnancy with diabetes

1.Classification
（1）Pregestational diabetes mellitus（PGDM）.

（2）Gestational diabetes mellitus（GDM）.

2.Characteristics of glucose metabolism in pregnancy

（1）Early and middle pregnancy: Fasting blood glucose decreases by about 10%.

（2）Middle and late pregnancy
- Antagonistic insulin-like substances increase in pregnant women, and demand for insulin increases correspondingly.
- Insulin secretion of pregnant women is limited.

3.Interaction between pregnancy and diabetes mellitus

（1）Effects of pregnancy on diabetes mellitus
- Aggravation of diabetes mellitus.
- Hypoglycemia.

（2）Effects of diabetes mellitus on pregnancy
- Effects on pregnant women
  - Abnormal embryonic development or death.
  - Hypertensive disorders of pregnancy.
  - Infection.
  - Polyhydramnios.
  - Increased risk of dystocia, birth canal injury and surgical delivery.
  - Postpartum hemorrhage.
  - Diabetic ketoacidosis.
- Effects on fetus
  - Macrosomia.

- 胎儿宫内生长受限（FGR）。
- 流产和早产。
- 胎儿窘迫和胎死宫内。
- 胎儿畸形。
  - ■ 对新生儿的影响
    - 新生儿呼吸窘迫综合征。
    - 新生儿低血糖。

4.临床表现与诊断

（1）孕前糖尿病的诊断

- ■ 妊娠前已确诊为糖尿病。

- ■ 首次检查达到以下任何一项标准
  - 空腹血糖（FPG）≥7.0 mmol/L。
  - 口服葡萄糖耐量试验（OGTT）：口服75g葡萄糖后2小时血糖≥11.1 mmol/L。
  - 伴有典型的高血糖或高血糖危象症状，同时任意血糖≥11.1mmol/L。
  - 糖化血红蛋白≥6.5%。

（2）妊娠期糖尿病的诊断

- ■ 推荐医疗机构
  - 在妊娠24～28周及28周后，首次就诊行OGTT。
  - 75g OGTT的诊断标准
    ①空腹、服糖后1小时、2小时的血糖值：5.1mmol/L、10.0mmol/L、8.5mmol/L。

    ②任何一点血糖值：达到或超过上述标准。

- ■ 孕妇
  - GDM高危因素或者医疗资源缺乏地区建议
    ①妊娠24～28周首先检查FPG。

- Fetal growth restriction（FGR）.
- Abortion and premature delivery.
- Fetal distress and intrauterine fetal death.
- Fetal malformation.
  - ■ Effects on newborn
    - Neonatal respiratory distress syndrome.
    - Neonatal hypoglycemia.

4.Clinical manifestations and diagnosis

（1）Diagnosis of prenatal diabetes mellitus

- ■ Diabetes mellitus is diagnosed before pregnancy.

- ■ First inspection: Meet any of the following criteria
  - Fasting plasma glucose（FPG）≥7.0 mmol/L.
  - 75g oral glucose tolerance test（OGTT）: 2nd hour after taking sugar: blood sugar ≥11.1mmol/L.

  - Accompanied by typical hyperglycemia or hyperglycemia crisis symptoms, and arbitrary blood sugar ≥11.1mmol//L.
  - Glycated hemoglobin ≥6.5%.

（2）Diagnosis of gestational diabetes mellitus

- ■ Recommendation for medical institutions
  - OGTT for the first visit after 24 ～ 28 weeks and 28 weeks of gestation.
  - Diagnostic criteria for 75g OGTT
    ①Glucose level: The values of fasting, 1 hour and 2 hours after taking sugar are 5.1mmol/L, 10.0mmol/L, and 8.5 mmol/L.

    ②Blood sugar level at any point: Reaching or exceeding the above criteria.

- ■ Pregnant women
  - High-risk factors of GDM or suggestion for areas lacking medical resources
    ①FPG should be examined first at 24 ～ 28 weeks of gestation.

②FPG≥5.1mmol/L，可以直接诊断为GDM，不必行75g OGTT。

（3）GDM的高危因素

■ 孕妇因素：年龄≥35岁、妊娠前超重或肥胖、多囊卵巢综合征。

■ 家族史：糖尿病家族史。

■ 妊娠分娩史：不明原因的死胎、死产、流产史、巨大胎儿分娩史、胎儿畸形和羊水过多史、GDM史。

■ 本次妊娠因素：大于胎龄儿、羊水过多、反复外阴阴道假丝酵母菌病。

（4）糖尿病孕妇的管理

■ 妊娠期血糖控制目标（表8-2）

■ 医学营养治疗

• 每日摄入总能量
①妊娠早期：≥1500kcal/d（1kcal=4.184kJ）。
②妊娠晚期：≥1800kcal/d。

• 热量分配
①碳水化合物：占50%～60%。
②蛋白质：占15%～20%。
③脂肪：占25%～30%。

②FPG≥5.1mmol/L, directly diagnosed as GDM, without 75g OGTT.

（3）High risk factors of GDM

■ Pregnant women factors: Age≥35, overweight or obesity before pregnancy, polycystic ovary syndrome.

■ Family history: Family history of diabetes mellitus.

■ Pregnancy and childbirth history: Unknown fetus death, stillbirth, abortion, macrosomia, fetal malformation, polyhydramnios and GDM.

■ Pregnancy factors: Large for gestational age（LGA）, polyhydramnios, repeated vulvovaginal candidiasis.

（4）Management of diabetic pregnant women

■ Goals of blood sugar control during pregnancy（Table 8-2）

■ Medical nutrition therapy

• Total energy intake per day
①Early pregnancy: ≥1500kcal/d（1kcal=4.184kJ）.
②Late pregnancy: ≥1800kcal/d.

• Calorie allocation
①Carbohydrates: 50%～60%.
②Protein: 15%～20%.
③Fat: 25%～30%.

表8-2　妊娠期血糖控制目标

Table 8-2　Goals of blood sugar control during pregnancy

	餐前血糖（mmol/L） Preprandial blood glucose（mmol/L）	餐后2小时血糖（mmol/L） 2h Postprandial blood glucose（mmol/L）	夜间血糖（mmol/L） Night blood glucose（mmol/L）	糖化血红蛋白（%） Glycosylated hemoglobin（%）
妊娠期糖尿病 GDM	≤5.3	≤6.7	≥3.3	＜5.5
孕前糖尿病 PGDM	3.3～5.6	5.6～7.1	3.3～5.6	＜6.0

④ 早、中、晚三餐的能量：10%～15%、30%、30%。

⑤ 每次加餐的能量：占5%～10%，防止餐前过度饥饿。

■ 运动疗法

● 每餐30分钟后。

● 中等强度的运动。

● 对母儿无不良影响。

■ 药物治疗

● 首选胰岛素

① 普遍推荐方案：长效胰岛素和超短效或短效胰岛素联合使用。

② 睡前注射：长效胰岛素。

③ 三餐前注射：超短效或短效胰岛素。

④ 从小剂量开始，逐渐调整至理想血糖标准。

● 口服降糖药物：推荐二甲双胍。

■ 妊娠期糖尿病酮症酸中毒的处理

● 血糖过高（＞16.6mmol/L）：先给予胰岛素0.2～0.4U/kg一次性静脉注射。

● 胰岛素持续静脉滴注
· 0.9%氯化钠注射液＋胰岛素，按胰岛素0.1U/（kg·h）或4～6U/h的速度输入。

● 监测血糖

① 每小时监测血糖1次：从使用胰岛素开始。

② 根据血糖下降情况进行

④ Energy of three meals in the morning, at noon and in the evening: 10% ～ 15%, 30% and 30%.

⑤ Energy for each extra meal: 5% ～ 10%, prevent excessive hunger before meals.

■ Exercise therapy

● 30 minutes after each meal.

● Moderate intensity exercise.

● No adverse effects on gravida and fetus.

■ Medical treatment

● Insulin: Preferred

① Generally recommended regimen: Combination of long-acting insulin and ultra-short-acting or short-acting insulin.

② Pre-bedtime injection: Long-acting insulin.

③ Pre-meal injection: Ultra-short-acting or short-acting insulin.

④ Start with a small dose, and gradually adjust to the ideal blood sugar standard.

● Oral hypoglycemic drugs: Metformin is recommended.

■ Treatment of ketoacidosis in gestational diabetes mellitus

● Hyperglycemia（＞16.6mmol/L）: Insulin 0.2 ～ 0.4U/kg of one-time intravenous injection.

● Continuous intravenous insulin infusion
· 0.9% sodium chloride injection ＋ insulin, inject at the speed of 0.1U/（kg·h）or 4 ～ 6U/h

● Blood sugar monitoring

① Monitor blood sugar once an hour: Starting from insulin use.

② Adjust according to blood sugar drop.

调整。

（5）孕期母儿监护

- 孕前糖尿病（PGDM）
  - 每周检查1次直至妊娠第10周。
  - 妊娠中期：每两周检查1次。
  - 妊娠20周
    ①一般胰岛素需要量开始增加，须及时进行调整。

    ②每1～2个月测定肾功能及糖化血红蛋白含量，同时进行眼底检查。

  - 妊娠32周以后：每周产前检查1次。
    ①血压、水肿、尿蛋白。

    ②胎儿发育、胎儿成熟度、胎儿状况和胎盘功能等。
    ③必要时及早住院。
- 妊娠期糖尿病（GDM）：定期监测血糖、胎儿发育。

- 分娩时机
  - 妊娠期糖尿病：无需胰岛素治疗而血糖控制达标
    ①无母儿并发症：期待至预产期。
    ②终止妊娠：到预产期仍未临产，可引产。

  - PGDM及需胰岛素治疗的GDM
    ①血糖控制良好且无母儿并发症，严密监测

（5）Gravida and fetus care during pregnancy

- Pregestational diabetes mellitus（PGDM）
  - Check once a week until the 10th week of pregnancy.
  - Mid-trimester pregnancy: Check every two weeks.
  - 20 weeks of pregnancy
    ①Generally insulin demand begins to increase and needs to be adjusted in time.

    ②Renal function and glycosylated hemoglobin are measured every 1～2 months, with fundus examination performed at the same time.

  - After 32 weeks of pregnancy: Prenatal examination once a week.
    ①Blood pressure, edema, urinary protein.

    ②Fetal development, fetal maturity, fetal status and placental function, etc.

    ③Early hospitalization if necessary.
- Gestational diabetes mellitus（GDM）: Regular monitoring of blood sugar and fetal development.
- Timing of delivery
  - GDM: Blood sugar control reaches the standard without insulin treatment
    ①No maternal and fetal complications: To the expected date of delivery.

    ②Termination of pregnancy: To the expected date of delivery, has not yet been in labor which can be induced labor.

  - PGDM and GDM requiring insulin therapy
    ①With good blood sugar control and no maternal and fetal complications,

下，妊娠39周后可终止妊娠。

②血糖控制不满意或出现母儿并发症，应及时收入院观察，根据病情决定终止妊娠时机。

③糖尿病伴微血管病变或既往有不良产史者，需严密监护，终止妊娠时机应个体化。

■ 分娩方式：糖尿病不是剖宫产的指征。
  ● 阴道分娩
    ①制订分娩计划。
    ②产程中密切监测孕妇血糖、宫缩、胎心变化。

    ③避免产程过长。
  ● 选择性剖宫产手术指征
    ①糖尿病伴微血管病变及其他产科指征。
    ②如胎盘功能不良、胎位异常等。
    ③胎儿偏大（尤其估计胎儿体重≥4250g）或者既往有死胎、死产史者，应适当放宽剖宫产手术指征。
■ 分娩期处理
  ● 一般处理：注意休息、镇静、饮食。
  ● 严密观察血糖、尿糖及酮体变化。
  ● 及时调整胰岛素用量。

pregnancy can be terminated after 39 weeks of gestation under close monitoring.

②If the blood sugar control is not good or maternal and fetal complications occur, the patient should be admitted to the hospital in time for observation, and the termination of pregnancy should be decided according to the condition.

③Diabetic patients with microangiopathy or previous adverse birth history should be closely monitored and the timing of termination of pregnancy should be individualized.

■ Mode of delivery: Diabetes is not an indication of cesarean section.
  ● Vaginal delivery
    ①Make a delivery plan.
    ②Closely monitor the changes of blood sugar, uterine contraction and fetal heart rate during labor.
    ③Avoid prolonged labor.
  ● Indications for selective cesarean section
    ①Diabetes mellitus with microangiopathy and other obstetric indications.
    ②Placental dysfunction and abnormal fetal position.
    ③The indications for cesarean section should be relaxed if the fetus is too large (especially if the estimated fetal weight ≥4250g) or the patient has a history of dead fetus or stillbirth.
■ Delivery management
  ● General management: Rest, sedation and diet.
  ● Close observation of blood sugar, urine sugar and ketone body changes.
  ● Timely adjustment of insulin dosage.

- 加强胎儿监护。
- 产后处理
  - 大部分GDM患者在分娩后即不再需要使用胰岛素。
  - 仅少数患者仍需胰岛素治疗。
  - 糖尿病合并妊娠：胰岛素量减半或1/3量。
  - 妊娠期糖尿病：产后6～12周行OGTT。
  - 监测血糖。
- 新生儿出生时处理
  - 注意保暖和吸氧。
  - 重点：防止新生儿低血糖。
  - 应在哺乳同时定期滴服葡萄糖液。

重点专业词汇

1.妊娠期高血压
2.子痫前期
3.子痫
4.慢性高血压并发子痫前期

5.妊娠合并慢性高血压
6.糖尿病合并妊娠（PGDM）
7.妊娠期糖尿病（GDM）
8.空腹血糖（FPG）
9.胰岛素

练习题

1.妊娠期高血压疾病最基本的病理生理改变是：（B）

　A.前列腺素/血栓素A平衡失调

　B.全身小血管痉挛
　C.过度水钠潴留
　D.血液浓缩
　E.高凝状态

2.妊娠期高血压疾病最常见的产科并发症是：（A）

　A.胎盘早期剥离

- Enhanced fetal monitoring.
- Postpartum management
  - Most GDM patients no longer need insulin after delivery.
  - Only a few patients still need insulin therapy.
  - Diabetes mellitus with pregnancy: Half or a third of insulin.
  - Gestational diabetes mellitus: OGTT at 6～12 weeks postpartum.
  - Blood sugar monitoring.
- Neonatal management at birth
  - Keep warm and breathe oxygen.
  - Focus: Prevent neonatal hypoglycemia.
  - Regularly drip glucose solution while breastfeeding.

Key words

1.Gestational hypertension
2.Preeclampsia
3.Eclampsia
4.Chronic hypertension with superimposed preeclampsia
5.Pregnancy with chronic hypertension
6.Pregestational diabetes mellitus（PGDM）
7.Gestational diabetes mellitus（GDM）
8.Fasting plasma glucose（FPG）
9.Insulin

Exercises

1.The basic pathophysiological change in hypertensive disorder of pregnancy is:（B）

　A.Prostaglandin/thromboxane A balance disorder

　B.Systemic small blood vessels convulsions
　C.Excessive water-sodium retention
　D.Blood concentration
　E.Hypercoagulable state

2.The most common obstetric complication of hypertensive disorder of pregnancy is:（A）

　A.Early exfoliation of placenta

B.急性肾衰竭

C.心脏病

D.视网膜剥脱

E.HELLP综合征

3.24小时尿蛋白定量达到或超过_____列为重度子痫前期。（D）

A.1g

B.2g

C.3g

D.5g

E.10g

4.孕32周，近一周水肿加剧，尿量减少，不能平卧，并有头痛，血压180/120mmHg，尿蛋白（＋），心率140次/分，呼吸22次/分，有腹水征，胎心胎位正常，此时不宜采用何种治疗？（C）

A.降压

B.解痉

C.扩容

D.镇静

E.利尿

5.关于子痫，下列哪项不对？（D）

A.大多数子痫患者抽搐前有短暂的前驱症状

B.子痫的发生以产前期为最多见

C.抽搐频繁，昏迷不醒者大多病情严重

D.终止妊娠是治疗子痫最根本的方法，一旦分娩后子痫就不再发生

E.子痫发作时易致自伤及胎儿窘迫

6.糖尿病对妊娠的影响，下列哪项不恰当？（D）

B.Acute renal failure

C.Heart disease

D.Retinal detachment

E.HELLP syndrome

3.24-hour urine protein quantitation meets or exceeds _____ as severe pre-eclampsia.（D）

A.1g

B.2g

C.3g

D.5g

E.10g

4.A woman has 32 weeks of pregnancy. Findings on examination are: edema increased last week, urine output decreased, unable to lie supine, headache, blood pressure 180/120mmHg, urine protein（＋）, heart rate 140 beats/min, breathing 22 times/min, ascites sign, normal fetal heart and position. What treatment should not be used at this time?（C）

A.Pressure reduction

B.Spasmolysis

C.Expansion

D.Sedation

E.Diuretic

5.Regarding eclampsia, which of the following is incorrect?（D）

A.Most patients with eclampsia have transient prodromal symptoms before convulsions

B.The occurrence of eclampsia is most common in the prenatal period

C.Most patients with frequent convulsions, and in a coma are seriously ill

D.Termination of pregnancy is the most fundamental way to treat eclampsia, since eclampsia no longer occurs after delivery

E.Self-injury and fetal distress are easily caused during eclampsia

6.Which of the following is not appropriate about the effects of diabetes on pregnancy?（D）

A.孕期死胎发生率增高

B.易发生巨大儿

C.合并妊娠期高血压疾病的发生率增高

D.胎儿成熟较晚，故一般应待孕38周后终止妊娠

E.易并发胎儿畸形

7.诊断妊娠期糖尿病75g OGTT的实验室指标是：（A）

A.空腹血糖≥5.1mmol/L

B.空腹血糖＞7.0mmol/L

C.餐后1小时血糖＞9mmol/L

D.餐后2小时血糖＞6.7mmol/L

E.餐后3小时血糖＞7.5mmol/L

（路旭宏）

A.Increased incidence of stillbirth during pregnancy

B.Prone to macrosomia

C.Increased incidence of hypertensive disorder complicating pregnancy

D.Fetal maturity is late, so it is generally expected to terminate pregnancy after 38 weeks of pregnancy

E.Easy to be complicated with fetal malformations

7.The laboratory indicator for the diagnosis of gestational diabetes 75g OGTT is:（A）

A.Fasting plasma glucose≥5.1mmol/L

B.Fasting plasma glucose＞7.0mmol/L

C.1h postprandial plasma glucose＞9mmol/L

D.2h postprandial plasma glucose＞6.7mmol/L

E.3h postprandial plasma glucose＞7.5mmol/L

第9章 胎盘与胎膜异常

CHAPTER 9 Abnormal placenta and fetal membranes

第一节 前置胎盘

1.定义

■ 妊娠28周后，若胎盘附着于子宫下段、下缘达到或覆盖宫颈内口，位置低于胎先露部。

2.病因

（1）子宫内膜病变或损伤：剖宫产史、子宫手术和多次刮宫史、产褥感染、盆腔炎等。

（2）胎盘异常：多胎妊娠，副胎盘。

（3）受精卵滋养层发育迟缓：受精卵着床于子宫下段进而发育成前置胎盘。

3.分类（图9-1）

（1）完全性前置胎盘：胎盘组织完全覆盖宫颈内口。

（2）部分性前置胎盘：胎盘组织覆盖部分宫颈内口。

（3）边缘性前置胎盘：胎盘组织下缘达到宫颈内口。

（4）低置胎盘：胎盘附着于子宫下段，边缘距宫颈内口＜2cm。

4.临床表现

（1）症状：典型症状为妊娠晚

Section 1　Placenta previa

1.Definition

■ The placenta is implanted in the lower uterine segment of cervix after 28 weeks of gestation, and its lower margin reaches or covers the cervical os, lower than the presentation.

2.Etiology

（1）Endometrial lesion or injury: Previous cesarean delivery, the history of multiple curettage or uterine surgery, puerperal infection, pelvic inflammation and so on.

（2）Placental abnormality: Multiple pregnancy, accessory placenta.

（3）Trophoblastic retardation of fertilized ovum: The fertilized ovum was implanted in the lower uterine segment, and develops into placenta previa.

3.Classification（Figure 9-1）

（1）Complete placenta previa: The placenta completely covers the internal cervical os.

（2）Partial placenta previa: The placenta partially covers the internal cervical os.

（3）Marginal placenta previa: The placenta is implanted in the margin of the internal cervical os.

（4）Low-lying placenta: The placenta is implanted in the lower uterine segment and the margin from the internal cervical os is less than 2cm.

4.Clinical manifestations

（1）Symptoms: Typical symptom is no-

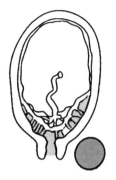

完全性前置胎盘
Complete placenta previa

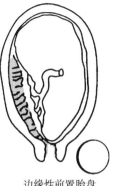

部分性前置胎盘
Partial placenta previa

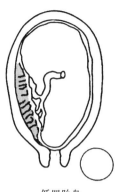

边缘性前置胎盘
Marginal placenta previa

低置胎盘
Low-lying placenta

图9-1 前置胎盘的分类

Figure 9-1 Classification of placenta previa

期或临产时，发生无诱因、无痛性反复阴道出血。

（2）体征

■ 一般情况与出血量有关，大量出血有休克表现。

■ 先露高浮或胎位异常。

■ 胎儿窘迫甚至胎死宫内。

■ 前壁前置胎盘，耻骨联合上方可闻及胎盘杂音。

■ 临产时宫缩为阵发性，间歇期子宫完全放松。

5.诊断

（1）病史：无痛性阴道出血，有多次刮宫、分娩史，子宫手术史，辅助生殖技术、多胎等。

（2）辅助检查

■ 超声（前壁胎盘要充盈膀胱），妊娠28周前称为胎盘前置状态。

■ 磁共振成像（MRI）。

6.对母儿影响

（1）产时、产后出血。

ninducing, painless recurrent vaginal hemorrhage during the third trimester of pregnancy or in labor.

（2）Signs

■ Related with the amount of bleeding, excessive bleeding may cause shock.

■ The presenting part high or abnormal fetal position.

■ Fetal distress, even dead fetus in uterus.

■ The placental souffle above the pubic symphysis can be heard for the anterior placenta previa.

■ The uterine contractions are paroxysmal during labor and the uterus is completely relaxed during the intermission.

5.Diagnosis

（1）Medical history: Painless hemorrhage, multiple curettage or birth history, history of uterine surgery, assisted reproductive technology, and multiple pregnancy.

（2）Auxiliary examination

■ Ultrasound（full bladder for anterior wall of placenta）, placenta previa occurs before 28 weeks of gestation.

■ Magnetic resonance imaging（MRI）.

6.Effects on gravida and fetus

（1）Bleeding of intrapartum or postpartum.

（2）植入性胎盘。

（3）产褥感染。

（4）围生儿预后不良。

7.治疗

原则：抑制宫缩、止血、纠正贫血和预防感染。

（1）期待疗法

■ 妊娠＜34周。

■ 胎儿体重＜2000g。

■ 胎儿存活。

■ 阴道出血量不多。

■ 一般情况良好的孕妇。

（2）一般处理

■ 侧卧位，绝对卧床休息。

■ 禁止性生活、阴道检查及肛查。

■ 胎儿电子监护。

■ 间断吸氧。

■ 纠正贫血。

（3）药物治疗

■ 必要时给予镇静药。

■ 应用广谱抗生素预防感染。

■ 妊娠35周前终止妊娠者，应促胎肺成熟。

（4）终止妊娠

■ 指征

　● 出血量大甚至休克，为挽救孕妇生命，无须考虑胎儿情况，应立即终止妊娠。

　● 出现胎儿窘迫等产科指征时，胎儿可存活，行急诊手术。

　● 临产后诊断前置胎盘，出血量多，短时间不能分娩者。

（2）Placenta increta.

（3）Puerperal infection.

（4）Poor perinatal outcomes.

7.Treatment

Principles: Inhibition of the uterine contractions, hemostasis, correction of anemia and infection prevention.

（1）Expected treatment

■ Gestation ＜ 34 weeks.

■ Fetal weight ＜2000g.

■ Fetus survival.

■ Less vaginal bleeding.

■ Good maternal general condition.

（2）General treatment

■ Lateral position, complete bed rest.

■ Sexual activity, vaginal examination and rectal examination are banned.

■ Fetal electronic monitoring.

■ Intermittent oxygen.

■ Correction of anemia.

（3）Medical treatment

■ Sedatives given when necessary.

■ Broad-spectrum antibiotics used to prevent infection.

■ Corticosteroids used to promote fetal lung maturation for termination of pregnancy before 35 gestational weeks.

（4）Termination of pregnancy

■ Indications

　● If excessive bleeding or even shock occurs, pregnancy should be terminated immediately to save the life of pregnant women whatever the fetal condition.

　● In case of obstetric indications, i.e. fetal distress, emergency surgery should be performed if the fetus is viable.

　● Placenta previa diagnosed after labor, much uterine bleeding, or unable to delivery in a short time.

- 无临床症状的前置胎盘根据类型决定分娩时机。
  - ①合并胎盘植入：妊娠36周及以上。
  - ②完全性前置胎盘：妊娠37周及以上。
  - ③边缘性前置胎盘：妊娠38周及以上。
  - ④部分性前置胎盘：适时终止妊娠。
- 手术管理：应当由技术娴熟的医师实施，做好分级手术管理，做好处理产后出血和抢救新生儿的准备。

- 阴道分娩：边缘性前置胎盘、低置胎盘、枕先露、阴道出血少，估计短时间内能结束分娩者。

重点专业词汇

1.完全性前置胎盘

2.部分性前置胎盘

3.边缘性前置胎盘

4.植入性胎盘

5.产褥感染

练习题

1.下列哪一项不是导致前置胎盘的高危因素？（D）

A.多次刮宫

B.多胎

C.副胎盘

D.身材矮小者

E.经产妇

2.下列哪一项是诊断前置胎盘最常用且准确的辅助检查？（D）

A.X线摄片

B.CT断层扫描

C.超声多普勒检查

- The timing of delivery depends on the type of asymptomatic placenta previa.
  - ①Combined with placental implantation: 36 weeks's gestation and above.
  - ②Complete placenta previa: 37 weeks' gestation and above.
  - ③Marginal placenta previa: 38 weeks' gestation and above.
  - ④Partial placenta previa: Timely termination of pregnancy.
- Surgery management: Operation should be performed by the skilled doctors, graded surgical management should be performed, be prepared to deal with postpartum hemorrhage and neonatal resuscitation.

- Vaginal delivery: Marginal placenta previa, low-lying placenta, occipital presentation, little vaginal bleeding, delivery estimated in a short time.

Key words

1.Complete placenta previa

2.Partial placenta previa

3.Marginal placenta previa

4.Placenta increta

5.Puerperal infection

Exercises

1.Which of the following is not a high risk factor for placenta previa?（D）

A.Multiple curettage

B.Multiple pregnancy

C.Accessory placenta

D.Short stature

E.Multipara

2.Which of the following is the most common and accurate auxiliary examination for diagnosis of placenta previa?（D）

A.X-ray

B.CT

C.Ultrasonic Doppler

D.超声

E.阴道检查

3.前置胎盘阴道出血的特点是：（C）

A.边缘性前置胎盘出血多发生在妊娠28周左右

B.出血量与前置胎盘类型关系不大

C.出血反复发作，无诱因和疼痛

D.出血时常伴腹痛

E.出血量与贫血程度不成正比

4.孕妇25岁，孕32周，无痛性少量阴道出血2天，胎心胎动好，无明显宫缩；超声检查提示前置胎盘，此病例最恰当的处理是：（A）

A.绝对卧床，给予镇静药，观察病情变化

B.立即行人工破膜

C.缩宫素静脉滴注引产

D.立即行剖宫产术

E.高危门诊继续随访观察

第二节　胎盘早剥

1.定义

■ 妊娠20周后或分娩期，正常位置的胎盘在胎儿娩出前，部分或全部从子宫壁剥离。

2.病因

（1）孕妇血管病变：妊娠期高血压疾病；仰卧位综合征。

（2）宫腔内压力骤减：胎膜早破；羊水过多；双胎妊娠分娩，第

D.Ultrasound

E.Vaginal examination

3.The characteristic of vaginal bleeding for placenta previa is：（C）

A.Vaginal bleeding usually occurs about 28 weeks' gestation for marginal placenta previa

B.The amount of bleeding has little relation with the classification of placenta previa

C.Recurrent bleeding, without inducement or pain

D.Bleeding with abdominal pain

E.The clinical findings of anemia is not consistent with the amount of vaginal bleeding

4.A 25-year-old pregnant woman has 32 weeks' gestation, and minor vaginal bleeding without pain for two days. The fetal heart rate and fetal movements are normal. No obvious uterine contractions are found; placenta previa is revealed by ultrasound. The best treatment for this case is：（A）

A.Complete bed rest, sedatives and observation of changes in the patient's condition

B.Immediate amniotomy

C.Induction of labor by oxytocin

D.Immediate cesarean section

E.Follow-up observation in high risk outpatient department

Section 2　Placental abruption

1.Definition

■ Defined as partial or full separation from the site of uterine implantation after 20 weeks' gestation or intrapartum.

2.Etiology

（1）Maternal vascular disease: Hypertensive disorders of pregnancy; supine position syndrome.

（2）Sudden decrease in intrauterine pressure: Premature rupture of membrane, polyhydramnios,

一胎儿娩出过快。

（3）机械性因素：外伤，脐带过短。

（4）其他高危因素：高龄孕妇，吸烟，子宫肌瘤，有胎盘早剥史。

3.病理及病理生理

（1）主要病理改变是底蜕膜出血并形成血肿，使胎盘从附着处分离。

（2）按病理分2种类型

■ 显性剥离。

■ 隐性剥离。

（3）子宫胎盘卒中，又称库弗莱尔子宫：血液浸入子宫肌层，引起肌纤维分离、断裂甚至变性。渗透至子宫浆膜层时，子宫表面呈现紫蓝色瘀斑。

（4）严重的胎盘早剥可引发弥散性血管内凝血等一系列病理生理改变。

4.临床表现及分类

Ⅰ度：外出血为主，胎盘剥离面积小，常无腹痛或腹痛轻微，贫血体征不明显，子宫软，胎位清楚，胎心率正常。

Ⅱ度：胎盘剥离面1/3左右，有突然发生的持续性腹痛、腰酸或腰背痛，贫血程度与阴道出血量不相符。子宫大于妊娠周数，胎盘附着处压痛明显，宫缩有间歇，胎儿存活。

Ⅲ度：胎盘剥离面超过胎盘面积1/2，出现休克症状，子宫硬如板状，宫缩间歇不能松弛，胎位扪不清，胎心消失。

twin pregnancy delivery, the first fetus delivered quickly.

（3）Mechanical factors: Trauma, excessively short umbilical cord.

（4）Other high risks: Advanced maternal age, smoking, uterine myoma, the history of placental abruption.

3.Pathology and pathophysiology

（1）The main pathological change is bleeding in decidua basalis and formation of hematoma, which causes the separation of the placenta.

（2）2 types based on pathology

■ Revealed abruption.

■ Concealed abruption.

（3）Uteroplacental apoplexy/Couvelaire uterus: Blood infiltrates the myometrium, resulting in myofiber separation, fracture, and, even degeneration. When blood arrives to the uterine serosa, the uterine surface presents purple-blue ecchymosis.

（4）Severe placental abruption can trigger a series of pathophysiological changes, such as disseminated intravascular coagulation.

4.Clinical manifestations and classification

Degree Ⅰ: External hemorrhage, small size of separations, no or mild abdominal pain, the sign of anemia being not obvious, uterus soft, fetal position clear and fetal heart rate normal.

Degree Ⅱ: The size of separations about one third, sudden and persistent abdominal pain, lumbago and backache, the clinical findings of anemia not consistent with the amount of vaginal bleeding, uterus larger than the gestational age, obvious tenderness of placental attachment, intermittent contractions and fetus alive.

Degree Ⅲ: The size of separations over one second, appearing shock symptoms, the uterus hard as a plate, intermittent uterine contractions not relaxed, fetal position unclear, fetal heart rate

5.辅助检查

（1）超声：阴性结果不能完全排除胎盘早剥，尤其是子宫后壁的胎盘。

（2）实验室检查：血常规、凝血功能检查。

6.并发症

（1）胎儿宫内死亡。

（2）弥散性血管内凝血（DIC）。

（3）产后出血。

（4）急性肾衰竭。

（5）羊水栓塞。

7.治疗

治疗原则：早期识别、积极处理休克、及时终止妊娠、控制DIC、减少并发症。

（1）纠正休克：建立静脉通路，迅速补充血容量，改善血液循环。

（2）及时终止妊娠

- 阴道分娩：Ⅰ度胎盘早剥患者，一般情况良好，病情较轻，估计短时间内可结束分娩。

- 剖宫产：Ⅰ度胎盘早剥，出现胎儿窘迫征象者；Ⅱ度胎盘早剥，不能短时间内结束分娩者；Ⅲ度胎盘早剥，孕妇病情恶化，胎儿已死，不能立即分娩；破膜后产程无进展者。

（3）并发症处理

- 产后出血：胎儿前肩娩出后立即给予子宫收缩药物。

- 凝血功能障碍：迅速终止妊

disappearing.

5.Auxiliary examination

（1）Ultrasound: Negative results cannot completely exclude placental abruption, especially the posterior wall of placenta.

（2）Laboratory examination: Blood routine examination, coagulation function test.

6.Complications

（1）Dead fetus in uterus.

（2）Disseminated intravascular coagulation（DIC）.

（3）Postpartum hemorrhage.

（4）Acute renal failure.

（5）Amniotic fluid embolism.

7.Treatment

Treatment principles: Early identification, active shock management, timely termination of pregnancy, control of the disseminated intravascular coagulation（DIC）, decrease in complications.

（1）Correction of shock: Establish intravenous access, replenish blood volume quickly, and improve blood circulation.

（2）Timely termination of pregnancy

- Vaginal delivery: Degree Ⅰ, the patient in good general and mild condition, and estimated to complete delivery in a short time.

- Cesarean section: Degree Ⅰ, with fetal distress; Degree Ⅱ, unable to deliver in a short time; Degree Ⅲ, the patient in deteriorated condition, the fetus dead, and unable to deliver immediately; no progress in labor after rupture of membrane.

（3）Management of complications

- Postpartum hemorrhage: Uterotonic agents are administered as soon as the infant's anterior shoulder delivered.

- Coagulation defects: Quick termination

娠、阻断促凝物质继续进入母血循环，纠正凝血机制障碍。

■ 肾衰竭：补充血容量，少尿予呋塞米静脉注射。出现尿毒症时应及时血液透析治疗。

重点专业词汇

1. 胎盘早剥
2. 显性剥离
3. 隐性剥离
4. 子宫胎盘卒中
5. 弥散性血管内凝血（DIC）

6. 产后出血
7. 羊水栓塞

练习题

1. 关于Ⅲ度胎盘早剥，下列哪项正确？（B）

A. 多发生在分娩期
B. 多见于妊娠高血压综合征

C. 胎盘剥离面积小于胎盘的1/3
D. 贫血程度与阴道出血量成正比
E. 主要临床表现为无痛性阴道出血

2. 重度子痫前期孕妇于孕晚期出现腹痛伴阴道出血，最可能的疾病是：（B）

A. 边缘性前置胎盘
B. 胎盘早剥
C. 子宫颈癌
D. 子宫破裂
E. 脐带帆状附着前置血管破裂

3. 以下哪项不是胎盘早剥的并发症？（C）

of pregnancy, blocking the procoagulant materials into the maternal blood circulation system, and the correction of the coagulopathy.

■ Renal failure: Supplement of blood volume, furosemide given by intravenous injection during oliguria. If uremia occurs, hemodialysis treatment should be timely.

Key words

1. Placental abruption
2. Revealed abruption
3. Concealed abruption
4. Uteroplacental apoplexy
5. Disseminated intravascular coagulation （DIC）

6. Postpartum hemorrhage
7. Amniotic fluid embolism

Exercises

1. Which of the following is correct for Degree Ⅲ placental abruption?（B）

A. Most occurs in intrapartum
B. More common in hypertensive disorders of pregnancy
C. The size of separations is less than one third
D. The clinical findings of anemia is consistent with the amount of vaginal bleeding
E. The main clinical manifestation is vaginal bleeding without abdominal pain

2. The pregnancies with severe preeclampsia develop vaginal bleeding with abdominal pain in the third trimester. The most likely disease is:（B）

A. Marginal placenta previa
B. Placental abruption
C. Cervical cancer
D. Rupture of uterus
E. Rupture of vasa previa with velamentous insertion

3. Which of the following is not the complication of placental abruption?（C）

A.弥散性血管内凝血（DIC）

B.产后出血

C.子宫破裂

D.羊水栓塞

E.急性肾衰竭

A.Disseminated intravascular coagulation （DIC）

B.Postpartum hemorrhage

C.Rupture of uterus

D.Amniotic fluid embolism

E.Acute renal failure

第三节　胎膜早破

Section 3　Premature rupture of membranes

1.定义

■ 临产前发生胎膜破裂；未达到37周发生者称为未足月胎膜早破。

1.Definition

■ Amniorrhexis prior to the onset of labor during any stage of gestation; not over 37 weeks' gestation called preterm premature rupture of membranes.

2.病因

（1）下生殖道感染。

（2）羊膜腔压力增高。

（3）胎膜受力不均。

（4）营养因素。

（5）其他：妊娠晚期性生活、羊膜穿刺不当。

2.Etiology

（1）Lower genital tract infection.

（2）Increased intra-uterine pressure.

（3）Uneven stress on membrane.

（4）Nutritional deficit.

（5）Others: Sexual intercourse especially in the third trimester, and improper amniocentesis.

3.临床表现

（1）90%患者突感有较多液体从阴道流出，有时混有胎脂及胎粪。少数患者仅感外阴湿润。

（2）阴道窥器检查见阴道后穹窿有羊水积聚或有羊水自宫口流出。

3.Clinical manifestations

（1）90% of patients feel gush of fluid from the vagina, sometimes mixed with vernix caseosa or meconium. The minority feel moist vulva only.

（2）The collection of amniotic fluid in the posterior fornix or amniotic fluid leakage from the cervix is revealed by the sterile speculum.

4.诊断

（1）胎膜早破诊断

■ 临床表现

■ 辅助检查

  • 阴道液pH测定：pH试纸变成蓝绿色，血液、宫颈黏液可能造成假阳性。

  • 阴道液涂片检查：可见羊齿状结晶或黄色脂肪小粒。

4.Diagnosis

（1）Diagnosis of PROM

■ Clinical manifestations

■ Auxiliary examination

  • Vaginal fluid pH measurement: pH test paper turns blue-green; blood and cervical mucus may cause the false positive.

  • Vaginal fluid smear: Fern-like pattern of crystallization or yellow fat granule.

- 胰岛素样生长因子结合蛋白-1检测。
- 超声检查。

（2）绒毛膜羊膜炎诊断

■ 临床表现

- 母体体温≥38℃。
- 阴道分泌物异味。
- 胎心率增快（胎心率基线≥160次/分）或母体心率增快（心率≥100次/分）。
- 母体外周血白细胞计数≥15×10^9/L。
- 子宫呈激惹状态、宫体有压痛。

母体体温升高的同时伴有上述的任何一项表现即可诊断。

■ 辅助检查

- 羊水检查：羊水涂片革兰染色检查，白细胞计数，细菌培养，临床较少使用。
- 胎盘、胎膜或脐带组织病理检查。

5.对母儿影响

（1）母亲方面：感染、胎盘早剥、剖宫产率增加。

（2）胎儿方面：早产、感染、脐带脱垂和受压、胎肺发育不良及胎儿受压。

6.治疗

（1）足月胎膜早破

■ 评估母胎状况。

■ 破膜超过12小时应预防性应用抗生素。

■ 破膜后2～12小时积极使用缩宫素引产。

■ 有明确剖宫产指征时宜行剖宫产终止妊娠。

- Insulin-like growth factor binding protein-1.
- Ultrasound examination.

（2）Diagnosis of chorioamnionitis

■ Clinical manifestations

- Maternal temperature ≥38℃ .
- Foul-smelling vaginal discharge.
- Fetal heart rate increase（baseline ≥ 160bpm）or maternal heart rate increase（heart rate ≥100bpm）.
- Maternal peripheral blood leukocyte count ≥15×10^9/L.
- Uterine irritability and tenderness.

Diagnosis can be made if maternal temperature increases along with any of the above manifestations.

■ Auxiliary examination

- Amniotic fluid examination: Amniotic fluid smear Gram staining, leukocyte count, bacterial cultivation, less used in clinic.
- Histopathological examination of placenta, fetal membrane or umbilical cord.

5.Effects on gravida and fetus

（1）Gravida: Infection, placental abruption, increased operative delivery rate.

（2）Fetus: Preterm birth, infection, prolapse and compression of umbilical cord, fetal pulmonary dysplasia and compression of the fetus.

6.Treatment

（1）Term premature rupture of membrane

■ Assessment of maternal and fetal conditions.

■ If rupture of membrane remains more than 12 hours, antibiotics should be used to prevent infection.

■ Oxytocin should be used to induce labor in 2 ～ 12 hours after rupture of membrane.

■ Operative delivery should be done to terminate pregnancy in case of obvious

（2）未足月胎膜早破

■ 引产

- 妊娠＜24周，胎儿存活率低、母胎感染风险大，引产为宜。

- 妊娠24～27⁺⁶周者，根据孕妇及家属意愿、医院对新生儿抢救能力决定。

■ 不宜继续妊娠，采取引产或剖宫产终止妊娠。

- 妊娠34～36⁺⁶周者。
- 无论孕周，明确诊断的绒毛膜羊膜炎、胎儿窘迫、胎盘早剥等。

■ 期待治疗

- 妊娠24～27⁺⁶周者，告知风险后仍要求期待治疗者。
- 妊娠28～33⁺⁶周无继续妊娠禁忌者，具体内容如下。
  ①一般处理：保持外阴清洁，监测感染情况。
  ②糖皮质激素：妊娠＜35周者。
  ③预防感染。
  ④抑制宫缩：应用48小时。

  ⑤胎儿神经系统保护：妊娠＜32周。

■ 分娩方式：无明确剖宫产指征时应阴道试产。阴道分娩时不必常规会阴切开。

indication of cesarean section.

（2）Preterm premature rupture of membranes

■ Induced labor

- Pregnancies prior to 24 weeks' gestation have extremely low rates of fetal salvage with considerable maternal risk. These patients should be induced labor.

- Between 24 and 27⁺⁶ weeks' gestation, induced labor should be decided by the will of the pregnant woman and her family and the ability to salvage newborns.

■ Not suitable to continue pregnancy, should be induced labor or done operative delivery.

- Between 34 and 36⁺⁶ weeks' gestation.
- Pregnancy with diagnosis of chorioamnionitis, fetal distress, placental abruption etc., should be terminated regardless of gestational weeks.

■ Expectant treatment

- Between 24 and 27⁺⁶ weeks' gestation, the patients ask for expectant treatment after being informed of the risks.
- Between 28 and 33⁺⁶ weeks' gestation, no contraindications for pregnancy. The specific methods are as follows.
  ①General treatment: Keep the vulva clean and monitor the infection.
  ②Corticosteroids: ＜35 weeks' gestation.
  ③Antibiotics.
  ④Tocolytics: Used for 48 hours' duration.
  ⑤Protection of the fetal nerve system: ＜32 weeks' gestation.

■ Delivery mode: If no clear indication of cesarean section, vaginal delivery is preferable to cesarean section. Episiotomy isn't conventional in vaginal delivery.

重点专业词汇

1.胎膜早破

2.绒毛膜羊膜炎

3.糖皮质激素

4.宫缩抑制剂

练习题

1.以下关于胎膜早破的定义，叙述正确的是哪项？（B）

A.胎膜在预产期前破裂

B.临产前胎膜破裂

C.妊娠未足月时胎膜破裂

D.妊娠满37周后，发生胎膜破裂

E.胎头娩出前，发生胎膜破裂

2.下列哪一项不是胎膜早破的并发症？（A）

A.早产

B.宫内感染

C.第二产程延长

D.脐带脱垂

E.胎儿窘迫

3.胎膜早破的期待疗法，下列哪项是错误的？（B）

A.适用于妊娠28～34周的患者

B.胎膜早破合并感染

C.胎膜早破不伴产科并发症

D.破膜12小时以上使用抗生素

E.给予地塞米松促胎肺成熟

（刘　芳）

Key words

1.Premature rupture of membranes

2.Chorioamnionitis

3.Corticosteroids

4.Tocolytics

Exercises

1.Which of the following is correct about the definition of premature rupture of membranes?（B）

A.Rupture of membranes prior to expected date of confinement

B.Rupture of membranes prior to the onset of labor

C.Rupture of membranes prior to preterm

D.Rupture of membranes after 37 weeks' gestation

E.Rupture of membranes prior to the fetal head delivery

2.Which of the following is not the complication of premature rupture of membranes?（A）

A.Preterm birth

B.Intrauterine infection

C.Protracted second stage

D.Prolapse of umbilical cord

E.Fetal distress

3.Which of the following is wrong about the expectant treatment of premature rupture of membranes?（B）

A.Suitable for patients with pregnancy of 28～34 weeks

B.Premature rupture of membrane with infection

C.Premature rupture of membranes without obstetrical complications

D.Antibiotics for premature rupture of membranes over 12 hours

E.Dexamethasone for maturity of the fetal lung

第10章 胎儿异常与多胎妊娠

第一节 巨 大 胎 儿

1.定义

■ 胎儿体重达到或超过4000g，欧美国家定义为胎儿体重达到或超过4500g。

2.高危因素

（1）孕妇肥胖。

（2）妊娠合并糖尿病，尤其是2型糖尿病。

（3）过期妊娠。

（4）经产妇。

（5）父母身材高大。

（6）高龄产妇。

（7）有巨大儿分娩史。

（8）种族、民族因素。

3.对母儿影响

（1）母亲方面：增加剖宫产率；肩难产；软产道损伤，子宫破裂；子宫收缩乏力、产程延长，易致产后出血；尿瘘或粪瘘。

（2）胎儿方面：手术助产，可引起颅内出血、锁骨骨折、臂丛神经损伤等产伤，严重时甚至死亡。

4.诊断

（1）病史及临床表现：存在高危因素，妊娠期体重增加迅速，腹部沉重等症状。

（2）腹部检查：腹部明显膨

Section 1　Macrosomia

1.Definition

■ Fetal weight is 4000g or more, and 4500g or more in European and American countries.

2.High risk factors

（1）Maternal obesity.

（2）Pregnancy complicated with diabetes, especially type 2 diabetes mellitus.

（3）Postterm pregnancy.

（4）Multiparity.

（5）Large stature of parents.

（6）Advanced maternal age.

（7）Previous macrosomia.

（8）Race and nation.

3.Effects on gravida and fetus

（1）Gravida: Increase of cesarean section rate, shoulder dystocia, lacerations, rupture of uterus, uterine atony, prolonged labor, vulnerable to postpartum hemorrhage, urinary fistula or fecal fistula.

（2）Fetus: Operative vaginal delivery leads to birth injury, such as intracranial hemorrhage, fracture of clavicle, brachial plexus injury etc, and even death.

4.Diagnosis

（1）Medical history and clinical manifestations: High risk factors, rapid weight gain during pregnancy, heavy abdomen.

（2）Abdominal examination: Obvious

隆，宫高＞35cm；先露部高浮，听胎心位置较高。

（3）超声检查：双顶径＞10cm须警惕。

5.治疗

（1）妊娠期：须排除糖尿病。

（2）分娩期
- 估计胎儿体重≥4000g且合并糖尿病者，建议行剖宫产终止妊娠。
- 无糖尿病者，可阴道试产，但需放宽剖宫产指征。
- 做好处理肩难产的准备工作，分娩后检查有无软产道损伤，并预防产后出血。

（3）新生儿处理：预防新生儿低血糖。

重点专业词汇

1.巨大胎儿

2.糖尿病

3.肩难产

4.子宫收缩乏力

5.臂丛神经损伤

6.双顶径

7.低血糖

练习题

1.下列哪一项不是发生巨大胎儿的高危因素？（C）

A.父母身材高大

B.孕妇糖尿病

C.脐带短而粗

D.过期妊娠

E.经产妇

2.巨大胎儿是指：（D）

A.胎儿体重2000～3000g

distended abdomen, the height of uterus more than 35cm, high position presentation, and high fetal heart position.

（3）Ultrasound examination: If the biparietal diameter ＞10cm, the macrosomia should be alerted.

5.Treatment

（1）Gestation period: Diabetes mellitus should be excluded.

（2）Delivery period
- If the fetal estimated weight ≥4000g and with diabetes mellitus, operative delivery is recommended.
- If without diabetes mellitus, vaginal trial delivery is possible but the operative indication is relaxed.
- Prepare for shoulder dystocia, check lacerations after delivery and prevent postpartum hemorrhage.

（3）Neonatal management: Prevent hypoglycemia.

Key words

1.Macrosomia

2.Diabetes mellitus

3.Shoulder dystocia

4.Uterine inertia

5.Brachial plexus injury

6.Biparietal diameter

7.Hypoglycemia

Exercises

1.Which of the following is not the high risk factor for macrosomia?（C）

A.Large stature of parents

B.Maternal diabetes

C.Short and thick umbilical cord

D.Postterm pregnancy

E.Multipara

2.Macrosomia is defined as:（D）

A.Fetal weight is between 2000 g and 3000 g

B.胎儿体重超过 2000g

C.胎儿体重超过 3500g

D.胎儿体重超过 4000g

E.胎儿体重超过 4500g

B.Fetal weight is greater than 2000 g

C.Fetal weight is greater than 3500 g

D.Fetal weight is greater than 4000 g

E.Fetal weight is greater than 4500 g

第二节 胎儿窘迫

Section 2　Fetal distress

1.定义

- 胎儿在子宫内因急性或慢性缺氧危及其健康和生命的综合症状。急性胎儿窘迫多发生在分娩期，慢性胎儿窘迫多发生在妊娠晚期。

1.Definition

- The comprehensive symptoms that acute or chronic anoxia of fetus in uterus endangers the fetal health and life. Acute fetal distress mostly occurs in the stages of labor, and chronic fetal distress mostly occurs in the late trimester of pregnancy.

2.病因

（1）胎儿急性缺氧

- 母胎间血氧运输及交换障碍或脐带血循环障碍所致。

- 常见因素
  - 前置胎盘、胎盘早剥。
  - 脐带异常：脐带缠绕、脐带真结、脐带扭转、脐带脱垂、脐带帆状附着等。

  - 母体严重血循环障碍致胎盘灌注急剧减少：母体休克。

  - 缩宫素使用不当：子宫收缩过强。
  - 孕妇应用麻醉药及镇静药过量。

（2）胎儿慢性缺氧

- 母体血液含氧量不足：先天性心脏病、肺部感染、重度贫血等。

2.Etiology

（1）Fetal acute anoxia

- Resulted from the obstacle of transportation and exchange of blood and oxygen between maternal and fetal or umbilical blood circulation disorders.

- Common factors
  - Placenta previa, and placental abruption.
  - Abnormal umbilical cord: Cord entanglement, true knotting of the umbilical cord, torsion of the umbilical cord, prolapse of the umbilical cord, cord velamentous insertion and so on.
  - The severe obstacle of maternal blood circulation results in the infusion to the placenta decreasing rapidly: Maternal shock.
  - Oxytocin misused: Tetanic contractions of uterus.
  - Excessive anaesthetics and sedatives for pregnant women.

（2）Fetal chronic anoxia

- Insufficient oxygen in maternal blood: Congenital cardiac diseases, pulmonary infection, severe anemia and so on.

- 子宫胎盘血管硬化、狭窄、梗死：妊娠期高血压疾病、糖尿病、过期妊娠等。

- 胎儿运输及利用氧能力下降：胎儿严重的心血管疾病、呼吸系统疾病，母儿血型不合，宫内感染、颅脑损伤。

3.临床表现及诊断

（1）急性胎儿窘迫

- 产时胎心率异常。

- 羊水胎粪污染：不是胎儿窘迫的征象，如果胎心监护正常，不需要进行特殊处理；如果胎心监护异常，存在宫内缺氧情况，会引起胎粪吸入综合征。

- 胎动异常：缺氧初期胎动频繁，继而减少。

- 酸中毒：胎儿头皮血进行血气分析，若pH＜7.2，PO_2＜10mmHg，PCO_2＞60mmHg，可诊断为胎儿酸中毒。

（2）慢性胎儿窘迫

- 胎动减少或消失。
- 产前胎儿电子监护异常。

- 胎儿生物物理评分（BPP）低。
- 脐动脉多普勒超声血流异常。

4.治疗

（1）急性胎儿窘迫：采取果断措施，改善胎儿缺氧状态

- 一般处理：左侧卧位、吸氧，停用缩宫素，阴道检查

- The blood vessel sclerosis, stenosis, infarction of uterus and placenta: Hypertensive disorders complicating pregnancy, diabetes mellitus, postterm pregnancy and so on.

- Decrease in fetal ability to transport and utilize oxygen: Severe Fetal cardiovascular diseases, diseases of respiratory system, maternal-fetal blood group incompatibility, intrauterine infection, and craniocerebral injury.

3.Clinical manifestations and diagnosis

（1）Acute fetal distress

- Intrapartum fetal heart rate abnormal.

- Meconium-stained amniotic fluid: It is not the sign of fetal distress, if the fetal heart monitoring is normal, no special treatment is needed. If the fetal heart monitoring is abnormal, the intrauterine anoxia may exist and result in meconium aspiration syndrome.

- Abnormal fetal movements: Fetal movements are frequent at the early stage and then decrease.

- Acidosis: Blood gas analysis of fetal scalp blood, if pH＜7.2, PO_2＜10mmHg, PCO_2＞60mmHg, fetal acidosis can be diagnosed.

（2）Chronic fetal distress

- Fetal movements decrease or disappear.
- Abnormal antenatal fetal heart electronic monitoring of fetus.
- Low fetal biophysical（BPP）score.
- Abnormal flow of umbilical artery Doppler ultrasound.

4.Treatment

（1）Acute fetal distress: Taking steps immediately to improve the fetal anoxia condition.

- General treatment: Left-lying position and inhaling of oxygen, oxytocin discontinuation,

除外脐带脱垂并评估产程进展。纠正脱水、酸中毒、低血压及电解质紊乱。

- 病因治疗：子宫收缩过强应抑制宫缩。
- 尽快终止妊娠：做好新生儿窒息复苏准备。
（2）慢性胎儿窘迫
- 针对病因，根据孕周、胎儿成熟度及胎儿缺氧程度决定处理方法。
  - 一般处理：全面检查评估母儿状况；左侧卧位，定时吸氧；积极治疗妊娠合并症及并发症；加强胎儿监护。
  - 期待疗法：孕周小，胎儿娩出后存活可能性小，尽量延长胎龄同时促胎肺成熟。
  - 终止妊娠。

重点专业词汇

1.急性胎儿窘迫

2.慢性胎儿窘迫

3.胎粪吸入综合征

练习题

1.导致慢性胎儿窘迫的原因是：（D）

A.脐带受压

B.胎盘早剥

C.孕妇休克

D.胎盘功能不全

E.宫缩过强或持续时间过长

2.关于胎儿窘迫，下列哪项描述正确？（C）

A.宫缩时胎心率为108次/分

vaginal examination to exclude prolapse of umbilical cord and assess the progress of labor stages. Correction of dehydration, acidosis, hypotension and electrolyte disturbance.

- Etiological treatment: Tetanic contraction of uterus should be inhibited.
- Termination of pregnancy as soon as possible: Preparation for neonatal resuscitation
（2）Chronic fetal distress
- According to the etiology, treatment determined by gestational age, fetal maturity and the degree of anoxia.
  - General treatment: Comprehensive examination and evaluation of maternal and fetal status, left lateral lying position, regular oxygen inhalation, treatment of complications, enhanced fetal monitoring.
  - Expectant management: Small gestational age, the survival rate is low after delivery, we should prolong the pregnancy at the same time mature the fetal lung.
  - Termination of pregnancy.

Key words

1.Acute fetal distress

2.Chronic fetal distress

3.Meconium aspiration syndrome

Exercises

1.Which of the following is the cause for chronic fetal distress?（D）

A.Umbilical cord compressed

B.Placental abruption

C.Maternal shock

D.Placental function insufficiency

E.Tetanic contraction of uterus or long duration

2.Which of the following is correct about fetal distress?（C）

A.Fetal heart rate is 108 bpm during uterine

B.临产后羊水有胎粪

C.多次出现晚期减速

D.20分钟胎动3次，每次胎动加速15～20次/分，持续20秒

E.胎儿头皮血pH为7.25

3.在子宫内胎儿缺氧早期表现为：（D）

A.胎动减弱

B.胎动次数减少

C.胎动增强

D.胎动频繁

E.以上都不是

4.胎儿窘迫的处理，错误的是：（E）

A.左侧卧位，吸氧

B.产程延长发生酸中毒应及时治疗

C.胎儿窘迫不见好转，需迅速终止妊娠

D.手术前不用镇静药物

E.积极寻找原因，不急于手术

第三节　多胎妊娠

1.定义

- 一次妊娠宫腔内同时有两个或两个以上胎儿时称为多胎妊娠，以双胎妊娠多见，本节主要讨论双胎妊娠。

2.分类及特点

（1）双卵双胎（图10-1）：两个卵子分别受精，占70%，遗传基因不完全相同，血型、性别可相同可不同；胎盘中间隔有两层羊膜、两层绒毛膜。

contractions

B.Meconium in amniotic fluid in labor

C.Late decelerations many times

D.There are 3 times fetal movements and every time the fetal heart rate increases 15 ～ 20 bpm and continues 20 seconds

E.The pH value of fetal scalp blood is 7.25

3.Which of the following is the clinical symptom of anoxia at the early stage?（D）

A.Fetal movements weaken

B.Fetal movements decrease

C.Fetal movements strengthen

D.Fetal movements are frequent

E.None of the above

4.Which of the following is wrong for the treatment of fetal distress?（E）

A.Left lateral lying position and inhaling oxygen

B.Fetal acidosis in prolonged labor should be treated timely

C.If fetal distress turns no better, termination of pregnancy is necessary

D.Sedatives are not used before operation

E.Searching for the reason actively, and no rush to surgery

Section 3　Multiple pregnancy

1.Definition

- Multiple pregnancy is defined as two or more than two fetuses in one pregnancy. Twin pregnancy is common, and will be discussed in this section.

2.Classification and characteristics

（1）Dizygotic twin（Figure 10-1）: Two separate ova are fertilized by two separate sperms, accounting for 70%. The genetic genes are not exactly the same, and the blood type and sex may be the same or different. There are two amnions

（2）单卵双胎

■ 一个受精卵分裂形成，具有相同的遗传基因。

■ 受精卵分裂时间不同，分为以下4种类型（图10-2）。

• 双绒毛膜双羊膜囊：分裂发生在桑葚期前，相当于受精后3日，形成2个独立的胚胎，两层绒毛膜，两层羊膜。

and two chorions in the intermediate dissepiment of placenta.

（2）Monozygotic twins

■ As a result of the division of a single fertilized ovum, monozygotic twins share the same genes.

■ Four types based on the different time of division of the fertilized ovum（Figure 10-2）.

• Dichorionic diamniotic: Division prior to the morula stage and differentiation of the trophoblast（the third day）results in 2 separate embryos, with 2 chorions, and 2 amnions.

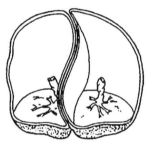 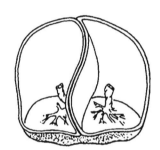

两个胎盘分开
Two separate placentas

两个胎盘融合
Two fused placentas

图10-1 双卵双胎
Figure 10-1 Dizygotic twins

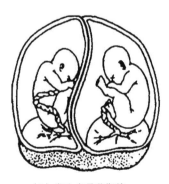 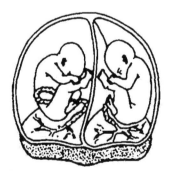 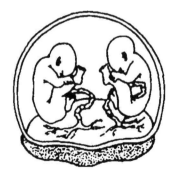

（1）发生在桑葚期前
Prior to morula stage

（2）发生在囊胚期
Blastula stage

（3）发生在羊膜囊已形成
Formation of amniotic sac

图10-2 受精卵在不同阶段形成单卵双胎的胎膜类型
Figure 10-2 Fetal types of membranes of monozygotic twins formed by zygote at different stages

- 单绒毛膜双羊膜囊：分裂发生在胚泡期，受精后第4～8日，一个胎盘，一层绒毛膜，两层羊膜。

- 单绒毛膜单羊膜囊：分别发生在受精后第9～13日，羊膜囊已形成，一个胎盘，共用一层绒毛膜，一层羊膜。

- 联体双胎：受精卵在第13日后分裂，机体不能完全分裂。

3.诊断

（1）病史及临床表现：家族史，使用促排卵药物或辅助生殖技术。

（2）产科检查：子宫大于停经周数，可以听到两个胎心。

（3）超声检查。

（4）绒毛膜性判断

- 妊娠6～10周通过孕囊数目进行判断。

- 妊娠10～14周，通过胎膜与胎盘插入点形状判断。

4.对母儿影响

（1）妊娠期高血压疾病：是单胎妊娠的3～4倍。

（2）妊娠期肝内胆汁淤积症：是单胎妊娠的2倍。

（3）贫血：是单胎妊娠的2.4倍。

（4）羊水过多。

（5）胎膜早破。

（6）宫缩乏力。

（7）胎盘早剥。

（8）产后出血。

- Monochorionic diamniotic: Division after differentiation of the trophoblast but before the formation of the amnion（4～8 days）yields a single placenta, a common chorion, and 2 amnions.

- Monochorionic monomniotic: Division after differentiation of the amnion（9～13 days）results in a single placenta, a common chorion, and a common amnion.

- Conjuncted twins: Division after the 13th day results in incomplete twinning.

3.Diagnosis

（1）Medical history and clinical manifestations: Family history, history of using drugs of ovulation induction or assisted reproduction technology.

（2）Obstetrical examination: Uterus is larger than amenorrhea weeks, and two fetal hearts can be heard.

（3）Ultrasound examination.

（4）Chorionic judgment

- The chorion judged by the number of gestational sacs between 6 and 10 weeks' gestation.

- The chorion judged by the shape of the insertion point of the membrane and placenta between 10 and 14 weeks' gestation.

4.Effects on gravida and fetus

（1）Hypertensive disorders of pregnancy: 3～4 times that of single pregnancy.

（2）Intrahepatic cholestasis of pregnancy: 2 times that of single pregnancy.

（3）Anemia: 2.4 times that of single pregnancy.

（4）Polyhydramnios.

（5）Premature rupture of membranes.

（6）Uterine inertia.

（7）Placental abruption.

（8）Postpartum hemorrhage.

（9）流产及早产：流产是单胎妊娠的2～3倍，早产发生率是单胎妊娠的7～10倍。

（10）单绒毛膜性双胎特有并发症：双胎输血综合征、选择性胎儿生长受限、动脉反向灌注序列、贫血多血质序列征。

5.治疗

（1）妊娠期监护

■ 补充足够营养。

■ 防止早产。

■ 及时防治并发症。

■ 监护胎儿生长发育情况及胎位变化。
  ● 双绒毛膜性双胎4周1次超声监测胎儿生长情况。

  ● 单绒毛膜性双胎2周1次超声监测胎儿生长发育从而早期发现特殊并发症。

（2）分娩时机

■ 无并发症及合并症的双绒毛膜性双胎可期待至孕38周时考虑分娩，最晚不超过孕39周。

■ 无并发症及合并症的单绒毛膜性双胎可在严密监测下至妊娠35～37周分娩。

■ 单绒毛膜单羊膜囊双胎的分娩孕周为32～34周。

（3）分娩期处理

■ 阴道分娩做好阴道助产及第

（9）Abortion and preterm birth: Abortion is 2～3 times that of single pregnancy, and preterm birth is 7～10 times that of single pregnancy.

（10）The specific complication of monochorionic twins: Twin to twin transfusion syndrome, selective intrauterine growth retardation, twin reversed arterial perfusion sequence, twin anemia polycythemia sequence.

5.Treatment

（1）Gestational monitoring

■ Nutrition supplementation.

■ Prevention of preterm birth.

■ Timely prevention and control of complications.

■ Monitoring the fetal development and the change of fetal position.
  ● An ultrasound evaluation should be performed to monitor the development of fetus once every 4 weeks for dichorionic twins.

  ● An ultrasound evaluation should be performed to monitor the development of fetus once every 2 weeks for monochorionic twins and find specific complications.

（2）Timing of delivery

■ The dichorionic twins without complications are performed to deliver till 38 weeks' gestation but it's better to be not more than 39 weeks' gestation.

■ The monochorionic twins without complications are performed to deliver between 35 and 37 weeks' gestation under close monitoring.

■ Monochorionic monoamniotic twins should be delivered between 32 and 34 weeks' gestation.

（3）Delivery management

■ It's better to prepare for vaginal midwifery

二胎儿剖宫产术的准备。

■ 第一胎儿娩出后，胎盘侧脐带必须立即夹紧，以防第二胎儿失血。

■ 第一胎儿娩出后，助手在腹部固定第二胎儿为纵产式，并密切观察胎心、宫缩及阴道出血情况。

■ 第一胎儿娩出后，等待15分钟仍无宫缩，可行人工破膜并静脉滴注低浓度缩宫素。

■ 无论何种分娩方式，需积极防治产后出血。

重点专业词汇

1.多胎妊娠

2.双卵双胎

3.单卵双胎

4.双绒毛膜双羊膜囊

5.单绒毛膜双羊膜囊

6.单绒毛膜单羊膜囊

7.联体双胎

8.双胎输血综合征

练习题

1.双卵双胎的特点是：（C）

A.两个胎儿体重悬殊

B.发生率低于单卵双胎

C.两胎囊间的中间隔由两层羊膜和两层绒毛膜组成

D.有发生双胎输血综合征的可能

E.胎儿死亡率高于单卵双胎

and do the cesarean section for the second fetus if vaginal delivery performed.

■ The umbilical cord should be clamped promptly to prevent the second twin from blood loss after the delivery of the first twin.

■ The helper fixes the second fetal longitudinal lie on abdomen after the delivery of the first twin, and closely observes the fetal heart rate, uterine contractions and vaginal bleeding.

■ If no uterine contractions after the delivery of the first twin in 15 minutes, artificial rupture of fetal membrane and intravenous drip with low concentration oxytocin can be performed.

■ No matter what kind of delivery method, postpartum hemorrhage should be prevented actively.

Key words

1.Multiple pregnancy

2.Dizygotic twins

3.Monozygotic twins

4.Dichorionic diamniotic

5.Monochorionic diamniotic

6.Monochorionic monoamniotic

7.Conjuncted twins

8.Twin to twin transfusion syndrome

Exercises

1.The feature of dizygotic twins is:（C）

A.The weights of two fetuses have a wide difference

B.The incidence is less than monozygotic twins

C.There are two amnions and two chorions in the intermediate dissepiment of two fetal sacs

D.Likely to occur twin to twin transfusion syndrome

E.Fetal mortality is higher than that of

2.双胎妊娠不易发生哪种并发症？（E）

A.胎膜早破

B.妊娠期高血压疾病（HDP）

C.胎盘早剥

D.产后出血

E.过期妊娠

3.双胎妊娠第一胎儿娩出后，下列哪项是错误的？（A）

A.采取措施，尽快娩出第二胎儿

B.应立即断脐，防止第二胎儿失血

C.定时听胎心

D.立即行阴道检查，查明第二胎儿胎位

E.保持纵产式，固定胎儿位置

（刘　芳）

monozygotic twins

2.Which of the following complications is less likely to occur in twin pregnancy?（E）

A.Premature rupture of membranes

B.Hypertensive disorders of pregnancy（HDP）

C.Placental abruption

D.Postpartum hemorrhage

E.Postterm pregnancy

3.Which of the following is wrong after the delivery of the first twin?（A）

A.Take measures to deliver the second twin as soon as possible

B.The umbilical cord should be clamped promptly to prevent the second twin from blood loss

C.Listen regularly to the fetal heart

D.Vaginal examination should be carried out immediately to determine the position of the second twin

E.Keep the longitudinal lie and fix the second fetal position

第 11 章　羊水量异常

第一节　羊水过多

1.定义

- 妊娠期间羊水量超过2000ml。

2.病因

（1）特发性羊水过多。

（2）胎儿结构异常。

（3）多胎妊娠及巨大儿。

（4）胎盘脐带病变。

（5）妊娠合并症：糖尿病，母儿血型不合，重度贫血。

3.诊断

（1）临床表现

- 急性羊水过多
  - 较少见。
  - 多发于妊娠20～24周。
  - 急剧增加数日。
  - 压迫症状：呼吸困难，发绀，外阴水肿，静脉曲张。
- 慢性羊水过多
  - 较多见。
  - 多发生在妊娠晚期。
  - 数周内羊水缓慢增多。
  - 症状较缓和。

（2）超声检查

- 羊水指数（AFI）≥25cm。

Section 1　Polyhydramnios

1.Definition

- The amount of amniotic fluid during pregnancy exceeds 2000ml.

2.Etiology

（1）Idiopathic polyhydramnios.

（2）Abnormal fetal structure.

（3）Multiple pregnancy and macrosomia.

（4）Placental umbilical cord lesions.

（5）Pregnancy comorbidity: Diabetes, maternal and fetal blood group incompatibility and severe anemia.

3.Diagnosis

（1）Clinical manifestations

- Acute polyhydramnios
  - Relatively rare.
  - More common in 20～24 weeks of gestation.
  - Sharp increase for several days.
  - Compression symptoms: Dyspnea, cyanosis, vulvar edema, and varicose vein.
- Chronic polyhydramnios
  - More common.
  - Most common in late trimester of pregnancy.
  - Amniotic fluid increases slowly within a few weeks.
  - Mild symptoms.

（2）Ultrasound examination

- Amniotic fluid index（AFI）≥25cm.

■ 羊水最大暗区垂直深度
（AFV）≥8cm。

4.对母儿的影响

（1）产妇：妊娠期高血压、胎膜早破、早产、胎盘早剥、子宫收缩乏力、产后出血。

（2）胎儿：胎位异常、早产、脐带脱垂、胎儿窘迫。

5.处理

（1）羊水过多合并胎儿畸形

■ 严重的胎儿结构异常：应及时终止妊娠。

■ 非严重的胎儿结构异常：应评估胎儿情况及预后，新生儿外科救治技术。

■ 羊膜腔穿刺术：排除染色体疾病。

（2）羊水过多合并正常胎儿

■ 应寻找病因，治疗原发病。

■ 吲哚美辛治疗。

第二节　羊水过少

1.定义

■ 妊娠晚期羊水量＜300ml者称为羊水过少。

2.病因

（1）羊水产生减少。

（2）羊水外漏增加。

（3）部分羊水过少原因不明。

■ 胎儿结构异常。

■ 胎盘功能减退。

■ 羊膜病变。

■ 母体因素。

3.诊断

（1）临床表现

■ Maximum depth in amniotic fluid volume
（AFV）≥8cm.

4.Effects on gravida and fetus

（1）Gravida: Gestational hypertension, premature rupture of membrane, premature delivery, placental abruption, uterine inertia, and postpartum hemorrhage.

（2）Fetus: Abnormal fetal position, premature delivery, umbilical cord prolapse, and fetal distress.

5.Management

（1）Polyhydramnios with fetal malformation

■ Severe fetal structural abnormalities: Termination of pregnancy in time.

■ Non-severe fetal structural abnormalities: Fetal condition and prognosis should be assessed, and neonatal surgical treatment techniques should be used.

■ Amniocentesis: Exclusion of chromosomal diseases.

（2）Polyhydramnios with normal fetus

■ Search for the cause to treat primary disease.

■ Indomethacin treatment.

Section 2   Oligohydramnios

1.Definition

■ The amount of amniotic fluid ＜ 300ml in late trimester of pregnancy.

2.Etiology

（1）Decreased amniotic fluid production.

（2）Increased amniotic fluid leakage.

（3）The cause of partial oligohydramnios is unknown.

■ Abnormal fetal structure.

■ Placental dysfunction.

■ Amniotic lesions.

■ Maternal factors.

3.Diagnosis

（1）Clinical manifestations.

- 临床症状多不典型，伴有：
  - 胎儿生长受限。
  - 胎动时腹部不适。

  - 胎盘功能减退时胎动减少。

  - 子宫紧裹胎儿感。

- 阴道检查
  - 羊膜囊不明显。
  - 胎膜紧贴胎儿先露部。

  - 人工破膜时羊水流出极少。

（2）超声检查
- 羊水指数（AFI）≤5cm。
- 羊水最大暗区垂直深度（AFV）≤2cm。

4.对母儿的影响
（1）胎儿：围生期死亡率增高。
（2）产妇：增加手术概率和引产率。

5.处理
（1）羊水过少合并胎儿畸形
- 确诊胎儿为严重致死性结构异常：应尽早终止妊娠。
- 超声明确胎儿结构异常。
- 染色体异常检测：依赖于介入性产前诊断，评估结果与家属沟通。

（2）羊水过少合并正常胎儿
- 寻找并去除病因。
- 终止妊娠：足月，胎儿能宫外存活者。
- 严密观察：未足月，胎肺不成熟者。
- 可针对病因对症治疗，尽量延长孕周。

- Clinical symptoms atypical, combined with:
  - Fetal growth restriction.
  - Abdominal discomfort during fetal movements.
  - Decreased fetal movements in hypofunction of placenta.
  - Sensation of uterus tightly wrapping around the fetus.
- Vaginal examination
  - Amniotic sac not obvious.
  - Fetal membranes close to the fetal presenting part.
  - Minimal amniotic fluid out flow during artificial rupture of membranes.

（2）Ultrasound examination
- Amniotic fluid index（AFI）≤5cm.
- Maximum depth in amniotic fluid volume（AFV）≤2cm.

4.Effects on gravida and fetus
（1）Fetus: Increase in perinatal mortality.
（2）Gravida: Increase in chances of surgery and labor induction.

5.Management
（1）Oligohydramnios with fetal malformation
- Severe fatal structural abnormality of fetus: Early termination of pregnancy.
- Fetal structural abnormalities by ultrasound.
- Chromosomal abnormality detection: Depending on interventional prenatal diagnosis and communicating with family members about the evaluation results.

（2）Oligohydramnios with normal fetus
- Find and eliminate the cause.
- Termination of pregnancy: Full term, extrauterine fetal survival.
- Close observation: Preterm, the fetal lung immature.
- Treat according to the etiology and symptoms, try to prolong the gestational

■ 根据胎龄及胎儿宫内情况，必要时终止妊娠。

重点专业词汇

1.羊水过多

2.羊水过少

3.羊水指数（AFI）

4.羊水最大暗区垂直深度（AFV）

练习题

1.属于羊水过多的指标是：（B）

A.羊水指数＜25cm

B.羊水指数≥25cm

C.羊水指数＜8cm

D.羊水指数≥8cm

E.羊水最大暗区垂直深度≥6cm

2.超声诊断羊水过少的标准是羊水指数：（A）

A.≤5cm

B.≤3cm

C.≤8cm

D.≤10cm

E.≤12cm

3.关于急性羊水过多正确的是哪一项？（E）

A.多发生在妊娠晚期

B.胎心听诊清楚

C.自觉症状轻微

D.下肢及外阴水肿发生率不高

E.容易发生早产

（路旭宏）

period.

■ Terminate pregnancy according to fetal age and intrauterine condition if necessary.

Key words

1.Polyhydramnios

2.Oligohydramnios

3.Amniotic fluid index（AFI）

4.Maximum depth in Amniotic fluid volume（AFV）

Exercises

1.An indicator of excessive amniotic fluid is:（B）

A.AFI＜25cm

B. AFI≥25cm

C. AFI＜8cm

D. AFI≥8cm

E. AFV≥6cm

2.The standard for ultrasonic diagnosis of oligohydramnios is AFI:（A）

A.≤5cm

B.≤3cm

C.≤8cm

D.≤10cm

E.≤12cm

3.Which is true about acute polyhydramnios?（E）

A.More common in the third trimester of pregnancy

B. Clear fetal heart auscultation

C.Mild self-conscious symptoms

D.Low incidence of lower limb and vulval edema

E.Prone to preterm delivery

第12章 异常分娩

CHAPTER 12 Abnormal labor

第一节 概 述

1.异常分娩（又称难产）

（1）分娩的因素
- 产力。
- 产道。
- 胎儿。
- 社会心理因素。

这些因素相互影响，互为因果。

任何1个或1个以上的因素发生异常及4个因素间相互不能适应，而使分娩进程受到阻碍。

（2）最常见的异常是：
- 产力异常。
- 产道异常。
- 胎儿异常。

2.病因

（1）产力异常的主要原因：子宫收缩力异常。

（2）产道异常，包括：
- 骨产道异常。
- 软产道异常。

以骨产道狭窄多见。

（3）胎儿异常
- 胎位异常
  - 头先露异常。
  - 臀先露。
  - 肩先露。
- 胎儿相对过大和胎儿发育

Section 1　Introduction

1. Abnormal labor（dystocia or abnormal delivery）

（1）Factors for labor
- Forces of labor.
- Birth canal.
- Fetus.
- Psychological factor.

These factors are both mutually influential and causal.

If one or more of the factors are abnormal and the four factors cannot adapt to each other, the delivery process is hindered.

（2）The most common abnormalities:
- Abnormal uterine action.
- Abnormal birth canal.
- Abnormal fetus.

2.Etiology

（1）The main cause of abnormal forces of labor: Abnormal uterine contractility.

（2）Abnormal birth canal, including:
- Abnormal bone birth canal.
- Abnormal soft birth canal.

Stenosis of bone birth canal are more common.

（3）Fetal abnormality
- Abnormal fetal position
  - Abnormal head presentation.
  - Breech presentation.
  - Shoulder presentation.
- Relatively large fetus and abnormal fetal

异常。

3.临床表现

（1）母体表现

产妇全身衰竭症状：

- 产妇烦躁不安。
- 体力衰竭。
- 进食减少。
- 脱水。
- 代谢性酸中毒。
- 电解质紊乱。
- 肠胀气。
- 尿潴留。

（2）产科情况

- 产程延长。
- 子宫收缩乏力。
- 过强/过频宫缩。

- 宫颈水肿。
- 宫颈扩张缓慢停滞。

- 胎先露下降：延缓停滞。

- 先兆子宫破裂甚至子宫破裂。
- 胎膜早破往往是异常分娩的征兆。
- 需要查明：有无头盆不称或胎位异常。

（3）胎儿表现

- 胎头未衔接或延迟衔接。
- 胎位异常

头位难产的首要原因：

- 胎方位衔接异常
  - 胎头高直位。
  - 前不均倾位。
- 内旋转受阻
  - 持续性枕后位。
  - 持续性枕横位。
- 胎头姿势异常

development.

3.Clinical manifestations

（1）Maternal manifestations

Symptoms of maternal systemic failure：

- Maternal restlessness.
- Physical exhaustion.
- Reduced food intake.
- Dehydration.
- Metabolic acidosis.
- Electrolyte disturbance.
- Intestinal flatulence.
- Urinary retention.

（2）Obstetric situations

- Prolonged labor.
- Uterine inertia.
- Hypertonic/over frequency uterine contraction.
- Cervical edema.
- Prolongation and stagnation of cervical dilation.
- Fetal presentation decline: Delayed or stagnated.
- Threatened uterine rupture or even uterine rupture.
- Premature rupture of membranes is often a sign of abnormal childbirth.
- Need to examine: Cephalopelvic disproportion （CPD）or abnormal fetal position.

（3）Fetal manifestations

- Non engaged or delayed fetal head.
- Abnormal fetal position

The primary cause of cephalic dystocia：

- Abnormal fetal engagement
  - Sincipital presentation.
  - Anterior asynclitism.
- Internal rotation obstruction
  - Persistent occipital posterior position.
  - Persistent occipital transverse position.
- Abnormal fetal head posture

- 胎头仰伸。
- 前顶先露。
- 额先露。
- 面先露。
- 胎头水肿或血肿。
- 胎儿颅缝过度重叠。
  - 预示：明显头盆不称。

- 胎儿窘迫。

（4）产程异常
- 潜伏期延长
  - 初产妇：超过20小时。
  - 经产妇：超过14小时。
- 活跃期异常，包括：
  - 活跃期延长
    - 定义：宫口扩张

初产妇：不超过0.5cm/h。

经产妇：不超过1cm/h。
  - 活跃期停滞
    - 当破膜且宫颈口扩张≥6cm，出现以下2种情况称为活跃期停滞。

    ①若宫缩好，宫颈口扩张停止≥4小时。
    ②若宫缩欠佳，宫颈口扩张停止≥6小时。
- 第二产程异常
  - 胎头下降延缓
    - 定义：胎儿头下降速度初产妇<1.0cm/h；经产妇<2.0cm/h。
  - 胎头下降停滞
    - 定义：胎头停留在原处不下降>1小时。
  - 第二产程延长
    - 定义

硬膜外镇痛分娩时：

初产妇>4小时。

- Extension of fetal head.
- Sincipital presentation.
- Brow presentation.
- Face presentation.
- Fetal head edema or hematoma.
- Excessive overlap of fetal cranial suture.
  - Indication: Obvious cephalopelvic disproportion.
- Fetal distress

（4）Abnormal labor stage
- Prolonged latent phase
  - Primipara: More than 20 hours.
  - Multipara: More than 14 hours.
- Active phase disorders, including:
  - Prolonged active phase
    - Definition: Dilation of internal os

Primipara: No more than 0.5 cm/h.

Multipara: No more than 1 cm/h.
  - Arrested active phase
    - After rupture of membrane, and cervical dilation ≥6cm, the following two situations are called active phase stagnation.
    ①If contractions normal, no cervical dilation ≥4h.
    ②If contractions abnormal, no cervical dilation ≥6h.
- Abnormal second stage
  - Protracted descent
    - Definition: Primipara, < 1.0cm/h; Multipara, < 2.0cm/h.
  - Arrested descent
    - Definition: Fetal head descending stops for > 1h.
  - Prolonged second stage
    - Definition

With epidural analgesic delivery:

Primipara: > 4 hours.

经产妇＞3小时。

无硬膜外镇痛分娩时：

初产妇＞3小时。

经产妇＞2小时。

- 急产
  - 初产妇总产程＜3小时。

4.处理

原则：应以预防为主。

综合分析决定分娩方式。

（1）阴道试产

无明显的头盆不称：原则上应尽量阴道试产。

- 应注意：
  - 第一产程
    - 宫颈扩张4cm之前，不应诊断难产。
    - 人工破膜和缩宫素使用后，方可诊断难产。

- 潜伏期延长
  - 潜伏期延长不是剖宫产的指征，可进行如下处理：

    - 哌替啶100mg：肌内注射。

    - 人工破膜。
    - 缩宫素静脉滴注。
- 活跃期延长
  - 评估
    - 人工破膜。
    - 缩宫素静脉滴注。
    - 手转胎头矫正胎方位。

- 活跃期停滞
  - 提示头盆不称。
  - 行剖宫产术。
- 第二产程异常
  - 要高度警惕头盆不称。

Multipara: ＞3 hours.

Without epidural analgesic delivery:

Primipara: ＞3 hours.

Multipara: ＞2 hours.

- Precipitate delivery
  - Total stage ＜3h for primipara.

4.Management

Principle: Prevention-oriented.

Comprehensive analysis determines the mode of delivery.

（1）Trial of labor

No obvious cephalopelvic disproportion: Try vaginal delivery.

- Attention should be paid to:
  - First stage of labor
    - Dystocia should not be diagnosed before cervical dilatation of 4 cm.
    - Only after artificial rupture of membranes and use of oxytocin, can dystocia be diagnosed.
- Prolonged latent phase
  - Prolonged latent phase is not an indication of cesarean section. It can be handled as follows:
    - Pethidine 100mg: Intramuscular injection.
    - Artificial rupture of membranes.
    - Intravenous drip of oxytocin.
- Prolonged active phase
  - Assessment
    - Artificial rupture of membranes.
    - Intravenous drip of oxytocin.
    - Rotate fetal head by hand to correct fetal position.
- Arrested active phase
  - Suggest cephalopelvic disproportion.
  - Perform cesarean section.
- Abnormal second stage.
  - Be highly alert to cephalopelvic

- 立即评估。
- 指导孕妇屏气用力。

- 徒手旋转胎头为枕前位。

- 胎头下降至≥S^{+3}水平：
  · 助产术
  ①产钳。
  ②吸引器。
- 胎头位置在≥S^{+2}水平以上：
  · 及时行剖宫产术

（2）剖宫产指征
■ 严重的胎位异常
  - 高直后位。
  - 前不均倾位。
  - 额先露。
  - 颏后位。
■ 骨盆绝对性狭窄
  - 胎儿过大。
  - 明显头盆不称。
  - 肩先露或臀先露，尤其是足先露。
■ 先兆子宫破裂
  - 应抑制宫缩。
  - 同时行剖宫产术，不论胎儿是否存活。
■ 胎儿窘迫而宫口未开全，也应考虑行剖宫产术。

第二节 产力异常

子宫收缩力是临产后贯穿于分娩全过程的主要动力。特点：具有节律性、对称性、极性及缩复作用。

产力异常定义：任何原因引发

disproportion.
- Immediate assessment.
- Guidance for pregnant women to hold their breath.

- Rotate fetal head with hands to keep occiput anterior position.
- Fetal head drops ≥ S^{+3} level:
  · Midwifery.
  ① Forceps.
  ② Fetal head aspirator.
- Position of fetal head ≥ S^{+2} level:

  · Cesarean section in time.

（2）Indications for cesarean section
■ Severe abnormal fetal position
  - Sincipital posterior presentation.
  - Anterior asynclitism.
  - Brow presentation.
  - Mentoposterior position.
■ Absolute pelvic stenosis
  - Oversized fetus.
  - Obvious cephalopelvic disproportion.
  - Shoulder or breech presentation, foot presentation especially.
■ Threatened uterine rupture
  - Suppress uterine contraction.
  - Perform cesarean section simultaneously no matter the fetus survives or not.
■ For fetal distress and incomplete cervical dilation, cesarean section should also be considered.

Section 2　Abnormal uterine action

Uterine contractility is the main motive force that runs through the whole process of delivery. Characteristics: Rhythm, symmetry, polarity and retraction.

Abnormal uterine action: The abnormal

的子宫收缩的节律性、对称性及极性不正常或收缩力的强度、频率变化均称为子宫收缩力异常，简称产力异常。

rhythm, symmetry and polarity of uterine contraction caused by any reason or the changes of intensity and frequency of contraction force are called abnormal uterine contraction force and abnormal uterine action for short.

1.分类

（1）子宫收缩乏力，简称宫缩乏力。

（2）子宫收缩过强，简称宫缩过强。

上述2个类型还分为：

- 协调性子宫收缩异常。

- 不协调性子宫收缩异常。

1.Classification

（1）Uterine atony, also called uterine inertia.

（2）Uterine over-efficiency, also called hyperuterine contraction.

The above two types are divided into:

- Coordinated uterine contraction abnormality.
- Uncoordinated uterine contraction abnormality.

2.病因

（1）子宫肌源性因素

- 子宫肌纤维过度伸展。

- 羊水过多。
- 巨大儿。
- 多胎妊娠。
- 子宫畸形。
- 子宫肌瘤。
- 子宫腺肌症。
- 经产妇。
- 高龄产妇。

（2）头盆不称或胎位异常。

（3）内分泌失调

- 减少体内乙酰胆碱、缩宫素及前列腺素合成及释放。
- 缩宫素受体量减少。
- 对宫缩物质的敏感性降低。

- 胎盘合成与分泌硫酸脱氢表雄酮量减少。
- 宫颈成熟度欠佳。

（4）精神源性因素

2.Etiology

（1）Myogenic factors of uterus

- Excessive stretching of uterine muscle fibers.
- Polyhydramnios.
- Macrosomia.
- Multiple pregnancy.
- Uterine malformation.
- Myoma.
- Adenomyosis.
- Multipara.
- Advanced maternal age.

（2）Cephalopelvic disproportion or abnormal fetal position.

（3）Endocrine dyscrasia

- Decrease in synthesis and release of acetylcholine, oxytocin and prostaglandin.
- Decrease in amount of oxytocin receptor.
- Decrease in sensitivity to uterine contractile substances.
- Reduction of synthesis and secretion of dehydroepiandrosterone sulfate in placenta.
- Poor cervical maturity.

（4）Psychogenic factors

■ 大脑皮质功能紊乱：对分娩有恐惧、紧张等精神心理障碍。

■ 待产时间久。

■ 过于疲劳、睡眠减少、体力过多消耗、膀胱过度充盈、水及电解质紊乱。

（5）其他：大剂量宫缩抑制剂及解痉、镇静、镇痛药。

协调性子宫收缩乏力

1.临床表现及诊断

（1）特点：子宫收缩节律性、对称性和极性均正常，仅收缩力弱，压力低于180Montevideo单位。

（2）宫缩

■ ＜2次/10分，持续时间短，间歇期较长。

■ 宫缩高峰，子宫无隆起。

■ 按压时子宫凹陷。

（3）根据宫缩乏力的发生时期，分为：

■ 原发性宫缩乏力：产程早期出现的宫缩乏力。

■ 继发性宫缩乏力
  ● 特点
    ①产程早期宫缩正常，第一产程活跃期后期或第二产程后，宫缩强度减弱。
    ②协调性宫缩乏力多为继发性宫缩乏力。

2.对产程及母儿的影响

（1）对产程的影响：产程进展缓慢甚至停滞。

（2）对孕妇的影响

■ 精神与体力消耗。

■ Cerebral cortex dysfunction: Maternal psychological disorders such as fear and tension in childbirth.

■ Long waiting time for delivery.

■ Excessive fatigue, sleep loss, excessive physical consumption, bladder over filling, water and electrolyte disorders.

（5）Others: Large doses of uterine contraction inhibitor and antispasmodic, sedative and analgesic.

Coordinated uterine inertia

1.Clinical manifestations and diagnosis

（1）Characteristics: Normal rhythm, symmetry, and polarity, but weak contraction force with pressure less than 180 Montevideo units.

（2）Uterine contractions

■ ＜2 times/10 minutes, short duration and long intermission period.

■ At the peak of contraction, no uterine eminence.

■ Uterus depressed when pressed.

（3）Classification according to occurrence period of uterine inertia:

■ Primary uterine inertia: Uterine inertia in the early stage of labor.

■ Secondary uterine inertia
  ● Characteristics
    ①Normal in the early stage of labor, uterine contraction intensity decreased in late active phase of labor or after the second stage of labor.
    ②Coordinated uterine inertia is mostly secondary uterine inertia.

2.Effects on labor process and gravida and fetus

（1）Effects on labor process: Delivery progresses slowly or even stagnates.

（2）Effects on gravida

■ Mental and physical exhaustion.

- 进食减少。
- 排尿困难及肠胀气。
- 产妇脱水。
- 酸中毒。

（3）对胎儿的影响

- 胎儿窘迫。
- 新生儿窒息。
- 产伤。
- 颅内出血。
- 吸入性肺炎。

3.处理

应首先明确病因。

第一产程

（1）一般处理

- 解除心理顾虑与紧张情绪。

- 指导休息及大小便。
- 及时补充膳食营养及水分等。

（2）强镇静剂：哌替啶100mg或吗啡10mg肌内注射。

（3）加强宫缩

- 人工破膜。
- 缩宫素静脉滴注。
  - 原则：最小浓度获得最佳宫缩。
  - 使用缩宫素注意事项：
    · 应有医师或助产士在床旁守护。
    · 监测宫缩、胎心、血压及产程进展等状况。

    · 评估宫缩强度的方法：触诊子宫；电子胎心监护。

    · 不良反应：高血压、尿少、水中毒。
    · 禁忌证：明显产道梗阻

- Decrease in food intake.
- Dysuria and intestinal distention.
- Maternal dehydration.
- Acidosis.

（3）Effects on fetus

- Fetal distress.
- Neonatal asphyxia.
- Birth injury.
- Intracranial hemorrhage.
- Aspiration pneumonia.

3.Management

The etiology should be clarified first.

First stage of labor

（1）General treatment

- Elimination of psychological worries and tension.

- Guidance of rest, and defecation.
- Timely supplement of dietary nutrition and water etc.

（2）Strong sedatives: Pethidine 100 mg or morphine 10 mg intramuscular injection.

（3）Strengthening contractions

- Artificial rupture of membranes.
- Oxytocin intravenous drip.
  - Principle: Get the best contraction at the minimum concentration.
  - Notes on use of oxytocin:
    · Doctors or midwives should be at the bedside.
    · Monitor uterine contraction, fetal heart rate, blood pressure and progress of labor etc.

    · Common methods to evaluate the intensity of uterine contraction: Palpation of uterus; electronic fetal heart rate monitoring.

    · Side effects: Hypertension, oliguria, and water intoxication.
    · Contraindications: Obvious obstruction

或瘢痕子宫。

第二产程

（1）评估有无头盆不称。

（2）静脉滴注缩宫素加强宫缩。

（3）指导产妇屏气用力。

（4）自然分娩。

（5）阴道助产。

（6）剖宫产术。

（7）胎头衔接不良。

（8）胎儿窘迫。

第三产程

（1）胎肩娩出后预防产后出血。

（2）预防感染指征

- 产程长。
- 破膜时间长。
- 手术产。

不协调性子宫收缩乏力

1.临床表现及诊断

（1）宫缩失去正常的节律性、对称性，尤其是极性。

（2）宫缩的兴奋点：来自子宫下段一处或多处。

（3）节律不协调、高频率的宫缩波：自下而上扩散，不能产生向下的合力。

（4）宫缩间歇期子宫不能很好地松弛。

（5）宫口扩张受限。

（6）胎先露不能如期下降。

（7）无效宫缩：此种宫缩多为原发性宫缩乏力。

2.处理

处理原则：调节子宫不协调收缩，使其恢复正常节律性及极性。

of birth canal or scarred uterus.

Second stage of labor

（1）Evaluation of cephalopelvic disproportion.

（2）Intravenous injection of oxytocin.

（3）Guidance for puerpera to hold breath.

（4）Natural delivery.

（5）Vaginal midwifery.

（6）Cesarean section.

（7）Poor fetal head engagement.

（8）Fetal distress.

Third stage of labor

（1）Prevention of postpartum hemorrhage after delivery of fetal shoulder.

（2）Indications for prevention of infection

- Long course of labor.
- Long time of rupture of membranes.
- Operative delivery.

Uncoordinated uterine inertia

1.Clinical manifestations and diagnosis

（1）Loss of normal rhythm and symmetry, especially polarity.

（2）Excitation point of uterine contraction: Coming from one or more parts of the lower part of the uterus.

（3）Irregular rhythm and high frequency uterine contraction wave: Diffusion from the bottom to the top and no downward resultant force.

（4）No good uterine relaxation during the intermission of contraction.

（5）Restricted dilatation of the uterine orifice.

（6）Failure to descend as scheduled for fetal presentation.

（7）Ineffective contraction: Mostly primary uterine inertia.

2.Management

Principle of treatment: Regulate uterine incongruous contraction and restore normal rhythm and polarity.

（1）哌替啶100mg或吗啡10mg肌内注射。

（2）宫缩仍较弱：按协调性宫缩乏力处理。

（3）在未恢复为协调性宫缩之前，严禁使用缩宫素。

（4）剖宫产指征

- 胎儿窘迫。
- 头盆不称。
- 用镇静剂后宫缩仍不协调。

子宫收缩过强

1.临床表现及诊断

（1）协调性子宫收缩过强

- 子宫收缩的节律性、对称性及极性均正常，仅子宫收缩力过强、过频。
- 急产：初产妇总产程＜3小时分娩者。
- 产道梗阻。
- 病理缩复环。
- 子宫破裂。

（2）不协调性子宫收缩过强

- 强直性子宫收缩。
- 子宫痉挛性狭窄环。

2.对母儿影响

（1）对产妇影响

- 急产。
- 胎盘嵌顿。
- 软产道裂伤。
- 子宫破裂。

（2）对胎儿的影响

- 胎儿窘迫。
- 新生儿窒息。

3.处理

（1）预防为主，寻找原因。

（1）Intramuscular injection of pethidine 100mg or morphine 10mg.

（2）Still weak contraction: To treat as coordinated uterine inertia.

（3）Before returning to coordinated contraction, uterine contraction agents should be strictly forbidden.

（4）Indications for cesarean section

- Fetal distress.
- Cephalopelvic disproportion.
- Uncoordinated contraction remaining after sedation.

Uterine over-efficiency

1.Clinical manifestations and diagnosis

（1）Coordinated uterine over-efficiency

- Normal rhythm, symmetry and polarity, but strong and frequent contraction force.

- Precipitate delivery: Total stage of labor ＜ 3 hours for primiparas.
- Obstruction of the birth canal.
- Pathological contraction ring.
- Uterine rupture.

（2）Uncoordinated uterine over-efficiency

- Tetanic contraction of uterus.
- Constriction ring of uterus.

2.Effects on gravida and fetus

（1）Effects on gravida

- Precipitate delivery.
- Placental incarceration.
- Soft birth canal laceration.
- Uterine rupture.

（2）Effects on fetus

- Fetal distress.
- Neonatal asphyxia.

3.Management

（1）Prevention centered, and searching for reasons.

（2）宫缩抑制剂

■ 缓慢静脉注射：25%硫酸镁20ml加入5%葡萄糖液20ml。

■ 哌替啶100mg肌内注射：适用于4小时内胎儿不会娩出者。

（3）密切观察胎儿安危：提前做好接产及抢救新生儿窒息的准备。

（4）子宫痉挛性狭窄环：应当停止阴道内操作及缩宫类药物。

第三节　产道异常

概述
（1）产道异常包括
■ 骨产道异常。
■ 软产道异常。
■ 胎儿娩出受阻。
（2）产科检查：明确狭窄骨盆的类型和程度。
（3）评估
■ 结合产力、胎儿等因素。

■ 综合判定来决定分娩方式。

骨产道异常

1.分级（表12-1）
（1）骨盆入口平面狭窄
■ 单纯扁平骨盆。
■ 佝偻病性扁平骨盆。
（2）中骨盆平面狭窄
（3）骨盆出口平面狭窄
■ 漏斗骨盆。
■ 横径狭窄骨盆。
（4）均小骨盆。

（2）Contraction inhibitors.

■ Slow intravenous injection: Adding 25% magnesium sulfate 20 ml to 5% glucose 20 ml.

■ Pethidine 100mg, intramuscular injection: Suitable for those who will not deliver the fetus within 4 hours.

（3）Close observation of fetal safety: Preparing for delivery and rescue of neonatal asphyxia.

（4）Constriction ring of uterus: Intravaginal operation and uterine contraction drugs should be stopped.

Section 3　Abnormal birth canal

Introduction
（1）Abnormal birth canal includes
■ Abnormal bony birth canal.
■ Abnormal soft birth canal.
■ Obstructed fetal delivery.
（2）Obstetric examination: Define the type and degree of narrow pelvis.
（3）Assessment
■ Combined with factors such as forces of labor and fetus.

■ Comprehensive judgment to determine the mode of delivery.

Abnormal bony birth canal

1.Classification （Table 12-1）
（1）Contracted pelvic inlet
■ Simple flat pelvis.
■ Rachitic flat pelvis.
（2）Contracted midpelvis
（3）Contracted pelvic outlet
■ Funnel shaped pelvis.
■ Transversely contracted pelvis.
（4）Generally contracted pelvis.

表 12-1　骨盆三个平面狭窄的分级

Table 12-1　Grading of three planes pelvic stenosis

分级 Grading	入口平面 Pelvic inlet	中骨盆平面 Midpelvis	出口平面 Pelvic outlet		
	对角径 Diagonal conjucate（DC）	坐骨棘间径 Interspinous diameter	坐骨棘间径＋ 中骨盆后矢状径 Interspinous diameter ＋Posterior sagittal diameter of midpelvis	坐骨结节 间径 Transverse outlet（TO）	坐骨结节间径 ＋出口后矢状径 Transverse outlet ＋Posterior sagittal diameter
Ⅰ级临界性 Level Ⅰ Criticality	11.5 cm	10 cm	13.5 cm	7.5 cm	15.0 cm
Ⅱ级相对性 Level Ⅱ Relativity	10.0 ～ 11.0 cm	8.5 ～ 9.5 cm	12.0 ～ 13.0 cm	6.0 ～ 7.0 cm	12.0 ～ 14.0 cm
Ⅲ级绝对性 Level Ⅲ Absoluteness	≤9.5 cm	≤8.0 cm	≤11.5 cm	≤5.5 cm	≤11.0cm

（5）畸形骨盆。

2.临床表现

（1）骨盆入口平面狭窄

■ 胎先露异常。

■ 胎方位异常。

■ 潜伏期延长。

■ 活跃期延长。

■ 其他

● 胎膜早破。

● 脐带脱垂。

● 先兆子宫破裂。

（2）中骨盆平面狭窄

■ 胎方位异常：持续性枕后（横）位。

■ 产程进展异常：继发性宫缩乏力。

（3）骨盆出口平面狭窄

■ 常与中骨盆平面狭窄并存。

■ 继发性宫缩乏力。

■ 第二产程延长。

■ 不宜强行阴道助产。

（5）Deformed pelvis.

2.Clinical manifestation

（1）Contracted pelvic inlet

■ Abnormal fetal presentation.

■ Abnormal fetal position.

■ Prolonged latent phase.

■ Prolonged active phase.

■ Others

● Premature rupture of membranes.

● Prolapse of umbilical cord.

● Threatened uterine rupture.

（2）Contracted midpelvis

■ Abnormal fetal position: Persistent occipital（transverse）position.

■ Abnormal progress of labor: Secondary uterine inertia.

（3）Contracted pelvic outlet

■ Often coexisting with contracted midpelvis.

■ Secondary uterine inertia.

■ Prolonged second stage.

■ Not suitable for forced vaginal midwifery.

3.诊断

（1）病史

■ 询问。

■ 佝偻病。

■ 脊柱和髋关节结核。

■ 经产妇询问有无难产或阴道助产。

（2）全身检查：观察孕妇体形、步态。

（3）腹部检查

■ 跨耻征阴性。

■ 跨耻征可疑阳性。

■ 跨耻征阳性。

（4）骨盆测量：通过产科检查评估骨盆大小（图12-1）。

（5）胎位及产程：动态监测。

4.对产程及母儿的影响

（1）对产程的影响：产程延长及停滞。

（2）对产妇的影响

■ 胎位异常。

■ 持续性枕横位或枕后位。

（3）对胎儿及新生儿的影响

3.Diagnosis

（1）Medical history

■ Inquiry.

■ Rickets.

■ Spinal and hip tuberculosis.

■ Dystocia or vaginal midwifery for multipara.

（2）General examination: Observation of the shape and gait of pregnant women.

（3）Abdominal examination

■ Negative span-pubis sign.

■ Suspicious positive span-pubis sign.

■ Positive span-pubis sign.

（4）Pelvic measurement: Assessing pelvic size by obstetric examinations（Figure 12-1）.

（5）Fetal position and delivery process: Dynamic monitoring.

4.Effects on delivery process, gravida and fetus

（1）Effects on delivery process: Prolongation and stagnation of labor.

（2）Effects on gravida

■ Abnormal fetal position.

■ Persistent occipital transverse/posterior position.

（3）Influences on fetus and newborn

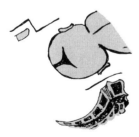 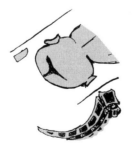 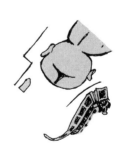

（1）头盆相称
Cephalopelvic proportion

（2）头盆可能相称
Possible cephalopelvic disproportion

（3）头盆不称
Cephalopelvic disproportion

图12-1 检查头盆相称程度

Figure 12-1 Cephalopelvic proportionality

■ 胎膜早破。

■ 脐带先露。

■ 脐带脱垂。

■ 新生儿产伤。

5.分娩处理

（1）骨盆入口平面狭窄

■ 绝对性骨盆入口狭窄

　● 剖宫产。

■ 相对性骨盆入口狭窄

　● 根据宫口扩张程度，试产。

　● 胎膜未破者，在宫口扩张
　　≥3cm时人工破膜。

（2）中骨盆平面狭窄

宫口开全

■ 若双顶径达坐骨棘水平或
　更低

　● 手转胎头。

　● 等待自然分娩。

　● 行产钳助产或胎头吸引术
　　助产。

■ 剖宫产指征

　● 若胎头双顶径未达坐骨棘
　　水平。

　● 胎儿窘迫征象。

（3）骨盆出口平面狭窄：阴道
试产应谨慎

■ 临床上常用评估出口大小的
　方法：坐骨结节间径与后矢
　状径之和。

■ 若两者之和＞15cm，多数经
　阴道分娩；有时需行产钳助
　产术或胎头吸引术。

■ 若两者之和≤15cm，足月胎
　儿不易经阴道分娩，应行剖
　宫产术结束分娩。

（4）均小骨盆

■ Premature rupture of membranes.

■ Presentation of umbilical cord.

■ Prolapse of umbilical cord.

■ Neonatal birth injury.

5.Childbirth treatment

（1）Contracted pelvic inlet

■ Absolute contracted pelvic inlet

　● Cesarean section.

■ Relative contracted pelvic inlet

　● The dilatation of the cervical os: Trial
　　delivery.

　● Unruptured membranes, dilatation of
　　cervical os ≥3cm, artificial rupture of
　　membranes.

（2）Contracted midpelvis

Complete dilatation of the cervical os

■ If the biparietal diameter reaches the level
　of ischial spine or below

　● Manual rotation of fetal head.

　● Waiting for natural delivery.

　● Midwifery by forceps or by aspiration.

■ Indications for cesarean section

　● Biparietal diameter not reaching the level
　　of sciatic spine.

　● Fetal distress signs.

（3）Contracted pelvic outlet: Vaginal trial
should be careful.

■ Commonly used method to evaluate the size
　of pelvic outlet: The sum of ischial tubercle
　diameter and posterior sagittal diameter.

■ If the sum ＞15cm, most deliveries are
　through vagina; sometimes forceps or
　suction is required.

■ If the sum ≤15cm, it is not easy for a full-
　term fetus to deliver through vagina and
　cesarean section should be performed to
　end the delivery.

（4）Generally contracted pelvis

- 若胎儿不大，产力、胎位及胎心均正常，头盆相称，可以阴道试产。

- 若胎儿较大，头盆不称，应及时行剖宫产术。

（5）畸形骨盆
- 根据以下情况具体分析：

  - 畸形骨盆的种类
  - 狭窄程度
  - 胎儿大小
  - 产力
- 若畸形严重，明显头盆不称，应及时行剖宫产。

第四节 胎位异常

胎位异常是造成难产的主要因素。包括：头先露、臀先露、肩先露。

以胎头为先露的难产，又称头位难产。

持续性枕后位、枕横位

1.定义
- 若充分试产，胎头枕部不能转向前方，仍位于母体骨盆后方或侧方（图12-2）。

发生率约占分娩总数的5%。

2.病因
（1）骨盆异常与胎头俯屈不良

- 男型骨盆。
- 类人猿型骨盆。

- If the fetus is not large, with cephalopelvic proportion, and the labor force, fetal position and fetal heart rate are normal, vaginal trial can be performed.
- If the fetus is large, with cephalopelvic disproportion, cesarean section should be performed in time.

（5）Deformed pelvis
- Make analysis and diagnosis according to the following factors:

  - Types of malformed pelvis
  - Degree of stenosis
  - Fetal size
  - Force of labor
- If the deformity is serious with obvious cephalopelvic disproportion, cesarean section should be performed in time.

Section 4　Abnormal fetal position

Abnormal fetal position is the main cause of dystocia, including: Head presentation, breech presentation, and shoulder presentation.

Dystocia with fetal head as presentation is called cephalic dystocia.

Persistent occiput posterior/transverse position

1.Definition
- If full trial delivery, the occipital part of the fetal head can not be turned forward, but still located in the posterior or lateral part of the maternal pelvis（Figure 12-2）.

Incidence rate is about 5% of the total number of delivery.

2.Etiology
（1）Pelvic abnormalities and fetal head dysflexion

- Male pelvis.
- Ape-like pelvis.

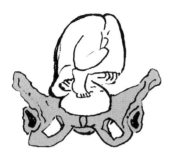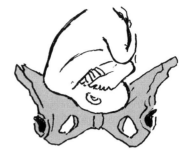

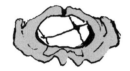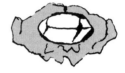

图12-2　持续性枕后位/持续性枕横位

Figure 12-2　Persistent occiput posterior/persistent transverse position

（2）其他

■ 宫颈肌瘤。

■ 头盆不称。

■ 前置胎盘。

■ 子宫收缩乏力。

■ 胎儿过大或过小。

■ 胎儿发育异常。

3.诊断

（1）临床表现。

（2）腹部检查。

（3）肛门检查及阴道检查。

（4）超声检查。

4.分娩机制

大多数枕后位及枕横位自然转为枕前位。

（1）枕后位

■ 俯屈较好。

■ 俯屈不良。

（2）枕横位

■ 一般能经阴道分娩。

■ 协助转胎位。

■ 手转胎头。

■ 胎头吸引器（产钳）。

（2）Others

■ Cervical myoma.

■ Cephalopelvic disproportion.

■ Placenta previa.

■ Uterine inertia.

■ Oversized or undersized fetus.

■ Abnormal fetal development.

3.Diagnosis

（1）Clinical manifestations.

（2）Abdominal examination.

（3）Anal examination and vaginal examination.

（4）Ultrasound examination.

4.Delivery mechanism

Most occipital posterior/transverse positions naturally turn to occipital anterior position.

（1）Occipital posterior position

■ Good flexion.

■ Poor flexion.

（2）Occipital transverse position

■ Delivery through vagina.

■ Assist in transposition.

■ Manual rotation of fetal head.

■ Fetal head aspirator（or forceps）.

5.对产程及母儿的影响

（1）第二产程

■ 胎头下降延缓。

■ 胎头下降停滞。

（2）对母体的影响

■ 继发性宫缩乏力。

■ 产程延长。

（3）对胎儿的影响

■ 胎儿窘迫。

■ 新生儿窒息。

■ 围生儿死亡率增高。

6.处理

（1）无头盆不称、胎儿不大时，可试产。

（2）应严密观察产程，注意：

■ 宫缩强弱。

■ 宫口扩张程度。

■ 胎头下降。

■ 胎心改变。

（3）第一产程

■ 潜伏期

　● 让产妇向胎儿肢体方向侧卧。

■ 活跃期

　● 不宜过早用力屏气。

（4）第二产程

　● 娩出困难助产或行剖宫产。

（5）第三产程

　● 做好抢救新生儿复苏准备，做好防止产后出血准备。

胎头高直位

1.概述（图12-3）

（1）定义：胎头以不屈不仰姿势衔接入盆，其矢状缝与骨盆入口前后径相一致。

5.Effects on delivery process, gravida and fetus

（1）Second stage of labor

■ Prolonged descent.

■ Arrested descent.

（2）Effects on gravida

■ Secondary uterine inertia.

■ Prolonged labor.

（3）Effects on fetus

■ Fetal distress.

■ Neonatal asphyxia.

■ Increased perinatal mortality.

6.Management

（1）If no cephalopelvic disproportion, no big fetus, trial delivery.

（2）Closely observe the delivery process and pay attention to:

■ Intensity of uterine contractions.

■ Degree of dilation of uterine orifice.

■ Descending of fetal head.

■ Change of fetal heart rate.

（3）First stage of labor

■ Latent phase

　● Have the puerpera lie on her side in fetal limbs direction.

■ Active phase

　● Do not hold breath too soon.

（4）Second stage of labor

　● If difficult delivery, midwifery or cesarean section.

（5）Third stage of labor

　● Getting ready for newborn resuscitation and prevention of postpartum hemorrhage.

Sincipital presentation

1.Introduction（Figure 12-3）

（1）Definition: Fetal head is connected to pelvis in a non-flexible position, and sagittal suture is consistent with anterior and posterior diameters

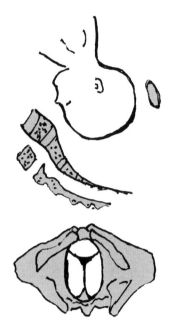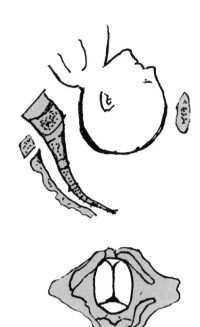

图12-3　高直后位／高直前位

Figure 12-3　Sincipital posterior/anterior presentation

（2）发病率国内报道为1.08%，国外资料为0.6% ～ 1.6%。

（3）包括：

■ 高直前位

● 胎头枕骨向前靠近耻骨联合，又称枕耻位。

■ 高直后位

● 胎头枕骨向后靠近骶岬，又称枕骶位。

（4）约占分娩者总数的1.08%。

（5）胎头高直位对母儿危害较大，应妥善处理。

2.诊断

（1）临床表现：入盆困难，胎头不下降。

（2）腹部检查

（3）阴道检查

of pelvic entrance.

（2）The incidence is 1.08% in China and 0.6% ～ 1.6% in foreign countries.

（3）Including:

■ Sincipital anterior presentation

● Occipital bone of fetus is anterior to the pubic symphysis, also known as occipito-pubic position.

■ Sincipital posterior presentation.

● Occpital bone of fetus is posterior to sacral promontory, also known as occipitosacral position.

（4）About 1.08% of total births.

（5）Sincipital presentation is harmful to gravida and fetus, and should be properly dealt with.

2.Diagnosis

（1）Clinical manifestations: Difficult to enter the pelvis, and no fetal head descent.

（2）Abdominal examination

（3）Vaginal examination

- 胎头嵌顿于骨盆入口。

- 宫口很难开全。

- 常停滞在3～5cm。

- 胎头矢状缝在骨盆入口的前后径上。

- 偏斜度不应超过15°。

（4）超声

- 高直位。

- 胎头双顶径均与骨盆入口横径一致。

3.处理

（1）高直前位

- 评估。

- 产力强。

- 无骨盆狭窄。

- 胎儿正常大小。

- 阴道试产

  ● 加强宫缩。

  ● 侧卧或半卧位。

  ● 促进胎头衔接和下降。

- 实施剖宫产术

  ● 试产失败。

  ● 伴明显骨盆狭窄。

（2）高直后位：应行剖宫产分娩。

前不均倾位

1.概述（图12-4）

（1）定义

- 枕横位入盆的胎头侧屈前顶骨先入盆，以前顶骨先入盆的一种异常胎位。

（2）发生率为0.5%～0.8%。

（3）病因

- Fetal head is incarcerated at the pelvic entrance.

- Uterine orifice is difficult to open completely.

- The opening often stagnates at 3～5 cm.

- The sagittal suture of the fetal head is located on the anterior and posterior diameters of the pelvic entrance.

- The deviation of sagittal suture should not exceed 15 degrees.

（4）Ultrasound

- Sincipital presentation.

- Biparietal diameter of fetal head is consistent with the transverse diameter of pelvic entrance.

3.Management

（1）Sincipital anterior presentation

- Assessment.

- Strong forces of labor.

- No pelvic stenosis.

- Normal size of fetus.

- Vaginal trial

  ● Strengthening uterine contractions.

  ● Lateral or semi-supine position.

  ● Promotion of fetal head engagement and decline.

- Perform cesarean section

  ● Trial delivery failure.

  ● With obvious pelvic stenosis.

（2）Sincipital posterior presentation: Cesarean section should be performed.

Anterior asynclitism

1.Introduction （Figure 12-4）

（1）Definition

- Cephalic lateral flexion with transverse occipital position enters into the pelvis, with the anterior parietal bone first.

（2）The incidence is 0.5%～0.8%.

（3）Etiology

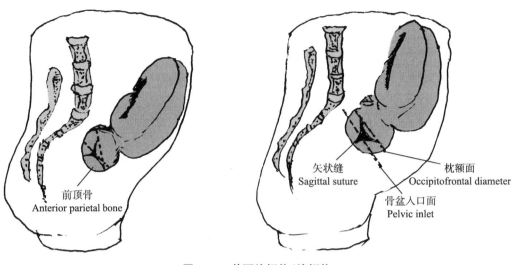

前顶骨
Anterior parietal bone

矢状缝
Sagittal suture

枕额面
Occipitofrontal diameter

骨盆入口面
Pelvic inlet

图12-4　前不均倾位 / 均倾位

Figure 12-4　Anterior asynclitism/synclitism

■ 头盆不称（CPD）。

■ 骨盆倾斜度过大。

■ 腹壁松弛。

2.诊断

（1）临床表现

■ 胎头下降停滞。

■ 产程延长。

■ 排尿困难。

■ 尿潴留。

（2）腹部检查

■ 随前顶骨入盆，后顶骨不能入盆。

■ 胎头折叠于胎肩之后。

■ 在耻骨联合上方不易触及胎头。

■ 形成胎头已衔接入盆的假象。

（3）阴道检查及肛门检查

■ 矢状缝与骨盆入口横径方向一致。

■ 矢状缝向后移靠近骶岬侧。

■ 后顶骨的大部分尚在骶岬之上，致使盆腔后半部空虚。

■ Cephalopelvic disproportion（CPD）.

■ Excessive pelvic tilt.

■ Abdominal wall relaxation.

2.Diagnosis

（1）Clinical manifestations

■ Arrested descent.

■ Prolonged labor.

■ Dysuria.

■ Urinary retention.

（2）Abdominal examination

■ Anterior parietal bone enters pelvis, but the posterior parietal bone does not enter pelvis.

■ Bend the fetal head near the shoulder.

■ Fetal head is not easily touched above pubic symphysis.

■ The illusion that the fetal head has been engaged to the pelvis.

（3）Vaginal and anal examinations

■ Sagittal suture is in line with the transverse diameter of the pelvic inlet.

■ Move backwards near the sacral promontory.

■ Most of the posterior parietal bones are still above the sacral promontory, resulting in emptiness of the posterior half of the pelvic cavity.

3.分娩机制

（1）前不均倾位。

（2）耻骨联合后面直而无凹陷。

（3）前顶骨紧紧嵌顿于耻骨联合后。

（4）胎头不能正常衔接入盆。

4.处理

（1）尽量避免胎头以前不均倾位衔接临产。

（2）产程早期产妇宜取坐位或半卧位。

（3）以减小骨盆倾斜度。

（4）一旦发现前不均倾位，应尽快以剖宫产结束分娩。

（5）除外以下情况

- 胎儿小。
- 骨盆宽大。
- 宫缩强。
- 短时间试产。

臀先露

1.概述

（1）臀先露占足月分娩总数的3%～4%。

（2）为最常见且容易诊断的异常胎位。

（3）臀先露以骶骨为指示点。

6种胎方位：

- 骶左（右）前位
- 骶左（右）横位
- 骶左（右）后位

2.病因

（1）胎儿发育

- 胎龄愈小发生率愈高。

3.Delivery mechanism

（1）Anterior asynclitism.

（2）Straight without depression behind pubic symphysis.

（3）Anterior parietal bone is closely incarcerated behind the pubic symphysis.

（4）Fetal head can not be properly engaged into the pelvis.

4.Management

（1）Avoid anterior asynclitism before labor.

（2）Take sitting position or semi-lying position in early stage of labor.

（3）In order to reduce pelvic inclination.

（4）Once anterior asynclitism found, cesarean section should be performed as soon as possible.

（5）Excluding

- Small fetus.
- Broad pelvis.
- Strong uterine contractions.
- Short-term trial delivery.

Breech presentation

1.Introduction

（1）Breech presentation accounts for 3%～4% of total full-term births.

（2）The most common and easily diagnosed abnormal fetal position.

（3）Breech presentation is indicated by sacrum.

Six fetal positions:

- Sacral left（right）anterior.
- Sacral left（right）transverse.
- Sacral left（right）posterior.

2.Etiology

（1）Fetal development

- The smaller the gestational age, the higher

■ 臀先露先天畸形发生率约为头先露的2.5倍。

（2）胎儿活动空间：过大或受限。

3.分类（图12-5）

■ 根据下肢的姿势分为：
- 单臀先露。
- 完全臀先露。
- 不完全臀先露。

4.诊断

（1）临床表现

■ 妊娠晚期：胎动时常有季肋部胀满感。

■ 临产
- 产程延长。
- 容易发生宫缩乏力。
■ 足先露。
- 胎膜早破。
- 脐带脱垂。

（2）腹部四步触诊

■ 宫底部：胎头圆而硬，按压时有浮球感。

■ 腹部一侧，触及宽而平坦的

---

the incidence.

■ The incidence of congenital malformation is about 2.5 times that of head presentation.

（2）Fetal activity space: Excessive or limited.

3.Classification（Figure 12-5）

■ According to lower limbs posture:
- Frank breech presentation.
- Complete breech presentation.
- Incomplete breech presentation.

4.Diagnosis

（1）Clinical manifestations

■ In the third trimester of pregnancy: Swollen feeling often occurs during fetal movements.

■ Labor
- Prolonged labor.
- Prone to uterine inertia.
■ Footling presentation.
- Premature rupture of membranes.
- Prolapse of umbilical cord.

（2）Abdominal four-step palpation

■ Bottom of uterus: Fetal head, round and firm, feeling like floating ball when palpated.

■ Abdominal side, palpating wide and flat

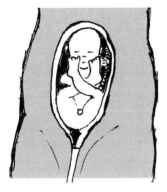 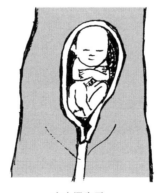 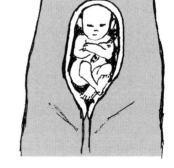

单臀先露
Frank breech presentation

完全臀先露
Complete breech presentation

不完全臀先露
Incomplete breech presentation

图12-5 臀先露分类
Figure 12-5 Breech presentation

胎背；对侧，可触及不平坦的小肢体。

- 在耻骨联合上方，若未衔接，可触及不规则、宽而软的胎臀。

- 若胎儿粗隆间径已入盆：胎臀相对固定不动。

- 胎心听诊
  - 通常在胎背侧。
  - 脐左（或右）上方响亮。
  - 衔接后
    · 胎心听诊：脐下最明显。

（3）阴道检查
- 触及胎臀。
- 触及肛门、坐骨结节。
- 与面先露相鉴别。
（4）超声
- 确定臀先露的类型。

- 估计胎儿大小。

5.对产程及母儿的影响

（1）对产程的影响
- 活跃期延长及停滞。
（2）对母体的影响
- 胎膜早破。
- 产褥感染。
- 继发性宫缩乏力。
- 产后出血。
- 手术产率增多。
（3）对胎儿及新生儿的影响
- 早产。
- 脐带脱垂。
- 低氧血症。
- 酸中毒。
- 新生儿窒迫。
- 新生儿出生后1分钟Apgar

back of fetus; the opposite side, palpating uneven small limbs.

- Above pubic symphysis, palpating irregular, wide and soft fetal buttock if not engaged.

- If intertrochanteric diameter of the fetus is already in the pelvis, fetal buttocks are relatively fixed.
- Fetal heart auscultation
  - Usually on dorsal side of fetus.
  - Loud, above the left（or right）navel.
  - After engagement
    · Fetal heart auscultation: Most obvious under umbilical cord.

（3）Vaginal examination
- Touching the buttock.
- Touching anal and sciatic tubercle.
- Differention from face presentation.
（4）Ultrasound
- Determination of types of breech presentation.
- Fetal size estimation.

5.Effects on delivery process，gravida and fetus

（1）Effects on delivery process
- Prolongation and stagnation of active phase.
（2）Effects on gravida
- Premature rupture of membranes.
- Puerperal infection.
- Secondary uterine inertia.
- Postpartum hemorrhage.
- Increased operative delivery rate.
（3）Effects on fetus and newborn
- Premature delivery.
- Prolapse of umbilical cord.
- Hypoxemia.
- Acidosis.
- Neonatal distress.
- Low Apgar score 1 minute after birth.

评分低。

6. 处理

（1）妇娠期

- 妊娠30周前大部分臀先露能自行转为头先露。
- 无须处理。
- 妊娠30周后仍为臀先露：矫正。
- 矫正方法（图12-6）：
  - 胸膝卧位。
  - 针灸或艾灸至阴穴。

  - 外倒转术（ECV）。

（2）分娩期

- 临产初期：根据下列因素决定正确的分娩方式。
  - 产妇年龄、本次妊娠经过、胎产次、骨盆类型、臀先露类型、胎儿大小、胎儿是否存活、发育是否正常及有无合并症等。
  - 择期剖宫产手术指征
    · 胎儿体重大于3500g、胎头仰伸位、脐带先露、不完全臀先露等。

  - 阴道分娩

6. Management

（1）Pregnancy period

- Most breech presentation turns to head presentation before 30 weeks of gestation.
- No need to deal with.
- Breech presentation after 30 weeks of gestation: Need to correct.
- Correction methods（Figure 12-6）:
  - Chest-knee position.
  - Acupuncture or moxibustion at point Zhiyin.
  - External cephalic version（ECV）.

（2）Delivery period

- Early parturition: Determine the correct mode of delivery based on the following factors.
  - Maternal age, the course of pregnancy, parity, pelvic type, breech presentation type, fetal size, fetal survival or not, development and complications etc.

  - Indications for elective cesarean section
    · Fetal weight more than 3500g, fetal head extension, umbilical cord presentation and incomplete breech presentation etc.

  - Vaginal delivery

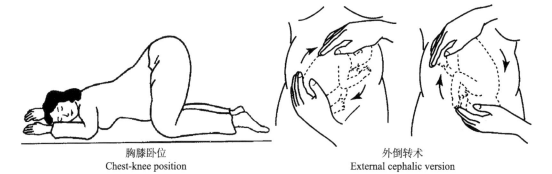

胸膝卧位
Chest-knee position

外倒转术
External cephalic version

图12-6 臀位纠正方法

Figure 12-6 Correction methods of breech presentation

第一产程
　①尽可能防止胎膜早破。

　②少做阴道检查。
　③不用缩宫素引产。
　④宫缩时："堵"。

　⑤待宫口开全、阴道充分扩张后，才能让胎臀娩出。
第二产程
　①做好接产前准备：导尿。
　②初产妇：会阴后侧切开术。
　③有3种娩出方式：a.臀助产术；b.臀牵引术；c.自然分娩。
第三产程
　①预防产后出血。
　②积极抢救新生儿窒息。
　③软产道损伤：应及时检查并缝合。
　④预防感染。

重点专业词汇

1.异常分娩

2.难产

3.潜伏期延长

4.活跃期延长

5.活跃期停滞

6.第二产程延长

7.胎头下降延缓

8.胎头下降停滞

9.产力异常

10.宫缩乏力

11.低张性子宫缩乏力

12.高张性子宫缩乏力

13.狭窄骨盆

14.头盆不称（CPD）

15.持续性枕后位

First stage of labor
　①Prevention of premature rupture of membranes.
　②Less vaginal examination.
　③Induction of labor without oxytocin.
　④During uterine contraction: "Closure".
　⑤Only after the uterine opening is complete and the vagina fully dilates can the fetal buttocks be delivered.
Second stage of labor
　①Preparing for delivery: Catheterization.
　②Primipara: Postero-lateral episiotomy.
　③Three modes of delivery: a. breech midwifery; b. breech traction; c. natural delivery.
Third stage of labor
　①Prevention of postpartum hemorrhage.
　②Active rescue of neonatal asphyxia.
　③Soft birth canal injury: Timely examination and suture.
　④Infection prevention.

Key words

1.Abnormal labor

2.Dystocia

3.Prolonged latent phase

4.Prolonged active phase

5.Arrested active phase

6.Prolonged second stage

7.Protracted descent

8.Arrested descent

9.Abnormal uterine action

10.Uterine inertia

11.Hypotonic uterine inertia

12.Hypertonic uterine inertia

13.Contracted pelvis

14.Cephalopelvic disproportion（CPD）

15.Persistent occiput posterior position

16.持续性枕横位

17.胎头高直位

18.前不均倾位

19.面先露

20.臀先露

21.肩先露

22.滞产

23.急产

24.外倒转术（ECV）

练习题

1.关于协调性宫缩乏力,下列哪一项正确？（B）

　　A.子宫收缩极性倒置

　　B.容易发生胎儿窘迫

　　C.不宜静脉滴注缩宫素

　　D.产程常延长

　　E.不易发生胎盘残留

2.关于不协调性子宫收缩乏力,下列哪一项正确？（B）

　　A.子宫肌肉不协调性收缩，致使宫腔内压力过低

　　B.为无效宫缩

　　C.孕妇于宫缩间歇期时安静，腹痛消失

　　D.子宫收缩极性倒置，但不影响宫口扩张

　　E.一般不会出现胎儿宫内窘迫

3.下列哪项易发生脐带脱垂?（A）

　　A.足先露，胎膜早破

　　B.部分性前置胎盘

　　C.脐带过长

　　D.双胎

　　E.枕后位

4.关于臀位,下列哪一项正确？（E）

16.Persistent occiput transverse position

17.Sincipital presentation

18.Anterior asynclitism

19.Face presentation

20.Breech presentation

21.Shoulder presentation

22.Prolonged labor

23.Precipitate delivery

24.External cephalic version（ECV）

Exercises

1.Which one of the following is correct about coordinated uterine inertia?（B）

　　A.Uterine contraction polarity inversion

　　B.Prone to fetal distress

　　C.Not suitable for intravenous drip of oxytocin

　　D.Often prolonged labor

　　E.Not prone to placenta residue

2.Which one of the following is correct about uncoordinated uterine?（B）

　　A.Uncoordinated contraction of uterine muscles, resulting in low intrauterine pressure

　　B.Ineffective contraction

　　C.The gravida is quiet during the intermittent period of contraction, and the abdominal pain disappears

　　D.The uterus contraction polarity is reversed, but the dilatation of cervical os is not affected

　　E.There will be no intrauterine distress generally

3.Which of the following is prone to umbilical cord prolapse?（A）

　　A.Footling presentation, and premature rupture of membranes

　　B.Partial placenta previa

　　C.Long umbilical cord

　　D.Twins

　　E.Occiput posterior position

4.Which one of the following is correct about breech position?（E）

A.胎体纵轴与母体纵轴垂直

B.完全臀位，指胎儿双髋关节屈曲，双膝关节伸直

C.胎心在母体脐下方听得最清楚

D.妊娠34周之前不必纠正胎位

E.胎儿脐带娩出后，胎头娩出时间最长不能超过8分钟

5.初产妇，孕1产0，足月临产12小时；宫口开大6cm，产程缓慢，胎心140次/分，胎头矢状缝与坐骨棘间径一致，枕骨在母体右侧S^{+1}。下列哪项诊断是正确的？（B）

A.右枕前位
B.持续性右枕横位
C.持续性左枕横位
D.持续性右枕后位
E.持续性左枕后位

（路旭宏）

A.The fetal longitudinal axis is perpendicular to the maternal's.

B.Complete breech position refers to the flexion of the sacroiliac joints of the fetus and the extension of the knee joints

C.The fetal heart can be heard most clearly below maternal umbilicus

D.It is not necessary to correct the fetal position before the 34th week of pregnancy

E.After the delivery of the umbilical cord of the fetus, the fetal head can be delivered for up to 8 minutes

5.A primipara has G1P0 and full-term labor for 12 hours; her cervix opening is up to 6cm, and the labor progresses slowly, her fetal heart rate is 140 bpm, sagittal suture of the fetal head is consistent with interspinous diameter, occipital bone on the maternal right side S^{+1}. Which of the following is correct?（B）

A.Right occipital anterior position
B.Persistent right occipital transverse position
C.Persistent left occipital transverse position
D.Persistent right occipital posterior position
E.Persistent left occipital posterior position

第13章 分娩并发症

CHAPTER 13 Complications of childbirth

第一节 产后出血

1.概述

产后出血（PPH）是全世界孕产妇死亡的主要原因，发生率为1%～3%。

（1）产后出血：指胎儿娩出后24小时内，阴道分娩者出血量≥500ml，剖宫产者≥1000ml。

（2）严重产后出血：指胎儿娩出后24小时内出血量≥1000ml。

（3）难治性产后出血
- 保守措施无法止血。

- 需要外科手术、介入治疗甚至切除子宫。

2.病因

这些原因可共存、相互影响或互为因果。

（1）子宫收缩乏力
- 是产后出血最常见的原因。
- 高危因素
  - 全身因素：产妇精神过度紧张。
  - 产科因素：产程延长、前置胎盘、胎盘早剥、妊娠期高血压疾病等。
  - 子宫因素
    · 子宫过度膨胀：多胎妊

Section 1　Postpartum hemorrhage

1.Introduction

Postpartum hemorrhage（PPH）is the leading cause of maternal death worldwide , with an incidence of 1%～3%.

（1）Postpartum hemorrhage: Defined as ≥500 ml of blood loss at time of vaginal delivery or ≥1000ml at cesarean section within 24 hours after delivery.

（2）Severe postpartum hemorrhage: Refers to the amount of bleeding ≥1000ml within 24 hours after delivery.

（3）Refractory postpartum hemorrhage
- Conservative measures can not stop bleeding.
- Surgery, interventional treatment or even hysterectomy are required.

2.Etiology

These causes can coexist, and are both mutually influential and causal.

（1）Uterine inertia
- The most common cause of PPH.
- High risk factors
  - Systemic factor: Maternal mental stress.
  - Obstetric factors: Prolonged labor, placenta previa, placental abruption, hypertensive disorders of pregnancy etc.
  - Uterine factors
    · Overexpansion of uterus: Multiple

娠、羊水过多、巨大儿。

·子宫肌壁损伤：剖宫产
史、肌瘤剔除术后、产
次过多。

·子宫病变：子宫肌瘤、
子宫畸形。

● 药物因素：镇静药、麻醉
药或宫缩抑制剂。

（2）胎盘因素

■ 胎盘滞留

● 定义：胎儿娩出后30分钟
胎盘仍未娩出。

● 常见原因
①膀胱充盈。
②胎盘嵌顿。
③胎盘剥离不全。

■ 胎盘植入

● 根据侵入深度

·胎盘植入分为粘连性、
植入性和穿透性。

● 根据胎盘粘连或植入的
面积

·分为部分性或完全性。

（3）软产道裂伤：阴道手术助
产、巨大儿、急产等。

（4）凝血功能障碍

■ 原发凝血功能异常

● 原发性血小板减少、再生
障碍性贫血、肝脏疾病等。

■ 继发凝血功能异常

● 胎盘早剥、死胎、羊水栓
塞、重度子痫前期等。

3.临床表现及诊断

产后出血原因常互为因果。

（1）阴道出血

■ 原因

● 软产道裂伤

pregnancy, polyhydramnios, macrosomia.

· Uterine muscle wall injury: History of cesarean section, myomectomy and excessive delivery.

· Uterine lesions: Uterine myoma, and uterine malformation.

● Drug factors: Sedatives, anesthetics or tocolytics.

（2）Placental factors

■ Retained placenta

● Definition: Placenta is not discharged 30 minutes after delivery of fetus.

● Common causes
①Bladder filling.
②Placental incarceration.
③Placental incompleteness.

■ Placental accreta

● Based on the depth of invasion

· Classification: Placenta accreta, placenta percreta, placenta increta.

● Based on the area of placental adhesion or implantation

· Classification: Partial or complete.

（3）Soft birth canal laceration: Vaginal midwifery, macrosomia, precipitate delivery etc.

（4）Coagulation defects

■ Primary coagulation dysfunction

● Primary thrombocytopenia, aplastic anemia, and liver diseases etc.

■ Secondary coagulation dysfunction

● Placental abruption, fetal death, amniotic fluid embolism, severe preeclampsia etc.

3.Clinical manifestations and diagnosis

The causes of postpartum hemorrhage are often both mutually causal.

（1）Vaginal bleeding

■ Causes

● Soft birth canal laceration

- 胎儿娩出后立即发生阴道出血，色鲜红。
  - 胎盘因素
    - 胎儿娩出后数分钟出现阴道出血，色暗红。

- 子宫收缩乏力或胎盘/胎膜残留
  - 胎盘娩出后阴道出血较多。
- 凝血功能障碍
  - 胎儿或胎盘娩出后阴道持续出血，且血液不凝。
- 隐匿性软产道损伤，如阴道血肿
  - 临床表现明显，伴阴道疼痛而阴道出血不多。

- 剖宫产
  ①主要表现：胎儿和胎盘娩出后，胎盘剥离面广泛出血。

  ②严重的子宫切口出血。
（2）低血容量及休克：头晕、面色苍白、烦躁、皮肤湿冷、脉搏细数等。
（3）正确测量和估计出血量。

■ 测量失血量的方法
- 称重法。
- 容积法。
- 面积法。
- 休克指数法（表13-1）
  - 休克指数＝脉率/收缩压（mmHg）。
- 血红蛋白测定
  - 血红蛋白每下降10g/L，

- Vaginal bleeding occurs immediately after delivery with bright red color.
  - Placental factor
    - Vaginal bleeding occurs several minutes after delivery with dark red color.

- Uterine inertia or placental residue/fetal membrane residue
  - More vaginal bleeding after placenta delivery.
- Coagulation dysfunction
  - Vagina bleeds continuously after the delivery of fetus or placenta and blood does not coagulate.
- Occult soft birth injury, such as vaginal hematoma
  - Clinical manifestations are obvious with vaginal pain and less vaginal bleeding.
- Cesarean section
  ① Main manifestation: Extensive bleeding on the detached surface of placenta after delivery of fetus and placenta.
  ② Severe uterine incision bleeding.
（2）Hypovolemia and shock: Dizziness, paleness, irritability, cold and moist skin, fine pulse etc.
（3）Correct measurement and estimation of bleeding volume.

■ Methods for estimating blood loss
- Weighing.
- Volumetric method.
- Area.
- Shock index（Table 13-1）
  - Shock index=pulse rate/systolic blood pressure（mmHg）.
- Hemoglobin measurement
  - For every 10 g/L decrease in hemoglobin,

表13-1 休克指数法

Table 13-1 Shock index

休克指数 Shock index（SI）	失血量（ml） Blood loss（ml）	失血量占全身血容量（%） Blood loss accounting for the whole body blood volume（%）
0.5	＜500	＜10
1.0	500～1500	10～30
1.5	1500～2500	30～50
2.0	2500～3500	50～70

失血量为400～500ml。

4.处理原则

针对出血原因

- 迅速止血。
- 补充血容量。
- 纠正失血性休克。
- 防止感染。

（1）子宫收缩乏力

- 加强宫缩
  - 导尿排空膀胱后可采用以下方法：

①按摩或按压子宫

a.腹部子宫按摩法（图13-1）。

b.腹部-阴道子宫按摩法（图13-2）。

②宫缩药

a.缩宫素。

b.麦角新碱。

c.前列腺素类药物：卡前列素氨丁三醇、米索前列醇、卡前列甲酯。

③宫腔填塞

包括：宫腔纱条填塞、宫腔球囊填塞。

④子宫压缩缝合术（图13-3）。

⑤结扎盆腔血管。

⑥经导管动脉栓塞术（TAE）。

blood loss is 400～500 ml.

4.Principles of management

Targeting the cause of bleeding

- Stop bleeding quickly.
- Supplement blood volume.
- Correct hemorrhagic shock.
- Prevent infection.

（1）Uterine inertia

- Strengthen uterine contraction
  - Following methods can be used after urinary catheterization and bladder emptying:

①Massage or press uterus

a.Abdominal uterine massage（Figure 13-1）.

b.Bimanual uterine massage（Figure 13-2）.

②Uterine contractile agents

a.Oxytocin.

b.Ergometrine.

c.Prostaglandin: Carboprost trometamol, misoprostol, carboprost methylate.

③Intrauterine tamponade

Including: Intrauterine gauze tamponade, intrauterine balloon tamponade.

④B-Lynch suture（Figure 13-3）.

⑤Ligation of pelvic vessels.

⑥Transcatheter arterial embolization（TAE）.

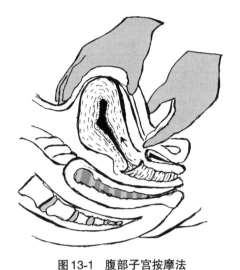

图13-1 腹部子宫按摩法

Figure 13-1　Abdominal uterine massage

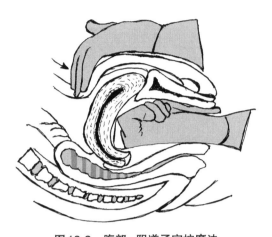

图13-2 腹部-阴道子宫按摩法

Figure 13-2　Bimanual uterine massage

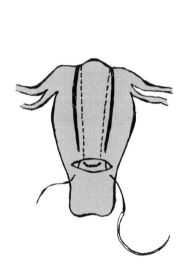
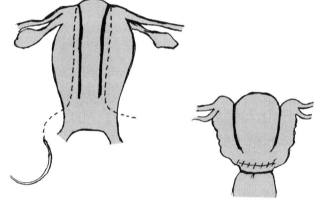

图13-3 子宫压缩缝合术

Figure 13-3　B-Lynch suture

⑦切除子宫：次全子宫切除或全子宫切除术。

（2）胎盘因素

■ 胎盘滞留

● 检查宫腔情况。

● 若胎盘已剥离，立即取出胎盘。

■ 胎盘植入

● 避免强行剥离。

⑦Hysterectomy: Subtotal hysterectomy or hysterectomy.

（2）Placental factors

■ Placental retention

● Examination of uterine cavity.

● If placenta has been detached, remove it immediately.

■ Placental implantation

● Avoid forcible stripping.

（3）软产道损伤

■ 应彻底止血，缝合裂伤。

■ 宫颈裂伤缝合。

■ 阴道裂伤缝合。

■ 会阴裂伤缝合。

■ 会阴血肿清除。

（4）凝血功能障碍

■ 尽快补充凝血因子并纠正休克。

■ 常用的血液制品
  ● 新鲜冷冻血浆（FFP）。
  ● 冷沉淀。
  ● 血小板。
  ● 其他：纤维蛋白原或凝血酶原复合物凝血因子等。

（5）失血性休克处理

■ 观察生命体征、保暖、吸氧、呼救、做记录。

■ 建立两条以上有效静脉通路，及时快速补充血容量。

■ 纠正低血压。

■ 纠正酸中毒。

■ 维持灌注，保证尿量，防治肾衰竭。

■ 必要时强心，保护心脏。

■ 预防感染
  ● 注意无菌操作。
  ● 合理使用广谱抗生素。

（6）输血治疗：通常给予成分输血。

■ 红细胞悬液
  ● 综合判断输血指征。
  ● 根据以下情况：出血量、临床表现、止血情况及继续出血风险

（3）Injury of soft birth canal

■ Bleeding should be stopped thoroughly and laceration should be sutured.

■ Suture of cervical laceration.

■ Suture of vaginal laceration.

■ Suture of perineal laceration.

■ Removal of perineal hematoma.

（4）Coagulation dysfunction

■ Replenish coagulation factors as soon as possible and correct shock.

■ Common blood products
  ● Fresh frozen plasma（FFP）.
  ● Cryoprecipitate.
  ● Platelet.
  ● Others: Fibrinogen or prothrombin complex coagulation factors etc.

（5）Treatment of hemorrhagic shock

■ Observe vital signs, keep warm, inhale oxygen, call for help and make records.

■ Establish more than two effective venous accesses and replenish blood volume promptly.

■ Correct hypotension.

■ Correct acidosis.

■ Maintain perfusion, ensure urine volume and prevent renal failure.

■ Strengthen heart when necessary, and protect heart.

■ Prevention of infection
  ● Aseptic operation.
  ● Rational use of broad-spectrum antibiotics.

（6）Blood transfusion treatment: Usually component transfusion.

■ Red blood cell suspension
  ● Comprehensive judgement of transfusion indications.
  ● According to amount of bleeding, clinical manifestations, hemostasis and risk of continued bleeding.

①血红蛋白＜60g/L：几乎均需要输血。

②血红蛋白＜70g/L：可考虑输血。

③若评估继续出血风险仍较大，可适当放宽输血指征至80g/L。

- 凝血因子：新鲜冷冻血浆、冷沉淀、血小板和纤维蛋白原等。

（7）大量输血方案（MTP）

- 最常用的推荐方案
  - 红细胞：血浆：血小板以1∶1∶1。
  - 例如
    ①10U红细胞悬液＋1000ml新鲜冷冻血浆＋1U机采血小板。
    ②有条件的医院：自体血液过滤后回输。

5.预防

（1）产前预防

- 加强围生期保健，纠正贫血，合理转诊。

（2）产时预防

- 积极处理第三产程。
- 最重要的是胎儿娩出后使用宫缩药。

（3）产后预防

- 产后严密监测，早期发现出血情况。

第二节　羊水栓塞

1.概述

（1）定义：羊水栓塞（AFE）是由于羊水进入母体血液循环，引

①Hemoglobin＜60g/L: Almost all require blood transfusion.

②Hemoglobin＜70g/L: Blood transfusion can be considered.

③Assessment: If the risk of continued bleeding is still high, the blood transfusion indication can be appropriately relaxed to 80g/L.

- Coagulation factors: Fresh frozen plasma, cryoprecipitation, platelet and fibrinogen etc.

（7）Massive transfusion protocol（MTP）

- Most common recommendations
  - Erythrocyte: plasma: platelet 1∶1∶1.
  - For instance
    ①Erythrocyte suspension 10U＋fresh frozen plasma 1000ml＋apheresis platelet 1U.
    ②Hospitals with the right conditions: Autologous blood filtration for reinfusion.

5.Prevention

（1）Prenatal prevention

- Strengthen perinatal health care, correct anemia, and make reasonable referral.

（2）Prevention during childbirth

- Actively deal with the third stage of labor.
- The most important is to use uterine contraction agents after delivery.

（3）Postpartum prevention

- Closely monitor, and detect bleeding early.

Section 2　Amniotic fluid embolism

1.Introduction

（1）Definition: Amniotic fluid embolism（AFE）is a series of pathophysiological changes

起的一系列病理生理变化的过程。

（2）病理生理改变

■ 肺动脉高压。

■ 低氧血症。

■ 循环衰竭。

■ 弥散性血管内凝血（DIC）。

■ 多器官功能衰竭。

（3）发病率为（1.9～7.7）/10万，死亡率为19%～86%。

（4）临床特点

■ 起病急骤。

■ 病情凶险。

■ 难以预测、病死率高。

（5）诱发因素

■ 高龄初产。

■ 经产妇。

■ 宫颈裂伤。

■ 急产。

■ 羊水过多。

■ 子宫收缩过强。

■ 胎膜早破。

■ 前置胎盘。

■ 剖宫产和刮宫术。

2.病因

■ 具体原因不明，可能与下列因素有关：

● 羊膜腔内压力过高。

● 血窦开放。

● 胎膜破裂。

3.病理生理

（1）过敏样反应

■ 羊水中的抗原成分引起Ⅰ型变态反应。

■ 肥大细胞脱颗粒、异常的花生四烯酸代谢产物

● 包括白三烯、前列腺素、血栓素等。

caused by amniotic fluid entering the maternal blood circulation.

（2）Pathophysiological changes

■ Pulmonary hypertension.

■ Hypoxemia.

■ Circulatory failure.

■ Disseminated intravascular coagulation （DIC）.

■ Multiple organs failure.

（3）Morbidity（1.9 ～ 7.7）/100 000, mortality 19% ～ 86%.

（4）Clinical features

■ Acute onset.

■ Dangerous condition.

■ Unpredictable and high mortality.

（5）Inducing factors

■ Older primipara.

■ Multipara.

■ Cervical laceration.

■ Precipitate delivery.

■ Polyhydramnios.

■ Uterine over-efficiency.

■ Premature rupture of membranes.

■ Placenta previa.

■ Cesarean section and curettage.

2.Etiology

■ The specific cause is unknown and may be related to the following factors:

● High intraamniotic pressure.

● Sinus opening.

● Rupture of membranes.

3.Pathophysiology

（1）Allergic reactions

■ Antigens in amniotic fluid cause type I allergy.

■ Mast cell degranulation and abnormal arachidonic acid metabolites

● Including: Leukotrienes, prostaglandins and thromboxane.

（2）肺动脉高压

■ 释放血管活性物质。

■ 肺血管反射性痉挛。

■ 血小板凝集、破坏后游离血清素被释放。

■ 羊水中的有形物质进入母体肺循环导致的机械性栓塞不是羊水栓塞的主要机制。

（3）炎症损伤：全身炎症反应综合征（SIRS）

（4）弥散性血管内凝血（DIC）

■ 羊水栓塞的临床特点之一。

■ 甚至是唯一的临床表现。

■ 常是最终死亡的主要原因。

4.发病机制

（1）羊水中含大量促凝物质类似于组织凝血活酶。

（2）进入母血后易在血管内产生大量的微血栓。

（3）消耗大量凝血因子及纤维蛋白原。

（4）炎性介质和内源性儿茶酚胺大量释放。

（5）触发凝血级联反应，导致DIC。

5.临床表现

（1）典型羊水栓塞

■ 特征

● 羊水栓塞三联征

①低氧血症。

②低血压。

③凝血功能障碍。

■ 前驱症状

● 非特异性。

（2）Pulmonary hypertension

■ Vasoactive substances released.

■ Pulmonary vascular reflex spasm.

■ Free serotonin released after platelet aggregation and destruction.

■ Mechanical embolism caused by the entry of visible substances in amniotic fluid into maternal pulmonary circulation is not the main mechanism.

（3）Inflammatory injury: Systemic inflammatory response syndrome（SIRS）

（4）Disseminated intravascular coagulation （DIC）

■ One of the clinical characteristics of amniotic fluid embolism.

■ Even the only clinical manifestation.

■ The leading cause of final death.

4.Pathogenesis

（1）Amniotic fluid contains a large amount of coagulant promoting substances similar to tissue thromboplastin.

（2）It is easy to produce a large number of microthrombus in blood vessels after entering maternal blood.

（3）Consume a large number of coagulation factors and fibrinogen.

（4）Release inflammatory mediators and endogenous catecholamines.

（5）Trigger coagulation cascade reaction, leading to DIC.

5.Clinical manifestations

（1）Typical amniotic fluid embolism

■ Characteristics

● Amniotic fluid embolism triad

①Hypoxemia.

②Hypotension.

③Coagulation dysfunction.

■ Prodromal symptoms

● Non-specificity.

- 呼吸急促。
- 胸痛。
- 憋气。
- 寒战。
- 呛咳。
- 头晕。
- 乏力。
- 心慌。
- 恶心。
- 呕吐。
- 麻木。
- 针刺样感觉。
- 焦虑。
- 烦躁和濒死感。
- 胎心减速。
- 胎心基线变异消失。

- 重视前驱症状有助于及时识别羊水栓塞。

- ■ 心肺功能衰竭和休克
  - 突发呼吸困难。
  - 发绀。
  - 心动过速。
  - 低血压。
  - 抽搐。
  - 意识丧失或昏迷。
  - 血氧饱和度下降。
  - 心电图ST段改变。
  - 右心受损。
  - 肺底部湿啰音。
  - 心搏骤停。
  - 心室颤动或室性心动过速。

  - 数分钟内猝死。
- ■ 凝血功能障碍
  - 子宫出血为主。
  - 全身出血倾向。
  - 临床表现

- Shortness of breath.
- Chest pain.
- Choking.
- Chills.
- Cough.
- Dizziness.
- Fatigue.
- Panic.
- Nausea.
- Vomiting.
- Numbness.
- Acupuncture-like sensation.
- Anxiety.
- Agitation and near-death experience.
- Deceleration of fetal heart rate.
- Variation and disappearance of fetal heart baseline.
- Attention to prodromal symptoms is helpful to identify amniotic fluid embolism in time.

- ■ Cardiopulmonary failure and shock
  - Dyspnea.
  - Cyanosis.
  - Tachycardia.
  - Hypotension.
  - Convulsion.
  - Loss of consciousness or coma.
  - Decrease of oxygen saturation.
  - ST segment changes of ECG.
  - Right heart damaged.
  - Moist rale at the bottom of lung.
  - Cardiac arrest.
  - Ventricular fibrillation or ventricular tachycardia.
  - Sudden death within minutes.
- ■ Coagulation dysfunction
  - Mainly uterine bleeding.
  - Tendency of systemic hemorrhage.
  - Clinical manifestations

①切口渗血。

②全身皮肤黏膜出血。

③针眼渗血。

④血尿。

⑤消化道大出血。

■ 急性肾衰竭

■ 全身脏器均可受损

● 最常见受损的器官：中枢神经系统和肾脏。

（2）不典型羊水栓塞

■ 临床表现

● 前驱症状。

● 当其他原因不能解释时，应考虑羊水栓塞。

6. 诊断

（1）排除性诊断。

（2）应根据临床表现和诱发因素进行诊断。

（3）目前尚无国际统一的羊水栓塞诊断标准和实验室诊断指标。

（4）常用的诊断依据

■ 临床表现。

■ 出现以下表现之一

①血压骤降或心搏骤停。

②急性缺氧如呼吸困难、发绀或呼吸停止。

③凝血功能障碍或无法解释的严重出血。

7. 处理

（1）羊水栓塞的处理原则是维持生命体征和保护器官功能。

（2）一旦怀疑羊水栓塞，立即按羊水栓塞急救流程实施抢救，分秒必争。

（3）推荐多学科密切协作，提

① Incision bleeding.

② Systemic skin and mucosal bleeding.

③ Needle-eye bleeding.

④ Hematuria.

⑤ Major gastrointestinal bleeding.

■ Acute renal failure

■ All organs can be damaged

● The most common organs damaged: Central nervous system and kidney.

（2）Atypical amniotic fluid embolism

■ Clinical manifestations

● Prodromal symptom.

● Amniotic fluid embolism should be considered when other reasons cannot be explained.

6. Diagnosis

（1）Exclusion diagnosis.

（2）Based on clinical manifestations and inducing factors.

（3）No international standard or laboratory diagnostic index for amniotic fluid embolism at present.

（4）Common diagnostic criteria

■ Clinical manifestations.

■ One of the following manifestations occurs

① Sudden blood pressure drop or cardiac arrest.

② Acute hypoxia such as dyspnea, cyanosis or respiratory arrest.

③ Coagulation dysfunction or unexplained severe bleeding.

7. Management

（1）Treatment principles: Maintaining vital signs and protecting organ function.

（2）Once amniotic fluid embolism is suspected, the first aid procedure for amniotic fluid embolism should be followed immediately.

（3）Close multi-disciplinary cooperation

高抢救成功率。

- 全面监测
  - 包括血压、呼吸、心率、血氧饱和度、心电图、中心静脉压、心排血量、动脉血气和凝血功能等。

- 增加氧合
  - 立即保持气道通畅。
  - 尽早实施面罩吸氧。

  - 气管插管。
  - 人工辅助呼吸。
- 血流动力学支持
  - 维持血流动力学稳定
    ①治疗的首选药物
    a.多巴酚丁胺。
    b.磷酸二酯酶-5抑制剂（米力农）。
    ②作用机制：强心和扩张肺动脉。
    ③低血压：去甲肾上腺素。
  - 解除肺动脉高压
    ①推荐特异性舒张肺血管平滑肌的药物：磷酸二酯酶-5抑制剂、一氧化氮（NO）等。
    ②其他：盐酸罂粟碱、阿托品、氨茶碱、酚妥拉明。
  - 液体管理
    ①注意管理液体出入量。
    ②避免左侧心力衰竭和肺水肿。
- 抗过敏
  - 应用大剂量糖皮质激素尚存在争议。
  - 基于临床实践的经验，早

is recommended to improve the success rate of rescue.

- All-round monitoring
  - Including blood pressure, respiration, heart rate, oxygen saturation, electrocardiogram, central venous pressure, cardiac output, arterial blood gas and coagulation function, etc.
- Increase in oxygenation
  - Maintain airway patency immediately.
  - Implement mask oxygen inhalation as soon as possible.
  - Endotracheal intubation.
  - Artificial assisted respiration.
- Hemodynamic support
  - Maintaining hemodynamic stability
    ① Preferred drugs for treatment
    a.Dobutamine.
    b.Phosphodiesterase-5 inhibitor (milrinone).
    ② Mechanism: Cardiac effect and pulmonary artery dilation.
    ③ Hypotension: Norepinephrine.
  - Relieving pulmonary hypertension
    ① Specific drugs recommended for relaxing pulmonary vascular smooth muscle: Phosphodiesterase-5 inhibitor, nitric oxide (NO), etc.
    ② Other drugs: Papaverine hydrochloride, atropine, aminophylline, and phentolamine.
  - Fluid management
    ① Management of liquid volume.
    ② Avoiding left heart failure and pulmonary edema.
- Anti-allergy
  - The use of high-dose glucocorticoids remains controversial.
  - The use of high-doses of glucocorticoids

期使用大剂量糖皮质激素或有价值。

■ 纠正凝血功能障碍

● 应积极处理产后出血。

● 及时补充凝血因子：输注大量的新鲜血、血浆、冷沉淀、纤维蛋白原等。必要时可静脉滴注氨甲环酸。

● 不推荐肝素治疗。

■ 产科处理

● 立即终止妊娠。

● 考虑紧急实施剖宫产。

● 必要时全子宫切除。

■ 器官功能受损的对症支持治疗

● 保护神经系统。

● 稳定血流动力学。

● 维持血氧饱和度和血糖。

● 支持肝脏功能。

● 适时应用血液透析。

● 积极防治感染。

● 维护胃肠功能。

8.预防

（1）正确使用缩宫素，防止宫缩过强。

（2）人工破膜在宫缩间歇期进行。

（3）避免产伤、子宫破裂、子宫颈裂伤等。

at early time may be valuable based on the experience of clinical practice.

■ Correcting coagulation dysfunction

● Postpartum hemorrhage should be treated actively.

● Timely replenishment of coagulation factors: Infusion of large amount of fresh blood, plasma, cryoprecipitate, fibrinogen, etc. Tranexamic acid can be infused intravenously if necessary.

● Heparin therapy is not recommended.

■ Obstetric management

● Immediate termination of pregnancy.

● Urgent cesarean section may be considered.

● Total hysterectomy if necessary.

■ Symptomatic supportive treatment for organ dysfunction

● Protecting nervous system.

● Maintaining stable hemodynamics.

● Maintaining oxygen saturation and blood glucose.

● Supporting liver function.

● Timely application of hemodialysis.

● Active prevention and treatment of infection.

● Maintaining gastrointestinal function.

8.Prevention

（1）Proper use of oxytocin to prevent excessive uterine contractions.

（2）Artificial rupture of membranes performed during the interval of uterine contractions.

（3）Avoiding birth injury, uterine rupture, cervical laceration, etc.

第三节 子宫破裂

概述

（1）定义：子宫破裂指在妊娠晚期或分娩期，子宫体部或子宫下段发生破裂。

（2）是直接危及产妇及胎儿生命的严重并发症。

1.病因

（1）子宫手术史（瘢痕子宫）。

（2）骨盆狭窄。

■ 先露部下降受阻。

（3）子宫收缩药物使用不当。

（4）产科手术损伤。

（5）子宫发育异常或多次宫腔操作。

2.临床表现

（1）多发生于分娩期，部分发生于妊娠晚期。

（2）按破裂程度

■ 分为完全性破裂和不完全性破裂。

（3）多数子宫破裂是渐进的。

■ 由先兆子宫破裂进展为子宫破裂。

（4）胎儿窘迫是最常见的临床表现。

（5）其他

● 电子胎心监护（EFM）异常。

● 宫缩间歇期仍有严重腹痛。

● 阴道异常出血。

● 血尿。

● 宫缩消失。

● 孕妇心动过速、低血压、晕厥或休克。

Section 3 Rupture of uterus

Introduction

（1）Definition: Rupture of uterus refers to the rupture of the uterus body or lower segment of the uterus in late pregnancy or childbirth.

（2）It is a serious complication that directly endangers the lives of pregnant woman and fetus.

1.Etiology

（1）History of uterine surgery（scarred uterus）.

（2）Pelvic stenosis.

■ Obstructed descent of presentation.

（3）Improper use of uterine contractile drug.

（4）Obstetric surgical injury.

（5）Abnormal uterine development or multiple uterine cavity operations.

2.Clinical manifestations

（1）Most occur during childbirth, and some occur in late pregnancy.

（2）Based on the degree of rupture

■ Classification: Complete rupture and incomplete rupture.

（3）Most uterine ruptures are gradual.

■ From threatened uterine rupture to uterine rupture.

（4）Fetal distress is the most common clinical manifestation.

（5）Others

● Abnormal electronic fetal heart rate monitoring（EFM）.

● Severe abdominal pain remaining during the intermittent period of contractions.

● Abnormal vaginal bleeding.

● Hematuria.

● Uterine contractions disappearing.

● Tachycardia, hypotension, syncope or shock in pregnant women.

- 胎先露异常
  - 腹部轮廓改变。

先兆子宫破裂

临床表现

（1）子宫呈强直性或痉挛性过强收缩。

（2）孕妇

■ 烦躁不安。

■ 呼吸、心率加快。

■ 下腹剧痛难忍。

（3）病理缩复环

（4）排尿困难及血尿

（5）无法触清胎体

■ 胎心率加快或减慢或听不清。

子宫破裂

1.不完全性子宫破裂

（1）定义：子宫肌层部分或全层破裂，但浆膜层完整，宫腔与腹腔不相通。

（2）多见于子宫下段剖宫产切口瘢痕破裂。

（3）急性大出血。

（4）阔韧带内血肿，多有胎心率异常。

2.完全性子宫破裂

（1）定义：子宫肌壁全层破裂，宫腔与腹腔相通。

（2）产妇突感：下腹撕裂样剧痛。

（3）子宫收缩骤然停止。

（4）全腹持续性疼痛。

■ 全腹压痛明显、有反跳痛。

（5）有低血容量、休克的征象。

- Abnormal fetal presentation
  - Abdominal contour change.

Threatened uterine rupture

Clinical manifestations

（1）Tonic or spastic over-efficiency of uterus.

（2）Gravida

■ Restlessness.

■ Rapid breathing and heart rate.

■ Severe pain in lower abdomen.

（3）Pathologic retraction ring.

（4）Dysuria and hematuria.

（5）Failure to touch the fetal body

■ Accelerated or decelerated or inaudible fetal heart rate.

Rupture of uterus

1.Incomplete uterine rupture

（1）Definition: Uterine myometrium partially or fully is ruptured, but the serosa is intact and the uterine cavity is not connected with abdominal cavity.

（2）More common in scar rupture of cesarean section incision in lower uterine segment.

（3）Acute massive hemorrhage.

（4）Hematoma in broad ligament with abnormal fetal heart rate.

2.Complete uterine rupture

（1）Definition: Uterine muscle wall is completely ruptured, and the uterine cavity is connected with the abdominal cavity.

（2）Sudden sensation of puerpera: Lacerationlike severe pain in the lower abdomen.

（3）Sudden cessation of uterine contraction.

（4）Persistent pain in the whole abdomen.

■ Obvious abdominal tenderness and rebound pain.

（5）Signs of hypovolemia and shock.

（6）腹壁下

■ 可清楚扪及胎体。

■ 子宫位于侧方。

（7）胎心胎动消失。

（8）阴道检查：可有鲜血流出。

（9）胎先露部升高。

（10）宫颈口缩小。

3.诊断

（1）典型的子宫破裂

■ 根据病史、症状、体征。

■ 容易诊断。

（2）不典型的子宫破裂

■ 综合判断。

■ 应结合
  ● 前次剖宫产史。
  ● 子宫下段压痛。
  ● 胎心异常。
  ● 胎先露部上升。
  ● 宫颈口缩小。
  ● 超声检查。

4.鉴别诊断

（1）胎盘早剥。

（2）难产并发宫内感染。

（3）妊娠临产合并急性胰腺炎。

5.处理

（1）先兆子宫破裂

■ 立即抑制子宫收缩。

■ 尽快手术。

（2）子宫破裂

■ 抢救休克。

■ 无论胎儿是否存活均应尽快手术治疗。

■ 根据术中情况选择术式：
  ● 破口修补术。
  ● 次全子宫切除术。
  ● 全子宫切除术。

（6）Under abdominal wall

■ Clearly palpate fetus.

■ Uterus is located on the side.

（7）Fetal heart and movements disappear.

（8）Vaginal examination: Fresh bleeding.

（9）Rise of fetal presentation.

（10）Reduction of cervical orifice.

3.Diagnosis

（1）Typical ruptures of uterus

■ According to medical history, symptoms and signs.

■ Easy to diagnose.

（2）Atypical ruptures of uterus

■ Comprehensive judgement.

■ Combined with
  ● Previous history of cesarean section.
  ● Tenderness of lower uterine segment.
  ● Abnormal fetal heart rate.
  ● Rise of fetal presentation.
  ● Reduction of cervical orifice.
  ● Ultrasound examination.

4.Differential diagnosis

（1）Placental abruption.

（2）Dystocia complicated with intrauterine infection.

（3）Acute pancreatitis during parturition.

5.Management

（1）Threatened uterine rupture

■ Immediate inhibition of uterine contraction.

■ Operation as soon as possible.

（2）Rupture of uterus

■ Shock rescue.

■ Surgical treatment should be performed as soon as possible regardless of whether the fetus is alive or not.

■ According to the intraoperative conditions:
  ● Rupture repair.
  ● Subtotal hysterectomy.
  ● Total hysterectomy.

- 控制感染
  - 足量。
  - 足疗程。
  - 广谱抗生素。
- （3）严重休克
  - 尽可能就地抢救。
  - 在输液、输血、抗休克后可转送。

6.预防

（1）做好产前保健。

（2）严密观察产程进展。

（3）严格掌握缩宫剂应用指征。

（4）正确掌握产科手术助产的指征及操作常规。

重点专业词汇

1.产后出血

2.子宫收缩乏力

3.胎盘滞留

4.凝血功能障碍

5.缩宫素

6.子宫压迫缝合术

7.大量输血方案（MTP）

8.羊水栓塞（AFE）

9.子宫破裂

10.病理缩复环

练习题

1.产后出血最常见的原因是：（A）

A.子宫收缩乏力

B.胎盘残留

C.胎盘植入

D.宫颈裂伤

E.凝血机制障碍

2.羊水栓塞的发生与下列哪项因素无关？（E）

A.宫缩过强致胎膜早破

B.高龄产妇

- Infection control
  - Adequate dosage.
  - Duration.
  - Broad-spectrum antibiotic.
- （3）Severe shock
  - On-site rescue as far as possible.
  - Transfer after infusion, blood transfusion and anti-shock.

6.Prevention

（1）Good prenatal care.

（2）Close observation of labor progress.

（3）Strict control of indications for uterine contraction agents.

（4）Good command of indication and routine of obstetric midwifery.

Key words

1.Postpartum hemorrhage

2.Uterine inertia

3.Retained placenta

4.Coagulation dysfunction

5.Oxytocin

6.B-Lynch suture

7.Massive transfusion protocol（MTP）

8.Amniotic fluid embolism（AFE）

9.Ruptures of uterus

10.Pathologic retraction ring

Exercises

1.The most common cause of postpartum hemorrhage is:（A）

A.Uterine inertia

B.Placental residue

C.Placental implantation

D.Cervical laceration

E.Coagulation mechanism disorder

2.Which of the following factors is irrelevant to the occurrence of amniotic fluid embolism?（E）

A.Uterine over-efficiency cause premature rupture of membranes

B.Advanced maternal age

C.急产

D.前置胎盘

E.臀位助产

3.下列哪种胎位易致子宫破裂？（E）

A.枕横位

B.枕后位

C.单臀位

D.枕前位

E.横位

4.导致子宫破裂的原因，错误的是：（B）

A.胎先露下降受阻

B.不适当的阴道助产手术

C.急性羊水过多

D.宫缩药使用不当

E.子宫壁瘢痕破裂

5.病理缩复环最常见于：（D）

A.女型骨盆

B.高张性宫缩乏力

C.软产道损伤

D.头盆不称

E.枕后位

（路旭宏）

C.Precipitate delivery

D.Placental previa

E.Breech midwifery

3.Which of the following fetal positions is prone to uterine rupture ?（E）

A.Occiput transverse position

B.Occiput posterior position

C.Single breech position

D.Occiput anterior position

E.Transverse position

4.The wrong cause of uterine rupture is:（B）

A.The descent of the presenting part is arrested

B.Inappropriate vaginal midwifery

C.Acute polyhydramnios

D.Improper use of uterotonics

E.Uterine wall scar rupture

5.Pathologic retraction ring is most common in:（D）

A.Female pelvis

B.Hypertonic uterine inertia

C.Soft birth canal injury

D.Cephalopelvic disproportion

E.Occiput posterior position

第14章 遗传咨询、产前筛查、产前诊断

第一节　遗传咨询

1.定义

■ 遗传咨询是由专业人员对咨询对象就其提出的家庭中遗传性疾病的相关问题予以解答，并提出医学建议的过程。

2.具体内容

（1）梳理家族史及病史。

（2）获取详细的临床表型。

（3）选择合理的遗传学检测方案。

（4）解读遗传检测结果。

（5）分析遗传机制。

（6）告知患者可能的预后和治疗方法。

（7）评估下一代再发风险并制订再生育计划。

3.遗传咨询的对象

（1）夫妇双方或一方家庭成员中有遗传病、出生缺陷、不明原因的癫痫、智力低下、肿瘤及其他与遗传因素密切相关的患者；曾生育过明确遗传病或出生缺陷儿的夫妇。

（2）夫妻双方或之一本身罹患智力低下或出生缺陷。

（3）不明原因的反复流产或有死胎、死产等病史的夫妇。

（4）孕期接触不良环境因素及患有某些慢性病的夫妇。

Section 1   Genetic counseling

1.Definition

■ Genetic counseling is the process in which a professional answers the questions about genetic diseases in the family and gives medical advice.

2.Content coverage

（1）Review of family history and medical history.

（2）Obtaining a detailed clinical phenotype.

（3）Choosing a reasonable genetic testing program.

（4）Interpretation of genetic test results.

（5）Analysis of genetic mechanisms.

（6）Informing patients of the possible prognosis and treatment.

（7）Assessing next generation recurrence risks and developing a re-fertility plan.

3.Subjects for genetic counseling

（1）Patients with genetic diseases, birth defects, unexplained epilepsy, mental retardation, tumors and other closely related to genetic factors in both or one family member of the couple; couples who have given birth to children with clear genetic diseases or birth defects.

（2）Both husband and wife or one of them suffering from mental retardation or birth defects.

（3）Couples with unexplained recurrent miscarriage or history of fetal death, stillbirth, etc.

（4）Couples exposed to adverse environmental factors during pregnancy and suffering from certain

（5）常规检查或常见遗传病筛查发现异常者。

（6）其他需要咨询者，如婚后多年不育的夫妇，或35岁以上的高龄孕妇。

（7）近亲婚配。

4.遗传咨询的类别

- 婚前咨询、孕前咨询、产前咨询、儿科相关遗传病咨询、肿瘤遗传咨询及其他专科咨询（如神经遗传病咨询、血液病咨询等）。

5.遗传咨询的原则

（1）自主原则。

（2）知情同意原则。

（3）无倾向性原则。

（4）守密和尊重隐私原则。

（5）公平原则。

6.遗传咨询的内容及基本流程

（1）帮助患者及家庭成员了解疾病的表型。

（2）以通俗易懂的语言向患者及家庭成员普及疾病的遗传机制。

（3）提供疾病治疗方案信息。

（4）提供再发风险的咨询。

（5）提供家庭再生育计划咨询。

7.人类遗传病的类型

（1）染色体疾病

- 例如21-三体综合征。

（2）基因组疾病

- 例如染色体7q11.23区域微缺失引起的Williams-Beuren综合征（WBS）。

（3）单基因遗传病

- 常染色体显性遗传（AD）。

chronic diseases.

（5）Abnormal persons found in routine examination or common genetic disease screening.

（6）Others who need counseling, such as couples who have been infertile for many years after marriage, or pregnant women over the age of 35.

（7）Marriage of close relatives.

4.Category

- Pre-marital counseling, pre-pregnancy counseling, prenatal counseling, pediatric-related genetic disease counseling, oncology genetic counseling, and other specialized counseling（such as neurogenetic disease counseling, blood disease counseling, etc.）.

5.Principles

（1）Principle of autonomy.

（2）Principle of informed consent.

（3）Principle of non-biases.

（4）Principle of confidentiality and respect for privacy.

（5）Principle of fairness.

6.Content and basic process

（1）Help patients and family members understand the phenotype of disease.

（2）Spread the genetic mechanism of disease to patients and family members in plain language.

（3）Provide information on treatment options.

（4）Provide advice on recurring risks.

（5）Provide family re-fertility planning consultation.

7.Types of human genetic diseases

（1）Chromosomal diseases

- Such as 21-trisomy syndrome.

（2）Genomic diseases

- Such as Williams-Beuren syndrome（WBS）caused by chromosome 7q11.23 regional microdeletion.

（3）Single gene genetic diseases

- Autosomal dominant inheritance（AD）.

- 常染色体隐性遗传（AR）。
- 性连锁显性遗传（XD）。
- 性连锁隐性遗传（XR）。
（4）多基因遗传病
- 例如糖尿病、哮喘。
（5）线粒体遗传病
- 例如Leber遗传性视神经病变。
（6）体细胞遗传病
- 例如癌症。

第二节 产前筛查

1.非整倍体染色体异常

（1）血清学筛查。

（2）超声遗传标志物筛查，又称为软指标。

- 例如胎儿颈项透明层厚度（NT）、颈部皮肤皱褶（NF）、肠管回声等。
- 无创产前检测技术（NIPT）。

2.神经管畸形（NTDs）

（1）高危因素
- 神经管畸形家族史。
- 暴露在特定的环境中。
- 与NTDs有关的遗传综合征和结构畸形。
- 神经管畸形高发地区。
- 在NTDs患者中发现，抗叶酸受体抗体的比例增高。

（2）诊断方法
- 血清学筛查：甲胎蛋白（AFP）。

- 超声筛查：妊娠中期超声诊断。
  - 时间：妊娠18～24周。
  - 诊断率几乎100%。
  - 鼻骨缺失。
  - 颅骨缺损。
  - 超声对NTDs的检出率为

- Autosomal recessive inheritance (AR).
- Sex-linked dominant inheritance (XD).
- Sex-linked recessive inheritance (XR).
(4) Polygenic genetic diseases
- Such as diabetes, and asthma.
(5) Mitochondrial genetic diseases
- Such as Leber's hereditary optic neuropathy.
(6) Somatic genetic diseases
- Such as cancers.

Section 2　Prenatal screening

1.Aneuploid chromosomal abnormality

(1) Serological screening.

(2) Ultrasound genetic marker screening, also called soft markers.

- Such as fetal nuchal translucency (NT); nuchal fold (NF); echogenic bowel, etc.

(3) Non-invasive prenatal test (NIPT).

2.Neural tube defects (NTDs)

(1) High risk factors
- Family history of neural tube defects.
- Exposure to a specific environment.
- Genetic syndrome and structural malformations associated with NTDs.
- High-risk areas of NTDs.
- Increased proportion of anti-folate receptor antibodies in patients with NTDs.

(2) Diagnostic methods
- Serological screening: Alpha-fetoprotein (AFP).

- Ultrasound screening: Mid-pregnancy ultrasound diagnosis.
  - Time: 18 ～ 24 weeks of pregnancy.
  - Diagnostic rate, almost 100%.
  - Absence of nasal bone.
  - Cranial defect.
  - Ultrasound detection rate of NTDs at

90%。

3.胎儿结构畸形筛查

（1）时间：妊娠20～24周。

（2）对象：所有产妇。

（3）检查目的：发现严重的结构畸形。

（4）检出率：50％～70%。

（5）漏诊的原因

- 影响因素：孕周、羊水、胎位、母体腹壁等。

- 部分胎儿畸形的产前超声检出率极低。
- 还有部分胎儿畸形目前还不能为超声所发现。

第三节 产 前 诊 断

1.定义

- 产前诊断又称宫内诊断。

2.产前诊断的对象

（1）羊水过多或羊水过少。

（2）胎儿发育异常。

（3）孕早期可能接触过导致胎儿先天缺陷的物质。

（4）夫妇一方患有先天性疾病或遗传性疾病，或有遗传病家族史。

（5）曾经分娩过先天严重缺陷婴儿。

（6）年龄≥35岁。

3.产前诊断的疾病

（1）染色体异常。

（2）性连锁遗传病。

（3）遗传性代谢缺陷病。

（4）先天性结构畸形。

4.产前诊断常用方法

- 观察胎儿的结构。

90%.

3.Fetal structural malformation screening

（1）Time: 20～24 weeks of pregnancy.

（2）Screening object: All gravida.

（3）Screening purpose: To discover serious structural abnormalities.

（4）Detection rate: 50%～70%.

（5）Reasons for missed diagnosis

- Influencing factors: Gestational age, amniotic fluid, fetal position, maternal abdominal wall, etc.

- Prenatal ultrasound detection rate of some fetal malformations is extremely low.
- Some fetal malformations can not be found by ultrasound currently.

Section 3   Prenatal diagnosis

1.Definition

- Prenatal diagnosis, also known as intrauterine diagnosis.

2.Subjects for prenatal diagnosis

（1）Polyhydramnios or oligohydramnios.

（2）Abnormal fetal development.

（3）Exposure to substances that may cause birth defects in early pregnancy.

（4）One of the couple has a congenital or hereditary disease, or has family history of hereditary disease.

（5）Those who have given birth to a baby with serious birth defect.

（6）Age≥35 years old.

3.Prenatal diagnosis of diseases

（1）Chromosomal abnormality.

（2）Sex-linked genetic disease.

（3）Hereditary metabolic deficiency.

（4）Congenital structural malformation.

4.Common methods of prenatal diagnosis

- Observation of fetal structure.

- 染色体核型分析。
- 基因检测。
- 检测基因产物。

（1）绒毛膜穿刺取样（CVS）

■ 时间：妊娠8～10周。

■ 方法
  - 经阴道。
  - 经腹。

■ 优点
  - 妊娠早期检查。
  - 诊断率为99%。
  - 流产率为1%。
  - 5～7天获得结果。

■ 缺点
  - 胚外组织。
  - 不能区分胎盘嵌合体。
  - 仅获得细胞，不能检测AFP。
  - 不能诊断NTD。

（2）羊膜腔穿刺术

■ 时间：妊娠15～17周。

■ 方法：经腹或经阴道。

■ 用途：细胞、染色体或AFP检测。

（3）经皮脐血穿刺

■ 时间：妊娠19～21周。

■ 超声引导下脐带穿刺，获取胎儿血
  - 指征
    ①要求快速。
    ②羊水穿刺失败。
    ③综合干预。

（4）胎儿组织活检。

5.实验室诊断技术

（1）荧光原位杂交技术（FISH）。

（2）染色体微阵列分析（CMA）。

（3）靶向基因测序。

（4）全外显子测序（WES）。

- Karyotype analysis.
- Genetic testing.
- Detection of gene products.

（1）Chorionic villus sampling（CVS）

■ Time: 8～10 weeks of pregnancy.

■ Methods
  - Transvaginal.
  - Transabdominal.

■ Advantages
  - Early pregnancy check.
  - Diagnosis rate 99%.
  - Abortion rate 1%.
  - Getting results in 5～7 days.

■ Disadvantages
  - Extraembryonic tissue.
  - Failure to distinguish placental mosaicism.
  - Only cells obtained, and failure to detect AFP.
  - Failure to diagnose NTD.

（2）Amniocentesis

■ Time: 15～17 weeks of pregnancy.

■ Methods: Transabdominal or transvaginal.

■ Uses: Cell, chromosome or AFP detection.

（3）Percutaneous cord blood puncture

■ Time: 19～21 weeks of pregnancy.

■ Ultrasound-guided umbilical cord puncture to obtain fetal blood
  - Indications
    ①Demand fast.
    ②Amniotic fluid puncture failed.
    ③Combined intervention.

（4）Fetal tissue biopsy.

5.Laboratory diagnostic technology

（1）Fluorescence in situ hybridization（FISH）.

（2）Chromosomal microarray analysis（CMA）.

（3）Targeted gene sequencing.

（4）Whole exome sequencing（WES）

6.超声产前诊断

- 超声诊断的出生缺陷的特点

  - 出生缺陷必须存在解剖异常。

  - 超声诊断与孕龄有关。

  - 胎儿非整倍体畸形往往伴有结构畸形。

7.磁共振产前诊断

（1）中枢神经系统
- 显示脑部的成熟与结构的关系。
- 诊断中枢神经系统的畸形。

（2）颈部肿块
- 评估胎儿气道，制订出生时的处理预案。

（3）胎儿胸部疾病：直接分辨肝脏疝入的部位和程度。

（4）胎儿腹腔畸形：有助于区分近端和远端小肠。

重点专业词汇

1.出生缺陷

2.遗传咨询

3.遗传筛查

4.产前筛查

5.颈项透明层厚度（NT）

6.鼻骨

7.皮肤皱褶

8.无创产前诊断技术（NIPT）

9.神经管畸形（NTDs）

10.产前诊断

11.宫内诊断

12.绒毛膜穿刺取样（CVS）

13.羊膜腔穿刺术

练习题

1.下列不属于遗传咨询的对

6.Ultrasound prenatal diagnosis

- Characteristics of birth defects diagnosed by ultrasound
  - Anatomical abnormalities exist in birth defects.
  - Ultrasound diagnosis is related to gestational age.
  - Fetal aneuploidy malformations are often accompanied by structural abnormalities.

7.Magnetic resonance imaging in prenatal diagnosis

（1）Central nervous system
- Showing the relationship between brain maturity and structure.
- Diagnosis of malformations of the central nervous system.

（2）Neck mass
- Assessing fetal airway and developing a treatment plan at birth.

（3）Fetal chest disease: Directly identify the location and extent of liver intrusion.

（4）Fetal abdominal malformation: Help distinguish the proximal and distal small intestine.

Key words

1.Birth defect

2.Genetic counseling

3.Genetic screening

4.Prenatal screening

5.Nuchal translucency（NT）

6.Nasal bone

7.Nuchal fold

8.Non-invasive prenatal test（NIPT）

9.Neural tube defects（NTDs）

10.Prenatal diagnosis

11.Intrauterine diagnosis

12.Chorionic villus sampling（CVS）

13.Amniocentesis

Exercises

1.Which of the following is not the subject for

象？（E）

A.夫妻双方或之一本身罹患智力低下或出生缺陷

B.不明原因的反复流产或有死胎、死产等病史的夫妇

C.孕期接触不良环境因素及患有某些慢性病的夫妇

D.常规检查或常见遗传病筛查发现异常者

E.30岁以上的高龄孕妇

2.超声遗传标志物筛查又称为软指标，不包括:（C）

A.胎儿颈项透明层（NT）

B.肠管回声

C.股骨长度

D.鼻骨缺失

E.颈部皮肤皱褶

3.下列哪项属于产前诊断？（A）

A.羊膜腔穿刺术

B.无创产前诊断技术（NIPT）

C.唐氏筛查

D.胎儿颈项透明层（NT）

E.颈部皮肤皱褶（NF）

4.羊膜腔穿刺术的时间:（A）

A.妊娠15～24周

B.妊娠24～28周

C.妊娠28～32周

D.妊娠＞32周

E.妊娠＞34周

5.下列哪项不是实验室诊断技术？（E）

A.荧光原位杂交技术（FISH）

B.染色体微阵列分析（CMA）

C.靶向基因测序

D.全外显子测序（WES）

E.唐氏筛查

（路旭宏）

genetic consultation?（E）

A.Both husband and wife or one of them suffers from mental retardation or birth defects

B.Couples with unexplained recurrent miscarriage or a history of fetal death, stillbirth, etc

C.Adverse environmental factors during pregnancy and couples with certain chronic diseases

D.Abnormal persons found in routine examination inspection or common genetic disease screening

E.Pregnant women over the age of 30

2.Ultrasound genetic marker screening is also known as soft markers, excluding:（C）

A.Nuchal translucency（NT）

B.Echogenic bowel

C.Femur length

D.Absence of nasal bone

E.Nuchal fold, NF

3.Which of the following belongs to prenatal diagnosis?（A）

A.Amniocentesis

B.Non-invasive prenatal test（NIPT）

C.Down's screening

D.Nuchal translucency（NT）

E.Nuchal fold（NF）

4.Timing of amniocentesis:（A）

A.15～24 weeks of pregnancy

B.24～28 weeks of pregnancy

C.28～32 weeks of pregnancy

D.＞32 weeks of pregnancy

E.＞34 weeks of pregnancy

5.Which of the following is not laboratory diagnostic technology?（E）

A.Fluorescence in situ hybridization（FISH）

B.Chromosomal microarray analysis（CMA）

C.Targeted gene sequencing

D.Whole exome sequencing（WES）

E.Down's screening

第 15 章 女性生殖系统炎症

CHAPTER 15 Inflammation of female reproductive system

第一节 概 述

1.种类

（1）外阴炎：非特异性外阴炎、前庭大腺炎、前庭大腺囊肿。

（2）阴道炎：滴虫性、念珠菌性（VVC）、细菌性阴道病（BV）、老年性阴道炎（萎缩性阴道炎）、婴幼儿外阴阴道炎。

（3）宫颈炎：急、慢性宫颈炎。

（4）盆腔炎：盆腔炎（PID），盆腔结核（TB）。

2.阴道正常菌群

正常阴道内有病原体寄居形成正常阴道菌群。

（1）革兰氏阳性需氧菌及兼性厌氧菌，如乳杆菌。

（2）革兰氏阴性需氧菌及兼性厌氧菌，如大肠埃希菌。

（3）专性厌氧菌。

（4）支原体及假丝酵母菌（念珠菌属）。

3.阴道微生态

（1）阴道上皮在卵巢分泌的雌激素影响下增生，增加对病原体侵入的抵抗力。同时上皮细胞中含有丰富糖原，在乳杆菌作用下分解为乳酸，维持阴道正常的酸性环境（pH≤4.5，多在3.8～4.4），使适

Section 1　Introduction

1.Types

（1）Vulvitis: Non-specific vulvitis, bartholinitis, Bartholin cyst.

（2）Vaginitis: Trichomonal, vulvovaginal candidiasis（VVC）, bacterial vaginosis（BV）, senile vaginitis（atrophic vaginitis）, infantile vaginitis.

（3）Cervicitis: Acute and chronic cervicitis.

（4）Pelvic inflammatory diseases: Pelvic inflammation disease（PID）, pelvic tuberculosis（TB）.

2.Vaginal normal flora

Pathogens living in normal vagina to form normal vaginal flora.

（1）Gram-positive aerobic bacteria and facultative anaerobic bacteria, such as lactobacillus.

（2）Gram-negative aerobic bacteria and facultative anaerobic bacteria, such as *Escherichia coli*.

（3）Obligate anaerobe.

（4）Mycoplasma and candida（monilia）.

3.Vaginal microecosystem

（1）Due to ovarian estrogen, vaginal epithelium proliferates,increasing resistance to pathogens, while epithelial cell are rich in glycogen which under the effect of lactobacillus decomposed into lactic acid to maintain normal vaginal acid environment（pH≤4.5, mostly 3.8 ～ 4.4）, so

应于弱碱性环境中繁殖的病原体受到抑制。

（2）影响阴道生态平衡因素。

（3）正常阴道内多种细菌存在，维持正常生态平衡。

（4）影响因素：雌激素、乳酸杆菌、阴道pH。

4.传播方式

（1）经性交直接传播。

（2）经公共浴池、浴盆、浴巾、游泳池、坐式便器、衣物等间接传播。

（3）医源性传播。

第二节　阴道炎症

1.滴虫阴道炎

（1）病原体

■ 阴道毛滴虫。

■ 消耗或吞噬阴道上皮细胞内的糖原，阻碍乳酸生成。

■ 50%～70%的阴道毛滴虫能被看见。

■ pH升高。

■ 使白细胞增加。

（2）临床表现

■ 外阴瘙痒、灼热、疼痛、性交痛。

■ 稀薄泡沫状白带增多。

■ 有细菌混合感染时，分泌物呈脓性，味臭。

■ 尿道感染：尿频、尿痛。

■ 妇科检查：阴道黏膜充血，严重者散在出血斑点，后穹窿多量白带。

that pathogens adapted to reproduction in the weak alkaline environment are inhibited.

（2）Factors affecting vaginal ecological balance.

（3）Multiple bacteria in normal vagina to maintain normal ecological balance.

（4）Influencing factors: Estrogen, lactobacillus, and vaginal pH.

4.Modes of transmission

（1）Direct transmission through sexual intercourse.

（2）Indirect transmission via public bath, bath basin, bath towel, swimming pool, sit type implement, clothings, etc.

（3）Iatrogenic transmission.

Section 2　Vaginitis

1.Trichomonal vaginitis

（1）Pathogens

■ Trichomonas.

■ Consumption or engulfment of glycogen in vaginal epithelial cells, thus impeding lactic acid production.

■ 50%～70% of trichomonas visible.

■ Increased pH.

■ Increase in leukocytes.

（2）Clinical manifestations

■ Vulval pruritus, burning, pain, sexual intercourse pain.

■ Thin foamy leucorrhea increase.

■ When coexisting with bacteria infection, the discharge is purulent, and smelly.

■ Urethral infection: Frequent urination and painful urination.

■ Pelvic examination: Vaginal mucosa hyperemia, petechiae in severe cases, excess leucorrhea in posterior fornix of the

（3）诊断

■ 阴道分泌物中找到滴虫可确诊。

■ 悬滴法；培养法。

（4）治疗

■ 甲硝唑，口服

• 局部用药。

• 甲硝唑泡腾片，阴道用。

■ 性伴侣同时治疗。

■ 治愈标准：3次月经后复查白带为阴性。

2.外阴阴道假丝酵母菌病

（1）病原体

■ 80%～90%为白假丝酵母菌。

■ 10%～20%为其他酵母属：光滑假丝、热带假丝等酵母菌。

■ 假丝酵母菌

• 适宜生长pH4.0～4.7。

• 条件致病：10%非孕妇和30%孕妇可被寄生。

• 不耐热，对干燥、紫外线、化学制剂抵抗。

（2）临床表现

■ 外阴瘙痒、灼痛。

■ 可有尿频、尿痛及性交痛。

■ 白色稠厚豆渣样或凝乳样白带。

■ 妇科检查：小阴唇内侧及阴道黏膜上附着白色膜状物，擦除后露出红肿黏膜面。

■ 急性期可见白色膜状物覆盖下有受损的糜烂面及浅溃疡。

vagina.

（3）Diagnosis

■ Trichomonas found in vaginal secretions.

■ Suspension; cultivation.

（4）Treatment

■ Metronidazole, take orally.

• Topical therapy

• Metronidazole effervescent tablet, vaginal use.

■ Simultaneous treatment of sexual partners.

■ Clinical cure standard: Leucorrhea negative after 3 periods.

2.Vulvovaginal candidiasis（VVC）

（1）Pathogens

■ 80%～90% *Candida albicans*.

■ 10%～20% others: *Candida glabrata*, *Candida tropicalis*, etc.

■ Candida

• pH 4.0～4.7 suitable for growth.

• Conditional pathogenesis: Parasitic in 10% non-pregnant women, and 30% pregnant women.

• No heat-resistant, resistant to dryness, ultraviolet rays and chemicals.

（2）Clinical manifestations

■ Vulval pruritus, burning pain.

■ Frequent urination, painful urination and pain in sexual intercourse.

■ White thick bean-dregs-like or curd-like leucorrhea.

■ Pelvic examination: White membrane attached to the inner side of the labia minora and vaginal mucosa with red and swollen mucosa exposed after erasing.

■ Acute phase marked by a white membrane covering with damaged erosive surfaces and superficial ulcers.

（3）诊断

- 阴道分泌物中找到白念珠菌可确诊。

- 悬滴法；培养法。

- 顽固病例应查血糖。

- 询问病史。

（4）治疗

- 消除诱因。

- 改变酸碱度：2%～4%碳酸氢钠液阴道冲洗。

- 局部用药
  - 咪康唑。
  - 克霉唑栓。
  - 制霉菌素。

3.细菌性阴道病

（1）病原体

- 加德纳菌属物。

- pH＞4.5。

- 由于阴道内乳酸杆菌减少，而其他细菌大量繁殖引起。

- 主要有加德纳菌、各种厌氧菌、不动杆菌、支原体引起的混合感染。

（2）临床表现

- 50%无症状。

- 难闻的"鱼腥味"分泌物。

- 瘙痒和炎症并不常见。

- 妇科检查：阴道黏膜无明显充血的炎症表现。

- 白带增多，灰白色、均匀一致的稀薄白带。

（3）诊断

- 下列标准中3条阳性者可确诊
  - 阴道分泌物为匀质稀薄的白带。
  - 阴道pH＞4.5。
  - 胺臭味试验阳性。
  - 线索细胞阳性。

（3）Diagnosis

- *Candida albicans* found in vaginal secretions.

- Suspension; cultivation.

- Blood sugar check for refractory cases.

- Inquiry for medical history.

（4）Treatment

- Eliminating the causes.

- pH value change: 2% ～ 4% sodium bicarbonate solution for vaginal irrigation.

- Topical therapy
  - Miconazole.
  - Clotrimazole suppository.
  - Nystatin.

3.Bacterial vaginosis

（1）Pathogens

- Gardnerella species.

- pH＞4.5.

- Lactobacillus in vagina reduced and other bacteria multiply.

- Mixed infection caused by gardnerella, various anaerobic bacteria, acinetobacter, and mycoplasma.

（2）Clinical manifestations

- 50% asymptomatic.

- Unpleasant secretions with "fishy smelling".

- Itching and inflammation uncommon.

- Pelvic examination: No obvious hyperemic inflammation in vaginal mucosa.

- Increase in leucorrhea, gray-white, homogeneous and thin leucorrhea.

（3）Diagnosis

- Diagnosis can be made if 3 of the following are positive.
  - Vaginal discharge is homogeneous and thin leucorrhea.
  - Vaginal pH＞4.5.
  - Positive for amine test.
  - Clue cell positive.

（4）治疗

- 甲硝唑，口服。
- 克林霉素，口服。
- 甲硝唑栓剂，阴道给药。

第三节 盆腔炎症

1.女性生殖道的自然防御功能

（1）两侧大阴唇自然合拢。

（2）盆底肌的作用。

（3）阴道口闭合，阴道前后壁紧贴。

（4）阴道自净。

（5）宫颈的自然防御功能。

（6）宫颈内口紧闭。

（7）宫颈管分泌黏液形成黏液栓。

（8）育龄妇女子宫内膜周期性剥脱。

（9）输卵管黏膜上皮细胞的纤毛蠕动。

（10）生殖道的免疫系统。

2.病原体

（1）外源性：主要为STD的病原体，如淋病奈瑟菌，衣原体，支原体。

（2）内源性：来自寄居于阴道的菌群，包括需氧菌及厌氧菌。

3.感染途径

（1）沿生殖器黏膜上行蔓延，淋病奈氏菌、沙眼衣原体及葡萄球菌沿此途径扩散。

（2）经淋巴系统蔓延，是产褥感染、流产后感染及放置宫内节育器后感染的主要传播途径，多见于链球菌、大肠埃希菌、厌氧菌感染。

（4）Treatment

- Metronidazole, take orally.
- Clindamycin, take orally.
- Metronidazole suppositories, vaginal use.

Section 3 Pelvic inflammatory diseases

1.Natural defense of female reproductive tract

（1）Natural close of labia majora on both sides.

（2）The action of pelvic floor muscles.

（3）Vaginal closing, with the anterior and posterior walls of the vagina tightly attached.

（4）Vaginal self-purification.

（5）The natural defense of the cervix.

（6）The inner cervix closed.

（7）Mucus plugs formed by cervical canal secretion.

（8）Periodic exfoliation of endometrium in women of childbearing age.

（9）Ciliary peristalsis of epithelial cells of the oviduct mucosa.

（10）The immune system of the reproductive tract.

2.Pathogens

（1）Exogenous: STD pathogens, such as *Neisseria gonorrhoeae*, chlamydia, mycoplasma.

（2）Endogenous: Bacteria from vagina, including aerobic and anaerobic bacteria.

3.Route of infection

（1）Spreading along the genital mucosa, including *Neisseria gonorrhoeae*, *Chlamydia trachomatis*, and *Staphylococcus*.

（2）Spreading through the lymphatic system, the main route of transmission after puerperal infection, post-abortion infection and placement of intrauterine devices. More common in *Streptococcus*, *Escherichia coli*, and anaerobic infections.

（3）经血循环传播，为结核菌感染的主要途径。

（4）直接蔓延：腹腔其他脏器感染后，直接蔓延到内生殖器，如阑尾炎可引起右侧输卵管炎。

4.发病率

（1）急性盆腔炎发生在1%～2%的年轻、性活跃的女性。

（2）16～25岁妇女最常见的严重感染。

（3）在性活跃的女性中，约85%的感染是自发的。

（4）15%的感染发生在宫颈黏液屏障被破坏的过程中，这使得阴道菌群有机会在上生殖道定植。

5.高危因素

（1）年龄。

（2）性活动。

（3）下生殖道感染。

（4）宫腔内手术操作后感染。

（5）性卫生不良。

（6）邻近器官炎症直接蔓延。

（7）盆腔炎再次发作。

（8）诱发因素。

（9）月经期。

（10）不洁性交。

（11）流产。

（12）刮宫。

（13）子宫输卵管造影。

（14）试管婴儿。

6.类型

（1）子宫内膜炎。

（2）输卵管卵巢脓肿（TOA）与卵巢炎。

（3）盆腔腹膜炎。

（4）结缔组织炎。

（3）Transmission though blood circulation, the main route of tuberculosis infection.

（4）Direct spread: Spread directly to internal genitals after infection of other organs in abdominal cavity. For example, appendicitis can cause right salpingitis.

4.Morbidity

（1）Acute pelvic inflammatory disease occurs in 1% to 2% of young and sexually-active women.

（2）The most common severe infection among women aged 16 to 25.

（3）About 85% of infections spontaneous in sexually-active females.

（4）15% of infections occur during the destruction of the cervical mucus barrier, which gives the vaginal flora the opportunity to colonize the upper genital tract.

5.High-risk factors

（1）Age.

（2）Sexually-active women.

（3）Female lower genital tract infection.

（4）Infection after the intrauterine operation.

（5）Poor sexual hygiene.

（6）Direct spread of adjacent organs inflammation.

（7）Recurrent attacks.

（8）Inducing factors.

（9）Menses.

（10）Dirty sex.

（11）Abortion（miscarriage）.

（12）Curettage.

（13）Hysterosalpingography.

（14）In vitro fertilization.

6.Types

（1）Endometritis.

（2）Tubo-ovarian abscess（TOA）& oophoritis.

（3）Pelvic peritonitis.

（4）Pelvic cellulitis.

（5）败血症与脓毒血症。

（6）肝周围炎。

7.诊断

（1）病史和体检

■ PID的症状包括3个或以上的体征：腹痛（通常为双侧和下象限），与月经有关的疼痛发作。

（2）月经过多。

（3）白带增多（脓性）。

（4）排尿困难。

（5）发热和（或）寒战。

（6）恶心呕吐。

（7）双合诊时子宫和附件区的压痛。

（8）血象检查，白细胞和红细胞沉降率。

（9）病原体检查。

8.临床表现

（1）可因炎症轻重及范围大小而有不同的临床表现。

（2）有发热、头痛、食欲缺乏、血白细胞增高等全身表现。

（3）伴有明显下腹痛、阴道脓性分泌物增多、尿频、里急后重。

（4）急性病容，体温升高、心率快、腹胀、下腹压痛、反跳痛、肌紧张、肠鸣音先强后减弱。

（5）阴道有大量脓性分泌物，宫体可略增大、变软、压痛阳性、活动受限，子宫两侧压痛，可增厚或触及明显压痛的包块。

9.诊断标准（2015年美国疾病预防和控制中心，CDC）

（1）最低标准

■ 宫颈或宫体举痛或摇摆痛或

（5）Sepsis & septicopyemia.

（6）Fitz-Hugh-Curtis syndrome.

7.Diagnosis

（1）Medical history and examination

■ Symptoms suggestive of PID include 3 or more signs: Abdominal pain（usually bilateral and in the lower quadrants）and, menstrual-related pain.

（2）Menometrorrhagia.

（3）Vaginal discharge（purulent）.

（4）Dysuria.

（5）Fever, and/or chills.

（6）Nausea or vomiting.

（7）Tenderness of the uterus and adnexa area, during bimanual examination.

（8）Blood test: WBC, ESR.

（9）Pathogens.

8.Clinical manifestations

（1）Being different due to the severity and extent of inflammation.

（2）Being systemic manifestations such as fever, headache, loss of appetite, and increased white blood cells.

（3）With obvious lower abdominal pain, increased vaginal purulent discharge, frequent urination, and tenesmus.

（4）Acute illness, high body temperature, fast heart rate, abdominal distension, lower abdominal tenderness, rebound tenderness, muscle tension, guarding bowel sounds first strong and then weakened.

（5）A lot of purulent secretions in the vagina. The uterus slightly enlarged, softened, tenderness positive, activity limited, tenderness on both sides of the uterus, thickening or palpable tenderness mass.

9.Diagnostic criteria（2015 Center for Disease Control and Prevention, CDC）

（1）Minimum criteria

■ Cervical or uterine body lifting pain, swing

附件区压痛。

（2）附加标准

■ 体温超过38℃。

■ 子宫颈脓性分泌物。

■ 阴道分泌物有大量白细胞。

■ 宫颈分泌物培养或革兰氏染色涂片淋病奈氏菌阳性或沙眼衣原体阳性。

■ 红细胞沉降率（ESR）升高。

■ 血C反应蛋白升高。

（3）特异标准

■ 子宫内膜活检组织学证实子宫内膜炎。

■ 超声或磁共振检查发现盆腔脓肿或炎性包块。

10.腹腔镜检查的诊断标准

（1）输卵管表面明显充血。

（2）输卵管壁水肿。

（3）输卵管伞端或浆膜面有脓性渗出物。

11.鉴别诊断

（1）阑尾炎。

（2）宫外孕。

（3）黄体囊肿破裂伴出血。

（4）感染性流产。

（5）卵巢囊肿扭转。

（6）肌瘤变性。

（7）子宫内膜异位症。

12.治疗

（1）支持疗法

■ 卧床休息，半卧位有利于脓液积聚于直肠子宫陷凹而使炎症局限。

■ 药物治疗

● 敏感抗生素。

● 兼顾厌氧菌和需氧菌，联

pain or tenderness in the adnexa area.

（2）Additional criteria

■ Body temperature over 38℃.

■ Purulent secretions in the cervix.

■ A lot of WBC in vagina discharge.

■ Cervical secretion culture or Gram stain smear positive for *Neisseria gonorrhoeae* or *Chlamydia trachomatis*.

■ Elevated erythrocyte sedimentation rate （ESR）.

■ Elevated blood C-reactive protein.

（3）Specific criteria

■ Endometritis confirmed by endometrial biopsy.

■ Pelvic abscess or inflammatory mass found by ultrasound or MRI.

10.Diagnostic criteria for laparoscopy

（1）Obvious hyperemia on oviduct surface.

（2）Oviduct wall edema.

（3）Purulent exudate at the fimbrial portion or serosal surface of fallopian tube.

11.Differential diagnosis

（1）Appendicitis.

（2）Ectopic pregnancy.

（3）Ruptured corpus luteum cyst with hemorrhage.

（4）Infected septic abortion.

（5）Torsion of ovarian cyst.

（6）Myoma degeneration.

（7）Endometriosis.

12.Treatment

（1）Supporting treatment

■ Bed rest, semi-decumbent position conducive to the accumulation of pus in rectouterine pouch and the limitation of inflammation.

■ Medical treatment

● Antibiotics.

● Considering both anaerobic and aerobic

合用药配伍合理。

- 抗生素要足量、足时，给药以静脉滴注收效快。
- 病情好转后，应巩固治疗10～14日。

（2）手术指征

■ 药物治疗无效：药物治疗48～72小时，体温不降、症状加重、包块增大者。

■ 输卵管积脓或输卵管卵巢脓肿（TOA）持续存在。

■ 脓肿破裂。

（3）中医治疗。

（4）性伴侣同时治疗。

13.预防

（1）安全性知识教育。

（2）使用避孕套和屏障方法避孕。

（3）其他的预防。

（4）高危人群筛查衣原体和淋病。

（5）性活跃女性的病原体筛查。

（6）提高敏感性诊断。

（7）治疗性伴侣。

（8）积极施教预防复发。

14.盆腔炎性疾病后遗症

（1）病理变化

■ 输卵管阻塞、增粗。

■ 输卵管卵巢肿块。

■ 输卵管炎、输卵管积水、输卵管卵巢炎及输卵管卵巢脓肿。

■ 盆腔结缔组织炎。

（2）盆腔炎性疾病主要后遗症

■ 宫外孕。

bacteria, with reasonable combination of drugs.

- Sufficient antibiotics for enough time, intravenous drip for quick results.
- Consolidated treatment for 10 ～ 14 days after improvement.

（2）Surgical indications

■ Drug treatment ineffective: Drug treatment for 48 ～ 72 hours, no decrease in body temperature, worsening symptoms, and increased mass.

■ Pyosalpinx or tubo-ovarian abscess（TOA）.

■ Abscess rupture.

（3）Traditional Chinese medicine.

（4）Simultaneous treatment of sexual partners.

13.Prevention

（1）Safe sex practices education for adolescents.

（2）Promoting use of condoms and chemical barrier methods.

（3）Other preventions.

（4）Screening of women at high risk for chlamydia and gonorrhea.

（5）Pathogen screening for sexually active women.

（6）Improved sensitivity diagnosis.

（7）Treatment of sexual partners.

（8）Education to prevent recurrent infection.

14.Sequelae of pelvic inflammatory disease

（1）Pathologic changes

■ Tubal obstruction and thickening.

■ Tubal ovarian mass.

■ Salpingitis, hydrosalpinx, salpingo-ovaritis and tubo-ovariay abscess.

■ Pelvic connective tissue inflammation.

（2）Major sequelae of PID

■ Ectopic pregnancy.

■ 慢性盆腔痛。

■ 不孕。

（3）临床表现

■ 慢性盆腔痛：下腹坠胀、疼痛；腰骶部酸痛，性交及月经前后加剧。

■ 不孕及异位妊娠。

■ 盆腔炎反复发作。

■ 全身症状：多不明显，有时低热、疲乏、精神不振、失眠及急性发作。

（4）妇科检查：子宫活动受限，子宫两旁增厚及轻压痛，形成囊肿时触及明显边界清或不清的囊性肿物。

（5）治疗

■ 原则：多种方法综合治疗。

 ● 一般治疗：增加营养，锻炼身体，以提高抵抗力。

 ● 中药治疗：清热利湿，活血化瘀。

 ● 物理治疗：超短波、微波等促进血液循环、以助炎症吸收消退（结核除外）。

 ● 药物治疗：抗生素。

 ● 手术治疗：以消除病灶彻底治愈为原则。

■ 对年轻的女性应尽量保留卵巢功能。

重点专业词汇

1.外阴炎

2.非特异性外阴炎

3.前庭大腺炎

■ Chronic pelvic pain.

■ Infertility.

（3）Clinical manifestations

■ Chronic pelvic pain: Abdominal distention, and pain; lumbosacral pain, aggravated before and after sexual intercourse and menstruation.

■ Infertility and ectopic pregnancy.

■ Pelvic inflammatory disease recurrent attacks.

■ Systemic symptoms: Less obvious, sometimes low fever, fatigue, lethargy, insomnia and acute attack.

（4）Pelvic examination: Uterine activity limited, thickened and light tenderness on both sides of the uterus, palpating clear or unclear cystic masses when forming cysts.

（5）Treatment

■ Principle: Comprehensive treatment with multiple methods.

 ● General treatment: Strengthen nutrition and exercise to improve resistance.

 ● Traditional Chinese medicine: Clearing heat and dampness, promoting blood circulation and removing blood stasis.

 ● Physical therapy: Ultrashort wave, microwave, etc. to promote blood circulation and help inflammation absorption and regression（tuberculosis excluded）.

 ● Medical treatment: Antibiotics.

 ● Surgical treatment: Elimination of lesions and thorough cure.

■ Trying to preserve ovarian function for young women.

Key words

1.Vulvitis

2.Non-specific vulvitis

3.Bartholinitis

4.前庭大腺囊肿

5.阴道炎

6.滴虫阴道炎

7.外阴阴道假丝酵母菌病

8.细菌性阴道病

9.老年性阴道炎

10.婴幼儿外阴阴道炎

11.宫颈炎

12.盆腔炎

13.阴道正常菌群

14.宫外孕

15.慢性盆腔痛

16.不孕

17.淋病奈瑟菌

18.衣原体

19.性活跃女性

20.下生殖道感染

21.子宫内膜炎

22.输卵管卵巢脓肿与卵巢炎

23.盆腔腹膜炎

24.结缔组织炎

25.败血症与脓毒血症

26.肝周围炎

练习题

1.下列哪项导致阴道黏膜出现肉眼可辨认的斑点状出血（"草莓斑"）？（B）

　　A.白念珠菌

　　B.阴道毛滴虫

　　C.淋病奈瑟菌

　　D.细菌性阴道病

　　E.萎缩性阴道炎

2.下列哪种阴道炎因吞噬精子而引起不孕?（A）

　　A.滴虫阴道炎

　　B.真菌阴道炎

　　C.细菌性阴道病

　　D.萎缩性阴道炎

　　E.淋病奈瑟菌

4.Bartholin cyst

5.Vaginitis

6.Trichomonal vaginitis

7.Vulvovaginal candidiasis

8.Bacterial vaginosis

9.Senile vaginosis

10.Infantile vaginitis

11.Cervicitis

12.Pelvic inflammatory disease

13.Vaginal normal flora

14.Ectopic pregnancy

15.Chronic pelvic pain

16.Infertility

17.*Neisseria gonorrhoeae*

18.Chlamydia

19.Sexually active women

20.Lower genital tract infection

21.Endometritis

22.Tubo-ovarian abscess & oophoritis

23.Pelvic peritonitis

24.Pelvic cellulitis

25.Sepsis & septicopyemia

26.Fitz-Hugh-Curtis syndrome

Exercises

1.Which of the following causes production of the grossly recognizable vaginal mucosa with punctate hemorrhage（"strawberry spots"）?（B）

　　A.*Candida albicans*

　　B.Trichomonas vaginalis

　　C.*Neisseria gonorrhoeae*

　　D.Bacterial vaginosis

　　E.Atrophic vaginitis

2.Which of the following causes infertility by swallowing sperm?（A）

　　A.Trichomonal vaginitis

　　B.Vulvovaginal candidiasis

　　C.Bacterial vaginosis

　　D.Atrophic vaginitis

　　E.*Neisseria gonorrhoeae*

3.阴道内有大量脓性黄绿色呈泡沫状分泌物，最常见的疾病是：（C）

A.真菌性阴道炎

B.细菌性阴道病

C.滴虫阴道炎

D.萎缩性阴道炎

E.淋病奈瑟菌

4.下列哪项与阴道自净作用无关？（D）

A.雌激素

B.阴道内乳酸杆菌

C.阴道黏膜上皮糖原含量

D.宫颈黏液

E.阴道上皮增生

（王学慧）

3.There are a large number of purulent yellow-green foamy vaginal discharges, and the most common disease is:（C）

A.Vulvovaginal candidiasis

B.Bacterial vaginosis

C.Trichomonal vaginitis

D.Atrophic vaginitis

E.*Neisseria gonorrhoeae*

4.Which of the following has nothing to do with vaginal self-purification?（D）

A.Estrogen

B.Lactobacillus

C.Glycogen content in vaginal mucosa

D.Cervical mucus

E.Hyperplasia of vaginal epithelial cells

第 16 章 子宫肌瘤

子宫肌瘤为良性肿瘤，生育期女性发生率为20%～25%，病因不明。

Leiomyoma of uterus（fibromyoma, fibroid, myoma）being benign uterine tumor, with the incidence of 20% ～ 25% in women during childbearing period, and the etiology unknown.

1.发病相关因素

- 遗传、性激素（雌、孕激素）、表皮生长因子；胰岛素样生长因子-1。

2.分类（图16-1）

（1）根据肌瘤所在部位：宫体肌瘤、宫颈肌瘤。

（2）按肌瘤发展过程中与子宫肌壁间的关系。

- 肌壁间肌瘤。

1.Risk factors

- Heredity, ovarian hormone（estrogen, progestierone）, epithelial growth factor, insulin-like growth factor-1.

2.Classification（Figure 16-1）

（1）According to the myoma position: Corpus myoma, cervical myoma.

（2）According to the relationship between myoma development and uterine muscle wall.

- Intramural myoma.

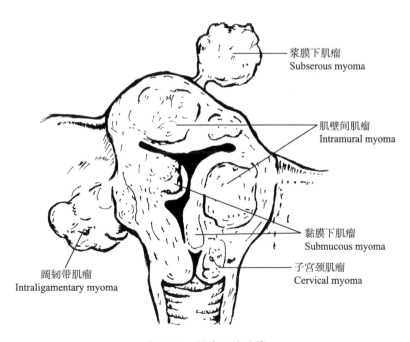

图 16-1　子宫肌瘤分类

Figure 16-1　Classification of uterine myoma

■ 浆膜下肌瘤。

■ 黏膜下肌瘤。

3.病理

■ 子宫平滑肌肿瘤通常是多发的。有子宫黏膜下，壁间和浆膜下的平滑肌瘤。

- 巨检
  ①很少单发，经常多发。
  ②分化良好，无包膜。
  ③假包膜完整。
  ④除非发生变性或出血，质硬。
  ⑤颜色：浅灰色或粉白色。
  ⑥切面：纵横交织或旋涡状的肌纤维排列成束，凸起。

- 镜检
  ①成分：平滑肌，结缔组织。
  ②无横纹的肌纤维排列成各种尺寸的束，这些束在多个方向上延伸。

4.变性

（1）玻璃样变。

（2）囊性变。

（3）红色变。

■ 偶发在妊娠相关的并发症（多在妊娠期及产褥期）。

■ 发病机制尚不清楚，可能是由于静脉阻塞导致肿瘤内血液积聚的结果。

■ 切面似生牛肉。

■ 临床表现：腹痛；发热；生长迅速，质软。

■ 一个较大的子宫肌瘤，经历了退行性变化，呈红色（所谓的"红色变性"）。

（4）肉瘤变

■ 少见：0.4% ～ 0.8%。

■ Subserous myoma.

■ Submucous myoma.

3.Pathology

■ Uterine smooth muscle tumors are usually multiple, including submucosal, intramural, and subserosal leiomyomata of the uterus.

- Gross appearance
  ①Rarely single, usually multiple.
  ②Well-differentiated, nonencapsulated.
  ③Pseudocapsule intact.
  ④Hard consistency except when degeneration or hemorrhage occurring.
  ⑤Color: Light gray or pinkish white.
  ⑥Section: Intertwining or whorl-like arrangement of muscle fibers, bulgy.

- Microscopic appearance
  ①Composition: Smooth muscle, connective tissue.
  ②The nonstriated muscle fibers arranged in bundles of various sizes that run in multiple directions.

4.Degeneration

（1）Hyaline degeneration.

（2）Cystic degeneration.

（3）Red degeneration.

■ Occasional pregnancy-related complications（mostly during pregnancy and puerperium）.

■ The pathogenesis is unknown, but may be the result of the blood accumulation in the tumor due to venous obstruction.

■ Section similar to raw beef.

■ Clinical manifestations: Abdominal pain; fever; rapid growth, tender.

■ A large leiomyoma, which has undergone degenerative changes, with red in color（so-called "red degeneration"）.

（4）Sarcomatous change

■ Rare: 0.4% ～ 0.8%.

- 多发生于40～50岁。
- 通常发生在肌纤维内。
- 生长迅速。
- 阴道出血。

（5）钙化性变性。

5.临床表现

（1）症状

- 贫血及经期延长，常见。

- 盆腔腹痛：发生于妊娠期的变性及肌瘤扭转时。其他：腹痛、腰酸、下腹坠胀。

- 子宫肌瘤通常无腹痛；浆膜下肌瘤蒂扭转，急性腹痛；肌瘤红色变性腹痛剧烈伴发热。

- 压迫症状：压迫膀胱，尿频、排尿障碍、尿潴留。压迫输尿管，肾盂积水。压迫直肠，便秘，排便困难，便意感。

- 自然流产、不孕。

（2）体征

- 腹部可触及包块。
- 妇科检查
  - 子宫：增大，不规则，硬。
  - 肌壁间肌瘤：子宫增大，表面不规则，单个或多个结节状突起。
  - 浆膜下肌瘤：可扪及质硬、球状块物与子宫有细蒂相连活动。
  - 黏膜下肌瘤：子宫多均匀增大，肌瘤可脱出于宫口内或阴道内，呈红色，实质表面光滑，伴感染时表面有渗液溃疡形成，排液有臭味。

- More common in 40 ～ 50 years old.
- Usually occur in muscle fibers.
- Rapid growth.
- Vaginal bleeding.

（5）Degeneration with calcification.

5.Clinical manifestations

（1）Symptoms

- Menorrhagia and prolonged menstrual period are common.

- Pelvic pain: Occurs in pregnancy if undergoing degeneration or torsion of a pedunculated myoma. Others: Abdominal pain, soreness of waist, and lower abdominal distension.

- Usually no abdominal pain. Acute abdominal pain if subserous myoma pedicle torsion. Red degeneration may cause severe abdominal pain and fever.

- Pelvic pressure symptoms: Pressure on bladder, urinary frequency, dysuresia, urinary retention. Pressure on ureter, hydronephrosis. Pressure on rectum, constipation, bowel difficulty, and tenesmus.

- Spontaneous abortion, infertility.

（2）Signs

- A palpable abdominal tumor.
- Pelvic examination
  - Uterus: Enlarged, irregular, and hard.
  - Intramural myoma: Uterus may be enlarged, having an irregular surface, and single or multiple nodular projections.
  - In case of subserous myoma, pelvic examination may palpate a hard, globular mass attached to the uterus by a pedicle.
  - Uterus with submucous myoma mostly evenly enlarged, with fibroids prolapsing from the cervix or vagina, red, and smooth. If infection, exudation of ulcers on the surface, with odor discharge.

6. 诊断

（1）病史。

（2）双合诊检查。

（3）超声检查。

（4）宫腔镜。

（5）腹腔镜。

（6）子宫造影术。

（7）辅助检查。

（8）诊断性刮宫。

（9）子宫输卵管造影（HSG）。

7. 鉴别诊断

（1）与恶性肿瘤相鉴别

■ 子宫肉瘤。

■ 子宫内膜癌。

■ 宫颈癌。

（2）与良性病变相鉴别

■ 妊娠子宫。

■ 卵巢肿瘤。

■ 子宫腺肌病。

■ 其他。

8. 治疗

（1）随诊和观察

■ 小的，无症状的不需要治疗，特别是近绝经期的，3～6个月复查一次。

（2）药物治疗

■ 促性腺激素释放激素激动剂。

■ 米非司酮。

（3）手术治疗

■ 适应证

 • 急性腹痛、肌瘤蒂扭转。

 • 月经失调导致贫血的。

 • 有压迫症状的。

 • 肌瘤造成的不孕或反复流产。

 • 疑有肉瘤变。

■ 方法

 • 肌瘤剔除术，非手术治

6.Diagnosis

（1）Medical history.

（2）Bimanual examination.

（3）Ultrasound examination.

（4）Hysteroscopy.

（5）Laparoscopy.

（6）Hysterography.

（7）Auxiliary examination.

（8）Diagnostic curettage.

（9）Hysterosalpingography（HSG）.

7.Differential diagnosis

（1）Malignant tumors

■ Sarcoma of uterus.

■ Endometrial carcinoma.

■ Cervical cancer.

（2）Benign tumors

■ Pregnancy.

■ Ovarian tumor.

■ Adenomyosis.

■ Others.

8.Treatment

（1）Follow up and observation

■ Small, and asymptomatic fibroids, no treatment needed, especially near menopause. Review every 3～6 months.

（2）Medical treatment

■ GnRH-a.

■ Mifepristone.

（3）Surgical treatment

■ Indications

 • Acute abdominal pain with torsion of pedunculated subserous myoma.

 • Anemia caused by menorrhagia.

 • Symptoms of compression.

 • Recurrent spontaneous abortion, or infertility.

 • Sarcomatous changes.

■ Methods

 • Myomectomy—conservative therapy;

疗；保留生育功能；有复发的风险。

- 子宫切除术，根治性治疗。
- 子宫次全切除术。

■ 手术路径

- 开腹。
- 经阴。
- 经腹腔镜或者宫腔镜手术。
- 提倡个体化治疗。

9.子宫肌瘤合并妊娠

（1）对妊娠的影响：流产。

（2）对分娩的影响

■ 早产。

■ 胎儿先露异常。

■ 胎盘残留。

■ 胎盘前置。

■ 手术助产

（产道阻滞）。

■ 产后出血。

（3）非手术治疗。

（4）药物治疗。

重点专业词汇

1.肌瘤

2.肌壁间肌瘤

3.浆膜下肌瘤

4.黏膜下肌瘤

5.变性

6.玻璃样变

7.囊性变

8.红色变性

9.肉瘤变

10.假包膜

11.宫腔镜

12.腹腔镜

13.子宫造影术

练习题

1.子宫肌瘤合并妊娠最常见的改变是什么？（C）

A.玻璃样变性

---

preserving fertility with risk of recurrence.

- Hysterectomy— radical therapy.
- Subtotal hysterectomy.

■ Approaches

- TA/trans-abdominal.
- TV/trans-vaginal.
- LH/laparoscopic or hysteroscopic.
- Individualized treatment.

9.Uterine leiomyomas with pregnancy

（1）Effects on pregnancy: Abortion.

（2）Effects on delivery

■ Premature labor.

■ Fetal malpresentation.

■ Retained placenta.

■ Placenta previa.

■ Surgical midwifery

（Birth canal obstruction）.

■ Postpartum hemorrhage.

（3）Conservative treatment.

（4）Medical treatment.

Key words

1.Myoma

2.Intramural myoma

3.Subserous myoma

4.Submucous myoma

5.Degeneration

6.Hyaline degeneration

7.Cystic degeneration

8.Red degeneration

9.Sarcomatous Change

10.Pseudocapsule

11.Hysteroscopy

12.Laparoscopy

13.Hysterography

Exercises

1.What is the most common change in uterine myoma complicated with pregnancy?（C）

A.Hyaline degeneration

B.囊性变性

C.红色变性

D.肉瘤样变

E.钙化

2.子宫肌瘤的临床症状与下列哪项联系最大？（C）

A.肌瘤大小

B.肌瘤数目

C.肌瘤部位

D.患者年龄

E.是否生育

3.子宫肌瘤最常见的症状是：（C）

A.不规则阴道出血

B.白带增多

C.经量增多

D.慢性盆腔痛

E.反复流产

4.子宫肌瘤最常见的并发症是：（B）

A.红色变性

B.继发性贫血

C.浆膜下肌瘤蒂扭转

D.肌瘤压迫输尿管引起肾盂积水

E.恶变

5.子宫肌瘤短期内迅速增大或伴有阴道出血应考虑下列哪项？（E）

A.感染

B.囊性变

C.红色变性

D.脂肪样变

E.肉瘤变

（王学慧）

B.Cystic degeneration

C.Red degeneration

D.Sarcomatous change

E.Degeneration with calcification

2.Which of the following is most related to the clinical symptom of uterine myoma?（C）

A.Tumor size

B.Tumor number

C.Tumor site

D.The age of patient

E.Childbearing or not

3.The most common symptom of uterine myoma is:（C）

A.Irregular vaginal bleeding

B.Increased leucorrhea

C.Menorrhagia

D.Chronic pelvic pain

E.Recurrent abortion

4.The most common complication of uterine myoma is:（B）

A.Red degeneration

B.Secondary anemia

C.Pedicle torsion of subserous myoma

D.Hydronephrosis caused by myoma compression of ureter

E.Malignant change

5.If uterine myoma rapidly increase in short term or with vaginal bleeding, which of the following should be considered?（E）

A.Infection

B.Cystic degeneration

C.Red degeneration

D.Steatosis

E.Sarcomatous change

第17章 子宫内膜癌

CHAPTER 17 Endometrial carcinoma

CHAPTER 17 Endometrial carcinoma

子宫内膜癌为女性三大恶性肿瘤之一，占女性生殖道恶性肿瘤的20%～30%，平均发病年龄为60岁，其中75%发生于50岁以上女性。

1.病因

（1）高危因素

■ 雌激素

● 多囊卵巢综合征（PCOS）、肿瘤、无排卵型子宫出血、外源性的雌激素、激素替代治疗（HRT）。

● 子宫内膜增生：不伴有不典型的增生（单纯性增生和复杂性增生），不典型增生（AH）子宫内膜上皮内瘤变（EIN）。

■ 体质

● 肥胖、未育、晚绝经、无雌激素抵抗、糖尿病。

■ 遗传

● 林奇综合征。

（2）类型

■ Ⅰ型雌激素依赖型

● 多见。

● 病理类型是腺癌。

● 分化好，孕激素受体阳性，雌激素受体阳性，预后好。

● 患者通常较年轻，肥胖，高血压，糖尿病，不育等。

■ Ⅱ型非雌激素依赖型

Endometrial carcinoma（cancer of the corpus uteri）, is one of the three major malignant tumors in women, accounting for 20% ～ 30% of female reproductive tract malignant tumors. The average age of onset is 60 years old, of which 75% occur in women over 50 years old.

1.Etiology

（1）High risk factors

■ Estrogen

● Polycystic ovary syndrome（PCOS）, tumor, anovulatory uterine bleeding, external estrogen, hormone replacement therapy（HRT）.

● Endometrial hyperplasia: Hyperplasia without atypia（simple hyperplasia and complex hyperplasia）, atypical hyperplasia（AH）, endometrioid intraepithelial neoplasia（EIN）.

■ Constitution

● Obesity, nulliparity, late menopause, unopposed estrogen stimulation, diabetes.

■ Heredity

● Lynch syndrome.

（2）Types

■ Type Ⅰ estrogen-dependent

● More common.

● Pathology: Adenocarcinoma.

● Well differentated, PR（＋）, ER（＋）, good prognosis.

● Patients usually young, with obesity, hypertension, diabetes, infertility, etc.

■ Type Ⅱ non-estrogen-dependent

- 患者多为老年人，体型消瘦，病理类型特殊，浆乳癌等，治疗上按照卵巢癌来处理，预后差。

2.病理

（1）内膜样癌。

（2）浆液性癌。

（3）黏液性癌。

（4）透明细胞癌。

（5）癌肉瘤。

3.转移途径

（1）直接蔓延

- 癌灶可沿子宫内膜蔓延，向下至宫颈管及阴道，向上经宫角至输卵管，也可侵犯肌层至浆膜，并广泛种植在盆腔腹膜、道格拉斯陷凹和网膜。

（2）淋巴转移

- 为内膜癌的主要转移途径
  - 宫底部癌：沿阔韧带，骨盆漏斗韧带，卵巢，向上至腹主动脉旁淋巴结。

  - 宫角部癌：沿圆韧带，腹股沟淋巴结。
  - 子宫下段、宫颈管癌：沿主韧带宫旁、髂内、髂外、髂总淋巴结。

  - 后壁癌：沿子宫骶韧带，直肠淋巴结。
  - 子宫内膜癌还可累及膀胱和阴道。

（3）血行转移

- 少见，主要为晚期经血行转移。可转移至肺、肝、骨等处。

- Most patients elderly, emaciated, with special pathological type, and serous cancer, etc., treatment similar to that of ovarian cancer, poor prognosis.

2.Pathology

（1）Endometrioid carcinoma.

（2）Serous carcinoma.

（3）Mucinous carcinoma.

（4）Clear cell carcinoma.

（5）Carcinosarcoma.

3.Metastatic spread

（1）Direct spread

- Cancer focus can spread on the endometrium, down to cervix and vagina, up to fallopian tube through the uterine horn, even invade myometrium and serosa and widely implant on the pelvic peritoneum, pouch of Douglas and omentum.

（2）Lymphatic metastasis

- The chief metastatic path way.
  - Uterine fundus cancer: Along broad ligament, infundibulopelvic ligament, ovary, and up to paraaortic lymph nodes （LN）.

  - Uterine horn cancer: Along round ligament, inguinal lymph nodes （LN）.
  - Lower segment and cervical canal cancer: Along parauterine, internal iliac, external iliac and common iliac lymph nodes （LN）.

  - Posterior wall cancer: Along uterosacral ligament, rectal lymph nodes （LN）.
  - Endometrial cancer also affect bladder and vagina.

（3）Hematogenous spread

- Rare, mainly late stage. Possible transfer to lungs, liver, bone, ect.

4.临床分期

■ 手术－病理分期（表17-1）。

5.临床表现

■ 症状
  ● 极早期无明显症状。
  ● 阴道出血。
  ● 阴道排液。
  ● 腹痛。
  ● 全身症状。

6.诊断

（1）病史。
（2）症状。
（3）体征。

4.Clinical staging

■ Surgical-pathological staging（Table 17-1）.

5.Clinical manifestations

■ Symptoms
  ● No symptoms in early stage.
  ● Vaginal bleeding.
  ● Vaginal discharge.
  ● Abdominal pain.
  ● Systemic symptoms.

6.Diagnosis

（1）Medical history.
（2）Symptoms.
（3）Signs.

表17-1　子宫内膜癌手术－病理分期（FIGO，2009年）

Table 17-1　Surgical-pathological staging of cancer of the corpus uteri（FIGO, 2009）

Ⅰ期	肿瘤局限于子宫体 Tumor confined to the corpus uteri
ⅠA	肿瘤浸润深度＜1/2肌层 No or less than half myometrial invasion
ⅠB	肿瘤浸润深度≥1/2肌层 Invasion equal to or more than half of the myometrium
Ⅱ期	肿瘤侵犯宫颈间质，但无宫体外蔓延 Tumor invades cervical stroma, but does not extend beyond the uterus
Ⅲ期	肿瘤局部和（或）区域扩散 Local and/or regional spread of the tumor
ⅢA	肿瘤累及子宫浆膜和（或）附件 Tumor invades the serosa of the corpus uteri and/or adnexa
ⅢB	肿瘤累及阴道和（或）宫旁组织 Vaginal involvement and/or parametrial involvement
ⅢC	盆腔淋巴结和（或）腹主动脉旁淋巴结转移 Metastases to pelvic and/or para-aortic lymph nodes
ⅢC1	盆腔淋巴结转移 Positive pelvic nodes
ⅢC2	腹主动脉旁淋巴结转移伴（或不伴）盆腔淋巴结转移 Positive para-aortic nodes with or without positive pelvic lymph nodes
Ⅳ期	肿瘤侵及膀胱和（或）直肠黏膜，和（或）远处转移 Tumor invades bladder and/or bowel mucosa, and/or distant metastases
ⅣA	肿瘤侵及膀胱和（或）直肠黏膜 Tumor invasion of bladder and/or bowel mucosa
ⅣB	远处转移，包括腹腔内和（或）腹股沟淋巴结转移 Distant metastasis, including intra-abdominal metastases and/or inguinal nodes

（4）辅助检查。

■ 超声检查。

■ 诊断性刮宫，这是确诊内膜癌最常用的刮取内膜组织的方法。

■ 细胞学检查。

■ 宫腔镜检查。

■ CA125、CT、MRI。

7.鉴别诊断

（1）老年性阴道炎。

（2）黏膜下肌瘤。

（3）内膜息肉。

（4）原发性输卵管癌。

（5）宫颈癌、子宫肉瘤。

8.治疗

（1）手术

■ Ⅰ期：筋膜外全子宫切除术及双附件切除术，具有以下情况之一者，应行盆腔及腹主动脉旁淋巴结取样和（或）清扫术：

  ● 病理类型为透明细胞癌、浆液性癌。

  ● G3内膜样癌。

  ● 侵犯肌层深度＞1/2。

  ● 肿瘤＞2cm。

■ Ⅱ期：广泛子宫切除术及双侧盆腔淋巴结及腹主动脉旁淋巴结清扫术。术中取腹水查找癌细胞。

（2）手术加放疗

■ Ⅰ期：患者腹水中找到癌细胞或深肌层已有癌浸润，淋巴结已有转移，手术后均需加用放射治疗。

■ Ⅱ、Ⅲ期：根据病灶大小，可在术前加用外照射或腔内照射。放疗结束后1～2周进行手术。

（4）Auxiliary examination

■ Ultrasound examination.

■ Diagnostic curettage, the most common method for the diagnosis of endometrial cancer.

■ Cytology.

■ Hysteroscopy.

■ CA125, CT, MRI.

7.Differential diagnosis

（1）Senile vaginitis.

（2）Submucous myoma.

（3）Endometrial polyp.

（4）Primary carcinoma of fallopian tube.

（5）Cervical cancer, uterine sarcoma.

8.Treatment

（1）Surgery

■ Stage Ⅰ: Pelvic and para-aortic lymph node sampling and/or dissection performed in cases of total extrafascial hysterectomy and bilateral adnexectomy:

  ● The pathological types were clear cell carcinoma and serous carcinoma.

  ● G3 endometrial carcinoma.

  ● Invasion of muscular depth ＞ 1/2.

  ● The tumor ＞ 2 cm.

■ Stage Ⅱ: Extensive hysterectomy and bilateral pelvic lymph nodes and para-aortic lymph nodes dissection. Intraoperative ascites were taken to look for cancer cells.

（2）Surgery & radiotherapy

■ Stage Ⅰ: Cancer cells found in patients' ascites or deep muscularis carcinoma infiltration, lymph node metastasis, radiation treatment after surgery.

■ Stage Ⅱ and Ⅲ: Preoperative external or intracavitary irradiation, depending on the size of the lesion. Surgery performed within 1 ～ 2 weeks after radiotherapy.

（3）放疗

- 老年或有严重合并症不能耐受手术。
- Ⅲ、Ⅳ期病例不宜手术者均可考虑放射治疗。

（4）孕激素治疗

- 对晚期或复发癌患者，不能手术切除或年轻、早期、要求保留生育功能者，均可考虑孕激素治疗。

（5）化疗

- 晚期不能手术或治疗后复发者考虑使用化疗。常用的化疗药物有5-氟尿嘧啶（5-FU）、环磷酰胺（CTX）、丝裂霉素（MMC）。

9.随访

10.预防

重点专业词汇

1.子宫内膜癌

2.老年性阴道炎

3.黏膜下肌瘤

4.内膜息肉

5.原发性输卵管癌

6.子宫肉瘤

7.阴道出血

8.阴道排液

9.腹痛

10.雌激素依赖

11.腺癌

12.子宫内膜过度增生

13.体质因素

14.延迟绝经

15.分段诊刮

16.临床分期

17.子宫内膜不典型增生

练习题

1.早期诊断子宫内膜癌最可靠、

（3）Radiotherapy

- Old age, or with severe complications, no tolerance of surgery.
- Radiotherapy for patients in stage Ⅲ and Ⅳ, who are not suitable for surgery.

（4）Progesterone therapy

- For patients with advanced or recrudescent cancer who are not suitable for surgical excision, and who are young, at early stage and asking to preserve reproductive function.

（5）Chemotherapy

- For patients who cannot undergo surgery or relapse after treatment in the advanced stage. Commonly used chemotherapy drugs include 5-fluorouracil（5-FU）, cyclophosphamide（CTX）and mitomycin（MMC）.

9.Follow up

10.Prevention

Key words

1.Endometrial carcinoma（cancer of the corpus uteri）

2.Senile vaginitis

3.Submucous myoma

4.Endometrial polyp

5.Primary carcinoma of fallopian tube

6.Uterine sarcoma

7.Vaginal bleeding

8.Vaginal discharge

9.Abdominal pain

10.Estrogen-dependent

11.Adenocarcinoma

12.Over hyperplasia of endometrium

13.Constitutional factors

14.Postponed menopause

15.Fractional curettage

16.Clinical Staging

17.Atypical hyperplasia of endometrium

Exercises

1.Which is the most reliable and simplest

最简单的方法是什么？（B）

A.阴道涂片及细胞学检查

B.子宫分段刮宫及组织病理检查

C.宫内冲洗及细胞学检查

D.宫腔镜检查

E.超声

2.绝经2年，阴道不规则出血半个月。阴道未见充血，宫颈光滑，子宫略大，经刮宫，发现子宫内膜豆渣样。下列哪项是最可能的诊断？（B）

A.围绝经期月经紊乱

B.子宫内膜癌

C.生殖器结核

D.黏膜下肌瘤

E.子宫内膜息肉

3.治疗ⅠA期子宫内膜癌的最佳方法是什么？（A）

A.手术

B.放疗

C.化疗

D.化疗＋手术

E.孕激素治疗

4.下列哪一种子宫内膜疾病恶性程度最高？（A）

A.腺癌

B.腺鳞癌

C.腺瘤样增生

D.腺囊性增生

E.子宫内膜息肉

5.子宫内膜癌晚期患者和复发患者应选择哪种治疗方案？（D）

A.化疗

B.手术

C.放疗

method used to diagnose endometrial carcinoma in early stage?（B）

A.Vaginal smear and cytologic examination

B.Fractional curettage of uterus and histopathological examination

C.Intrauterine douche and cytologic examination

D.Hysteroscopic examination

E.Ultrasound

2.A woman has been in menopause for 2 years, and irregular vaginal bleeding for half a month. No vaginal congestion, cervix smooth, uterine slightly larger, by curettage, bean dregs-like endometrium found. Which of the following is the most possible diagnosis?（B）

A.Perimenopausal menstral disorder

B.Endometrial carcinoma

C.Genital tuberculosis

D.Submucous myoma

E.Endometrial polyp

3.Which is the best method to treat endometrial carcinoma of stage ⅠA?（A）

A.Surgery

B.Radiotherapy

C.Chemotherapy

D.Chemotherapy ＋ surgery

E.Progesterone therapy

4.Which of the following endometrial disorders is the most malignant?（A）

A.Adenocarcinoma

B.Adenosquamous carcinoma

C.Adenomatous hyperplasia

D.Cystic glandular hyperplasia

E.Endometrial polyp

5.Which kind of treatment chosen for endometrial carcinoma patients in late stage or a relapsed one?（D）

A.Chemotherapy

B.Surgery

C.Radiotherapy

D.孕激素治疗

E.化疗加手术

6.局限于子宫体的子宫内膜癌的主要治疗方式是：（B）

A.放疗

B.子宫切除术和双侧输卵管卵巢切除术

C.化疗

D.孕酮治疗

E.宫腔镜治疗

7.患有子宫内膜癌的女性最常出现下列哪一种症状？（C）

A.腹胀

B.体重减轻

C.绝经后出血

D.阴道流液

E.腹痛

8.子宫内膜癌的癌前病变是什么？（A）

A.子宫内膜不典型增生

B.子宫内膜息肉

C.子宫内膜腺瘤样增生

D.子宫内膜囊性增生

E.子宫内膜过度增生

9.56岁老年女性，主诉：绝经4年，阴道流液半年，阴道不规则出血半个月。妇科检查：宫颈正常，子宫体略大。最可能的诊断是什么？（A）

A.子宫内膜癌

B.急性宫颈炎

C.宫颈肌瘤

D.宫颈癌

E.慢性宫颈炎

（王学慧）

D.Progestogen treatment

E.Chemotherapy ＋ surgery

6.The primary mode of treatment for endometrial carcinoma limited in the uterine corpus is:（B）

A.Radiotherapy

B.Hysterectomy and bilateral salpingo-oophorectomy

C.Chemotherapy

D.Progestin therapy

E.Hysteroscopy

7.Which of the following symptoms is most common among women with endometrial carcinoma?（C）

A.Bloating

B.Weight loss

C.Postmenopausal bleeding

D.Vaginal discharge

E.Abdominal pain

8.Which is the preneoplastic change of the endometrial carcinoma?（A）

A.Atypical hyperplasia of endometrium

B.Polyp of endometrium

C.Adenomatous glandular hyperplasia of endometrium

D.Cystic hyperplasia of endometrium

E.Over hyperplasia of endometrium

9.A 56-year-old woman complains of postmenopausal status for 4 years; serous vaginal discharge for half a year; irregular vaginal bleeding for half a month. Pelvic examination: Cervix normal, the body of uterus slightly enlarged. What is the most likely diagnosis?（A）

A.Endometrial carcinoma

B.Acute cervicitis

C.Cervical myoma

D.Cervical cancer

E.Chronic cervicitis

第18章 卵巢肿瘤

CHAPTER 18 Ovarian tumor

CHAPTER 18 Ovarian tumor

卵巢是肿瘤好发部位。卵巢恶性肿瘤是女性生殖器三大恶性肿瘤之一。发病率仅次于宫颈癌和子宫内膜癌而居第三位，但死亡率居首位。目前仍缺乏有效的早期诊断方法。5年生存率30%左右。

Ovary is the predilection site of tumor. Ovarian malignant tumor is one of the three malignant tumors of female genital organs. Although ovarian tumor ranks third in terms of morbidity, after cervical cancer and endometrial cancer, the mortality of ovarian tumor is in the first place. There is still no effective early diagnosis method. The 5-year survival rate is about 30%.

第一节 概 述

Section 1 Introduction

1. 概述

- 卵巢肿瘤是女性生殖器常见肿瘤之一。卵巢肿瘤组织学类型最多，良性、恶性、交界性均可发生，不易早期发现。

1.Introduction

- Ovarian tumor is one of the most common tumors in female genital organs. Ovarian tumors have the most histological types, which can be benign, malignant and borderline, and difficult to discover in the early stage.

2. 组织学分类

（1）卵巢上皮性肿瘤

- 上皮性肿瘤占原发卵巢肿瘤的50%～70%，占卵巢恶性肿瘤的85%～90%。来源于卵巢表面的生发上皮，即来自原始的体腔上皮，具有分化各种苗勒上皮的潜能。

（2）生殖细胞肿瘤

- 生殖细胞肿瘤占卵巢肿瘤的20%～40%；来源于生殖腺

2. Histological classification

（1）Epithelial ovarian tumors

- Epithelial tumors account for 50% ～ 70% of primary ovarian tumors, and account for 85% ～ 90% of the malignant ovarian tumors. The germinal epithelium derived from the surface of the ovary, that is from the primitive coelothelium, has the potential to differentiate into various Mullerian epithelium.

（2）Germ cell tumors

- Germ cell tumors account for 20% ～ 40% of ovarian cancers; they originate from

以外的内胚叶组织；生殖细胞有发生所有组织的功能。

（3）性索间质肿瘤

■ 性索间质肿瘤占卵巢肿瘤的5%；来源于原始体腔的间叶组织，可向男女两性分化；肿瘤有内分泌功能，又称为功能性卵巢肿瘤。

（4）转移性肿瘤

■ 转移性肿瘤占卵巢肿瘤的5%～10%；原发部位常为胃肠道、乳腺及生殖器官。

3.组织学分级

（1）WHO分级标准主要依据组织结构，并参照细胞分化程度而分为3级：

■ 分化1级：高度分化。
■ 分化2级：中度分化。
■ 分化3级：低度分化。

（2）组织学分级对预后的影响较组织学类型更重要，组织分化越差，预后越差。

4.临床表现

（1）良性肿瘤：发展缓慢，早期多无症状。

（2）恶性肿瘤

■ 常表现为腹胀，腹部肿块及腹水。

■ 恶性肿瘤症状的轻重决定于：

● 肿瘤的大小，位置，侵犯邻近器官的程度。

endodermal tissues other than genital glands. Germ cells have the function of developing into all tissues.

（3）Sex cord stromal tumors

■ Sex cord stromal tumors account for 5% of ovarian cancers; they derive from mesenchymal tissue of primitive body cavity, which can differentiate into male and female. The tumor has the function of endocrine, also called functional ovarian tumor.

（4）Metastatic tumors

■ Metastatic tumors account for 5% ～ 10% of ovarian cancers; the primary sites are usually gastrointestinal tract, breast and reproductive organs.

3.Histological grades

（1）The WHO standard of histological grading is chiefly based on tissue structure and falls into 3 grades according to the degree of cell differentiation:

■ Grade Ⅰ: Highly differentiated.
■ Grade Ⅱ: Moderately differentiated.
■ Grade Ⅲ: Poorly differentiated.

（2）The effect of histological grades on the prognosis is more important than that of histological types. The worse the tissue differentiation, and the worse the prognosis.

4.Clinical manifestations

（1）Benign ovarian tumors: Slow development, asymptomatic at the early stage.

（2）Malignant ovarian tumors

■ The most common manifestations are abdominal distention, abdominal mass and ascites.

■ Severity of the symptoms depends on:

● Tumor size, location and extent of invasion of adjacent organs.

- 肿瘤的组织学类型。
- 有无并发症。

5.并发症

（1）蒂扭转。

（2）破裂。

（3）感染。

（4）恶变。

6.恶性肿瘤转移途径

（1）转移特点：外观局限肿瘤，却在腹膜、大网膜、腹膜后淋巴结、横膈等部位已有亚临床转移。主要直接蔓延到腹膜和网膜种植；淋巴转移也是重要途径；血行转移少见，终末期可转移到肝、肺、脑。

（2）淋巴道转移途径：沿着卵巢血管的走行，从卵巢淋巴管向上达腹主动脉旁淋巴结。从卵巢门淋巴管达髂内、髂外淋巴结，经髂总淋巴结至腹主动脉旁淋巴结。沿圆韧带入髂外及腹股沟淋巴结。

7.恶性肿瘤临床分期

（1）根据临床，手术和病理来分期，用以估计预后和比较疗效。

（2）具体分期如下（美国国家综合癌症网络临床实践指南2016版）：

Ⅰ期：肿瘤限于卵巢。

Ⅰa：肿瘤局限于一侧卵巢，包膜完整，表面无肿瘤，腹水或腹腔冲洗液中不含恶性肿瘤细胞。

Ⅰb：肿瘤局限于两侧卵巢，包膜完整，表面无肿瘤，腹水或腹腔冲洗液中不含恶性肿瘤细胞。

Ⅰc：Ⅰa或Ⅰb肿瘤，伴有以下任何一种情况：包膜破裂，卵巢

- Histological type of the tumor.
- Any complications.

5.Complications

（1）Torsion.

（2）Rupture.

（3）Infection.

（4）Malignant change.

6.Metastatic path way of malignant tumors

（1）Metastatic features: Subclinical metastases in peritoneum, omentum majus, retroperitoneal LN and diaphragm although the tumor is localized on its appearance. The tumor cells may directly invade and implant on the peritoneum and omentum. Lymphatic metastasis is also an important metastatic way. Blood metastasis is rare, and may transfer to the liver, lung and brain at a very late stage.

（2）Lymphatic vessels metastasis: Spreading along the ovarian blood vessels to para-aortic LN through ovarian lymphatic vessels. From ovarian hilus lymphatic vessels to internal and external iliac LN, then from the common iliac LN to para-aortic LN. Along the round ligament into the external iliac and inguinal LN.

7.Clinical stage of malignant tumors

（1）Staging is based on clinical,surgical and pathological conditions to estimate prognosis and compare efficacy.

（2）Specific stages are as follows（NCCN 2016）:

Stage Ⅰ Tumor confined to ovaries.

Ⅰa Tumor limited to one ovary, capsule intact, no tumor on ovarian surface, no malignant cells in the ascites or peritoneal washings.

Ⅰb Tumor limited to both ovaries（capsules intact）, no tumor on ovarian surface, no malignant cells in the ascites or peritoneal washings.

Ⅰc Based on Ia or Ib, tumor on the surface（unilateral or bilateral）; or capsule ruptured; or

表面有肿瘤，腹水或腹腔冲洗液中含恶性肿瘤细胞。

Ⅱ期： 一侧或双侧卵巢肿瘤，伴盆腔内扩散。

Ⅱa： 蔓延和（或）转移到子宫和（或）输卵管。

Ⅱb： 蔓延到其他盆腔组织。

Ⅱc： Ⅱa或Ⅱb肿瘤，腹水或腹腔冲洗液中含恶性肿瘤细胞。

Ⅲ期： 一侧或双侧卵巢肿瘤，伴显微镜下证实盆腔外有腹膜转移和（或）区域淋巴结转移，肝表面转移定为Ⅲ期。

Ⅲa： 显微镜下证实的盆腔外的腹腔转移。

Ⅲb： 一侧或双侧卵巢肿瘤，腹腔转移灶直径≤2cm，LN阴性。

Ⅲc： 腹腔转移灶直径＞2cm和（或）区域淋巴结转移。

Ⅳ期： 远处转移，除外腹腔转移（胸腔积液有癌细胞，肝实质转移）。

8.诊断

（1）年龄。

（2）病史。

（3）体征。

（4）辅助检查：超声检查；腹腔镜检查；放射学诊断；细胞学检查；肿瘤标志物；hCG（对原发性卵巢绒癌有特异性）；性激素。

9.鉴别诊断

（1）卵巢良性肿瘤与恶性肿瘤的鉴别。

（2）卵巢良性肿瘤鉴别诊断

■ 卵巢瘤样病变、输卵管卵巢囊肿、子宫肌瘤、妊娠子宫、腹水等。

malignant cells in ascites or in peritoneal washings.

Stage Ⅱ Unilateral or bilateral ovarian tumor with pelvic metastasis.

Ⅱa Spread to uterus and/or fallopian tube.

Ⅱb Spread to other tissues in pelvis.

Ⅱc Based on the IIa or IIb, malignant cells in ascites or peritoneal washings.

Stage Ⅲ Unilateral or bilateral ovarian tumor. Microscopic extrapelvic peritoneal metastasis and/or regional LN positive, liver surface metastasis.

Ⅲa Microscopic extrapelvic peritoneal metastasis.

Ⅲb Unilateral or bilateral ovarian tumor, peritoneal metastasis ≤ 2cm in diameter, LN negative.

Ⅲc Peritoneal metastasis is ＞ 2cm in diameter and/or regional LN positive.

Stage Ⅳ Distant metastasis, excluding peritoneal metastasis（cancer cells in hydrothorax, and liver parenchyma metastasis）.

8.Diagnosis

（1）Age.

（2）Medical history.

（3）Signs.

（4）Auxiliary examination: Ultrasound; laparoscopy; radio-diagnosis; cytologic examination; tumor markers; hCG（specific to primary ovarian choriocarcinoma）; sex hormone.

9.Differential diagnosis

（1）Differential diagnosis between benign and malignant ovarian tumors.

（2）Differential diagnosis of benign ovarian tumors

■ Ovarian neoplastic lesions, tubo-ovarian cyst, uterine myoma, pregnant uterus, ascites, etc.

（3）卵巢恶性肿瘤的鉴别诊断

■ 子宫内膜异位症；盆腔结缔组织炎；结核性腹膜炎；生殖道以外的肿瘤，转移性卵巢肿瘤。

10. 治疗

（1）恶性肿瘤一经确诊，即应手术治疗。

（2）恶性肿瘤治疗原则以手术为主，加用化疗和放疗的综合治疗。

11. 恶性肿瘤的预后

■ 与患者年龄、临床分期、组织学类型及分级、治疗方式等有关。

12. 恶性肿瘤的随访

（1）随访时间：术后1年，每月1次；术后2年，每3个月1次；术后3年，每6个月1次；3年以上者，每年1次。

（2）监测内容：临床症状、体征、全身及盆腔检查；超声，必要时CT、MRI；肿瘤标志物的测定。

13. 预防

■ 高危因素的预防；开展普查普治；早期发现及处理。

14. 妊娠合并卵巢肿瘤

（1）卵巢囊肿合并妊娠常见，但恶性肿瘤很少妊娠。妊娠合并良性肿瘤，以成熟囊性畸胎瘤及浆液性或黏液性囊腺瘤居多。恶性者以无性细胞瘤及浆液性囊腺癌为多。

（2）卵巢肿瘤对妊娠的影响
■ 妊娠早期：流产。
■ 妊娠晚期：胎位异常。

（3）Differential diagnosis of malignant ovarian tumors

■ Endometriosis; pelvic connective tissue inflammation; TB peritonitis; extra-reproductive tract tumors, metastatic ovarian tumors.

10.Treatment

（1）Once a malignant tumor is diagnosed, surgery is the first option.

（2）The principle of treatment for malignant tumors is surgery, combined with chemotherapy and radiotherapy.

11.Prognosis of malignant tumors

■ Depending on age, clinical stages, histological types, and treating methods.

12.Follow-up of malignant tumors

（1）Time of follow-up: Once a month, 1 year after surgery; once every 3 months, 2 years after surgery; once every 6 months, 3 years after surgery, and once a year for those with over 3 years' surgery.

（2）Monitoring contents: Symptoms, signs, general and pelvic examinations, ultrasound, CT and MRI if necessary and tumor marker.

13.Prevention

■ Prevention of high risk factors; popularization of regular examination and treatment; early diagnosis and treatment.

14.Pregnancy with ovarian tumors

（1）Ovarian cysts are common in pregnancy, but malignant tumors are rare. Benign tumors in pregnancy are mostly mature cystic teratoma and serous or mucinous cystadenoma. Most malignant tumors are dysgerminoma and serous cystadenocarcinoma.

（2）The effect of ovarian tumor on pregnancy
■ First trimester of pregnancy: Abortion.
■ Third trimester of pregnancy: Abnormal fetal position.

■ 分娩：难产。

（3）妊娠对卵巢肿瘤的影响

■ 妊娠早期：多无影响。

■ 妊娠中期：肿瘤易发生蒂扭转。

■ 分娩：肿瘤易发生破裂。

■ 妊娠时盆腔充血，肿瘤可迅速增大，并促使恶性肿瘤扩散。

（4）妊娠合并卵巢肿瘤的处理

■ 早孕合并卵巢囊肿，妊娠3个月进行手术。

■ 妊娠晚期发现者，剖宫产同时切除肿瘤。

■ 诊断或疑为卵巢恶性肿瘤，应尽早手术。

第二节　卵巢上皮性肿瘤

卵巢上皮性肿瘤是最常见的卵巢肿瘤；发病年龄为30～60岁；有良性、交界性、恶性之分。

1.发病的高危因素

（1）持续排卵；内分泌因素。

（2）遗传因素和家族因素。

（3）环境因素及生活习惯。

2.病理

（1）浆液性囊腺瘤：常见，约占良性肿瘤25%。多为单侧，有单纯性和乳头性两型。①圆形薄壁囊肿，外表光滑。②内含透明清亮液。

（2）交界性黏液性囊腺瘤：多为双侧，乳头状向囊外生长；5年生存率90%以上。

■ Delivery: Dystocia.

（3）The effects of pregnancy on ovarian tumor

■ First trimester of pregnancy: No effects.

■ Second trimester of pregnancy: Tumor is prone to pedicle torsion.

■ Delivery: Tumor is prone to rupture.

■ Pelvic congestion during pregnancy, the tumor can rapidly be enlarged, and promote the spread of malignant tumors.

（4）Treatment of ovarian tumors in pregnancy

■ Early pregnancy with ovarian cysts, surgery at 3 months of pregnancy.

■ Third trimester of pregnancy, cesarean section should be performed simultaneously with removal of the tumor.

■ Diagnosed or suspected ovarian malignant tumor should be operated as soon as possible.

Section 2　Epithelial ovarian tumor

Epithelial ovarian tumor is the most common ovarian tumor which occurs between 30～60 years old, which includes benign, borderline and malignant tumors.

1.High risks factors of ovarian tumor

（1）Incessant ovulation; endocrine factors.

（2）Hereditary and family factors.

（3）Environmental factors and lifestyle.

2.Pathology

（1）Serous cystadenoma: Common, accounting for 25% of benign tumors. Mostly unilateral, has simple type and papillary type. ①Circular cyst with a smooth and thin wall. ②Containing transparent clear liquid.

（2）Borderline mucinous cystadenoma: Mostly bilateral, papillary growth out of the cyst. 5-year survival rate above 90%.

（3）浆液性囊腺癌：最常见的卵巢恶性肿瘤，占40%～50%；多为双侧，体积较大，半实质性；5年存活率仅为20%～30%。

（4）黏液性囊腺瘤：占良性肿瘤的20%；多单侧，体积较大。

（5）交界性黏液性囊腺瘤：多发生在40岁左右，预后较好。

（6）黏液性囊腺癌：占恶性肿瘤的10%；单侧常见，囊壁可见乳头，囊实混合，囊液浑浊或血性；5年存活率为40%～50%。

（7）卵巢内膜样肿瘤：良性肿瘤，少见。多为单房，表面光滑，囊壁似正常子宫内膜腺上皮。5年生存率为40%～50%。

3.治疗

（1）良性肿瘤

- 若肿块直径＜5cm，疑为卵巢瘤样病变，可短期观察。

- 单侧良性肿瘤：患侧附件切除术/卵巢切除术/卵巢肿瘤剥出术。
- 双侧肿瘤：卵巢肿瘤剥出术，保留部分卵巢组织。
- 绝经后女性：全子宫及双附件切除术。

（2）交界性肿瘤

- 早期（Ⅰ期和Ⅱ期）：全子宫及双附件切除术；保留卵巢及生育功能的Ⅰ期年轻患者可行患侧附件切除术/卵巢肿瘤剥出术。

- 晚期（Ⅲ期和Ⅳ期）：同晚

（3）Serous cystadenocarcinoma: The most common type of ovarian malignant tumor, accounting for 40% ～ 50%; Mostly bilateral, relatively large, semi-solid; 5-year survival rate only 20% ～ 30%.

（4）Mucinous cystadenoma: Accounting for 20% of benign tumors; mostly unilateral, and bulky.

（5）Borderline mucinous cystadenoma: More occurring at 40 years old, with better prognosis.

（6）Mucinous cystadenocarcinoma: Accounting for 10% of malignant tumors; mostly unilateral, and with papillae on the cyst wall, cystic-solid mixed, the cystic fluid turbid or bloody. 5-year survival rate 40% ～ 50%.

（7）Ovarian endometrioid tumor: Benign tumor, rare. Mostly single cyst, with smooth endometrioid wall. 5-year survival rate 40% ～ 50%.

3.Treatment

（1）Benign ovarian tumor

- If mass diameter ＜ 5cm, suspection of ovarian tumor-like lesions, short-term observation.

- Unilateral benign tumor: The ipsilateral dysgerminoma/oophorectomy/ovarian tumorectomy.

- Bilateral tumor: Ovarian tumorectomy, retaining part of ovarian tissue.

- Perimenopausal women: Total hysterectomy and bilateral adnexectomy.

（2）Borderline ovarian tumor

- Stage Ⅰ and Ⅱ: Total hysterectomy and bilateral adnexectomy. For young patients with stage Ⅰ tumor, who need to preserve ovarian and reproductive function, the ipsilateral adnexectomy and ovarian tumorectomy can be performed.

- Stage Ⅲ and Ⅳ: The same as that of advanced

期卵巢癌。

（3）恶性肿瘤

- 治疗原则以手术为主，加用化疗、放疗的综合治疗。
  - 手术：一经疑为恶性肿瘤，尽早剖腹探查。
    - 手术范围：Ⅰa、Ⅰb期：全子宫及双附件切除术。Ⅰc期及以上：同时行大网膜切除术。Ⅱ期及其以上：肿瘤细胞减灭术。现多主张常规行后腹膜淋巴结清扫术。
  - 化疗：用于预防复发、晚期不能手术者。方法：静脉化疗、腹腔内化疗。

第三节　卵巢非上皮性肿瘤

1.包括
（1）生殖细胞肿瘤。
（2）性索间质肿瘤。

2.卵巢生殖细胞肿瘤
（1）畸胎瘤：成熟畸胎瘤；未成熟畸胎瘤。
（2）无性细胞瘤。
（3）内胚窦瘤。

3.卵巢性索间质瘤
（1）颗粒细胞-间质细胞瘤（颗粒细胞瘤、卵泡膜细胞瘤）。
（2）纤维瘤。
（3）支持-间质细胞瘤。

4.治疗
（1）良性生殖细胞或性索间质瘤
- 单侧肿瘤：卵巢肿瘤剥出术。

ovarian cancer.

（3）Malignant tumor

- Principle: Surgery, combined with chemotherapy and radiotherapy.
  - Surgery: Once suspected malignant tumor, laparotomy as soon as possible.
    - Scope of surgery: Stage Ia or Ib: Hysterectomy and bilateral adnexectomy; Stage Ic or above: Omentectomy at the same time. Stage Ⅱ or above: Cytoreductive surgery. Now conventional retroperitoneal lymph node dissection is recommended.
  - Chemotherapy: For the prevention of recurrence, and for advanced inoperable patients. Methods: Intravenous chemotherapy and intraperitoneal chemotherapy.

Section 3　Nonepithelial ovarian tumor

1.Content
（1）Ovarian germ cell tumors.
（2）Ovarian sex cord stromal tumors.

2.Ovarian germ cell tumors
（1）Teratoma: Mature, and immature.
（2）Dysgerminoma.
（3）Endodermal sinus tumor.

3.Ovarian sex cord stromal tumors
（1）Granulosa-stromal cell tumor（granulosa cell tumor, theca cell tumor）.
（2）Fibroma.
（3）Sertoli-Leydig cell tumor.

4.Treatment
（1）Benign germ cell or sex cord stromal tumor
- Unilateral: Ovarian tumorectomy.

■ 双侧肿瘤：卵巢肿瘤剥出术，保留部分卵巢组织。

■ 围绝经期女性（＞50岁）：全子宫及双附件切除术。

（2）恶性生殖细胞及性索间质肿瘤

■ 手术治疗

● Ⅰ期希望生育的年轻患者：患侧附件切除术。

● Ⅰ期不希望生育：全子宫及双附件切除术。

● 晚期肿瘤：肿瘤减灭术。

■ 化疗。

■ 放疗

● 无性细胞瘤最敏感。

● 颗粒细胞瘤中度敏感。

5.转移性肿瘤

（1）手术：全子宫及双附件切除术，并切除其他部位容易切除的肿瘤原发病灶。

（2）化疗：根据原发肿瘤特征，辅以化疗。

重点专业词汇

1.蒂扭转

2.破裂

3.感染

4.恶变

5.畸胎瘤

6.无性细胞瘤

7.内胚窦瘤

8.卵巢性索间质瘤

9.颗粒细胞－间质细胞瘤

10.颗粒细胞瘤

11.卵泡膜细胞瘤

12.纤维瘤

13.支持－间质细胞瘤

14.卵巢转移性肿瘤

■ Bilateral tumor: Ovarian tumorectomy, retaining part of ovarian tissue.

■ Perimenopausal women（＞50 years old）: Total hysterectomy and bilateral adnexectomy.

（2）Malignant germ cell or sex cord stromal tumor

■ Surgery treatment

● Stage Ⅰ young patients with fertility needs: The ipsilateral adnexectomy.

● Stage Ⅰ young patients without fertility needs: Total hysterectomy and bilateral adnexectomy.

● Late stage tumor: Cytoreductive surgery.

■ Chemotherapy.

■ Radiotherapy

● Dysgerminoma, the most sensitive.

● Granulosa cells tumor, moderately sensitive.

5.Metastatic tumor

（1）Surgery: Total hysterectomy and bilateral adnexectomy, and resection of primary focus.

（2）Chemotherapy: Combined with chemotherapy according to the characteristics of primary tumor.

Key words

1.Torsion

2.Rupture

3.Infection

4.Malignant change

5.Teratoma

6.Dysgerminoma

7.Endodermal sinus tumor

8.Ovarian sex cord stromal tumor

9.Granulosa-stromal cell tumor

10.Granulosa cell tumor

11.Theca cell tumor

12.Fibroma

13.Sertoli-Leydig cell tumor

14.Ovarian metastatic tumor

15.卵巢上皮性肿瘤

16.肿瘤细胞减灭术

17.浆液性囊腺瘤

18.黏液性囊腺瘤

练习题

1.卵巢肿瘤最常见的来源：（A）

A.生发上皮

B.非特异间质

C.索间质

D.原始生殖细胞

E.生殖细胞

2.内胚窦肿瘤是通过分泌下列哪一种肿瘤标志物来识别的？（C）

A.hCG

B.CEA

C.AFP

D.CA125

E.CA199

3.Meigs综合征与下列哪一种肿瘤有关？（B）

A.盆腔结核

B.卵巢纤维瘤

C.浆膜下肌瘤

D.颗粒细胞瘤

E.卵泡膜细胞瘤

4.哪种卵巢肿瘤对放射治疗最敏感？（C）

A.畸胎瘤

B.浆液性囊腺癌

C.无性细胞瘤

D.黏液性囊腺癌

E.颗粒细胞瘤

5.以下哪种肿瘤不是卵巢体腔上皮来源的肿瘤？（E）

A.浆液性囊腺瘤

B.黏液性囊腺瘤

C.子宫内膜样肿瘤

15.Epithelial ovarian tumor

16.Cytoreductive surgery

17.Serous cystadenoma

18.Mucinous cystadenoma

Exercises

1.Ovarian neoplasms most commonly arise from:（A）

A.Germinal epithelium

B.Nonspecific mesenchyma

C.Sex cord stroma

D.Primitive germ cells

E.Germ cells

2.Endodermal sinus tumors identified by secretion from which of the following tumor marker?（C）

A.hCG

B.CEA

C.AFP

D.CA125

E.CA199

3.Which of the following tumors is associated with Meigs syndrome?（B）

A.Pelvic tuberculosis

B.Ovarian fibroma

C.Subserous myoma

D.Granulosa cell tumor

E.Theca cell tumor

4.Which of the ovarian tumors is the most sensitive to radiation therapy?（C）

A.Teratoma

B.Serous cystadenocarcinoma

C.Dysgeminoma

D.Mucinous cystadenocarcinoma

E.Granulosa cell tumor

5.Which of the following tumors is not from the epithelium of the ovary?（E）

A.Serous cystadenoma

B.Mucinous cystadenoma

C.Endometrioid tumor

D.透明细胞瘤

E.卵泡膜细胞瘤

6.哪种卵巢良性上皮肿瘤易恶变？（E）

A.黏液性囊腺瘤

B.浆液性囊腺瘤

C.子宫内膜样肿瘤

D.纤维上皮瘤

E.透明细胞瘤

7.病例：女，34岁，体检发现右附件区包块6个月，无自觉症状，超声提示右附件3cm×4cm包块，内为液性暗区。

问题：（1）该患者可能的诊断。

（2）如何处理？

（王学慧）

D.Hyaline cell tumor

E.Theca cell tumor

6.Which ovarian benign epithelial tumor is prone to malignant change?（E）

A.Mucinous cystadenoma

B.Serous cystadenoma

C.Endometrioid tumor

D.Fibroepithelioma

E.Hyaline cell tumor

7.Case: Female, 34 years old, physical examination revealed a mass in the right adnexal area for half a year, with no symptoms, ultrasound indicated a mass of 3cm×4cm in the right adnexal area with a liquid area.

Question:（1）Possible diagnosis for the patient.

（2）How to deal with?

第19章 子宫颈肿瘤

CHAPTER 19 Cervical tumor

第一节 子宫颈鳞状上皮内病变

宫颈鳞状上皮内病变（SIL）是与子宫颈浸润癌密切相关的一组子宫颈病变，常发生于25～35岁女性。

1.发病相关因素

（1）HPV感染：尤其与高危HPV16/18型相关。

（2）性行为及分娩次数：多个性伴侣、初次性生活＜16岁、早年分娩、多产。

（3）其他：吸烟可增加感染HPV效应。

2.组织学特点

■ 转化区（移行带）：因其位于子宫颈鳞状上皮与柱状上皮交界处，又称为鳞-柱状交接部，为SIL好发部位。

3.病理学诊断和分级

（1）根据感染的程度和部位进行分级，反映宫颈病变发生发展中的连续过程。

（2）SIL既往称为"子宫颈上皮内瘤变（CIN）"，现采用二级分类法，即（LSIL和HSIL）。

（3）CIN Ⅰ级：轻度异型。异形细胞＜上皮下1/3层，细胞排列稍

Section 1　Cervical squamous intraepithelial lesion

Cervical squamous intraepithelial lesion(SIL) is defined as a group of cervical lesions that are closely related to cervical invasive carcinoma, often occur in women aged 25～35.

1.Risk factors

（1）HPV infection: especially associated with high-risk HPV 16 or 18.

（2）Sexual activity and number of births: Multiple sexual partners, first sex＜16 years old, early delivery, and multiple births.

（3）Others: Cigarette smoking can increase the effect of HPV infection.

2.Cervical histology

■ Transformation zone: The junction between columnar mucous epithelium and nonkeratinized stratified squamous epithelium is called squamo-columnar junction, where SIL mostly occurs.

3.Pathological diagnosis and grading

（1）Grading depends on the degree and location of infection, which reflects the continuous process of cervical lesion.

（2）SIL traditionally referred to as CIN (cervical intraepithelial neoplasia), and secondary classification used at present（LSIL and HSIL）.

（3）CIN Ⅰ: Mild dysplasia, abnormal cells confined to the basal 1/3 of the epithelium, with

紊乱，细胞异形性轻。

（4）CINⅡ级：中度异型。异形细胞＜上皮下1/3～2/3，细胞排列紊乱，细胞异型明显。

（5）CINⅢ级：重度异型和原位癌。异形细胞＞2/3或全部上皮层。

（6）LSIL相当于CINⅠ，HSIL包括CINⅢ和大部分CINⅡ，CINⅡ用p16免疫组化染色，p16染色阴性按LSIL处理，p16染色阳性按HSIL处理。

4.临床表现

■ 无特殊症状。

5.诊断

（1）子宫颈细胞学检查：既往采用巴氏涂片法。现在采用液基细胞涂片法，SIL及早期子宫颈癌筛查的基本方法。

■ 筛查应该在性生活开始3年后开始，或21岁以后开始，并定期复查。

（2）高危型HPV-DNA检测。

（3）阴道镜检查。

（4）子宫颈活组织检查：确诊子宫颈鳞状上皮内病变的最可靠方法。任何肉眼可见病灶，均应做单点或多点活检。

6.治疗

（1）LSIL：低度病变，不足2年观察随访。

（2）HSIL：高度病变需治疗

■ 子宫颈锥切术。

■ 冷灼法。

■ 电环切除术（LEEP）。

slightly disordered cell arrangement.

（4）CINⅡ: Moderate to marked dysplasia, confined to the basal 1/3 ～ 2/3 of the epithelium, with cells disordered.

（5）CINⅢ: Severe dysplasia and carcinoma in situ, confined to ＞2/3 of the epithelium, and may involve the full thickness.

（6）LSIL is equivalent to CINⅠ, HSIL includes CINⅢ and most CINⅡ, CINⅡ uses p16 immunohistochemical staining, if p16 staining negative, the same treatment as that of LSIL; if p16 staining positive the same as HSIL.

4.Clinical manifestation

■ No typical symptoms.

5.Diagnosis

（1）Cervical cytology: Pap smear used in the past; at present, liquid-based cell smear, and basic screening methods for SIL and early cervical cancer are used.

■ Screening should begin 3 years after sexual activity or after the age of 21 with regular reexamination.

（2）High risk HPV-DNA detection.

（3）Colposcopy.

（4）Biopsy of cervix: The most reliable diagnosis method for SIL, single or multiple biopsies for any visible lesion.

6.Treatment

（1）LSIL: Mild dysplasia, observation and follow-up, if less than 2 years.

（2）HSIL: Treatment

■ Cervical conization.

■ Cryocautery.

■ Loop electrical excision procedure(LEEP).

第二节 子宫颈癌

1.概述

宫颈癌是最常见的妇科恶性肿瘤，发病年龄为50～55岁。

发病相关因素：同"SIL"。

流行病学：世界范围。

宫颈癌是导致女性癌症患者死亡的第四大肿瘤因素。在2012年，调查528 000名宫颈癌患者中有266 000名死亡。宫颈癌是仅次于乳腺癌的第二大女性常见癌症，导致约8%的总死亡率和女性癌症死亡率。宫颈癌患者中，约有80%存在于发展中国家。

2.病理

（1）鳞状细胞浸润癌：占子宫颈癌的75%～80%。

- 巨检
  - 外生型：最常见，菜花头。

  - 内生型：宫颈体积增大，质硬，呈桶状。
  - 溃疡型：可形成空洞，似火山口。
  - 宫颈管型：癌灶发生于颈管内。
- 镜检
  - 微小浸润癌

    ①原位癌基础上，在镜下发现癌细胞小团似泪滴状、锯齿状穿破基底膜，浸润间质。

    ② I A1间质浸润深度＜3 mm，水平扩散≤7 mm。

    ③ I A2间质浸润深度3～5 mm，水平扩散≤7 mm。

Section 2　Cervical cancer

1.Introduction

Cervical cancer is the most common gynecological malignancy. The age of onset is 50～55 years old.

Risk factors: See "SIL".

Epidemiology: Worldwide.

Cervical cancer is the fourth leading cause of cancer death in women. In 2012, 266 000 of the 528 000 cervical cancer patients surveyed died. It is the second most common cancer in women after breast cancer, causing about 8% of both total mortality and female cancer mortality. About 80% of cervical cancers occur in developing countries.

2.Pathology

（1）Invasive squamous cell carcinoma: Accounting for 75%～80% of cervical cancers.

- Gross appearance
  - Exophytic type: Most common, like a cauliflower top.
  - Entophytic type: Cervix enlarged, hard, and barrel-shaped.
  - Ulcerative type: Forming hollows, like craters.
  - Endocervical type: Carcinoma occurred in cervical canal.
- Microscopic appearance
  - Microinvasive carcinoma

    ①Microscopically, small clusters of cancer cells are teardrop-like and serrated, penetrating basement membrane and infiltrating stroma.

    ② I A1 depth of stromal invasion＜3 mm, and horizontal extension≤7 mm.

    ③ I A2 depth of stromal invasion 3～5 mm, and horizontal extension≤7 mm.

- 宫颈浸润癌
  - ① Ⅰ级——>角化性大细胞型，分化好，核分裂象＜2/HP。
  - ② Ⅱ级——>非角化性大细胞型，中度分化，细胞大小不一，核分裂象2～4/HP。
  - ③ Ⅲ级——>小细胞型，低分化，核分裂象＞4/HP。

（2）腺癌：占宫颈癌的20%～25%。

- 巨检
  - 来自颈管内，浸润管壁，形如桶状，或向宫颈外口突出生长。
- 显微镜检
  - 黏液腺癌：最常见。

  - 恶性腺癌：又名微腺癌，实际上是一种分化很高的黏液腺癌，内生性型，分泌大量黏液，扩散早，预后差。

  - 鳞腺癌：占宫颈癌的3%～5%。
  - 其他：如神经内分泌癌。

3.转移途径

（1）直接蔓延，最常见。

（2）淋巴转移

- 一级：包括宫旁，宫颈旁，闭孔，髂内、髂外、髂总、骶前淋巴结。

- 二级：包括腹股沟深浅淋巴结及腹主动脉旁淋巴结。

- Invasive carcinoma of cervix
  - ① Ⅰ — > Large-cell keratinized type, well differentiated, karyokinesis ＜ 2/HP.
  - ② Ⅱ — > Large-cell non-keratinized type, moderately differentiated, with cells varying in size, karyokinesis 2 ～ 4/HP.
  - ③ Ⅲ — > small cell type, poorly differentiated, karyokinesis ＞ 4/HP.

（2）Adenocarcinoma: Accounting for 20% ～ 25% of cervical cancers.

- Gross appearance
  - From inside the cervix, invading the wall of cervical canal, barrel-shaped, growing outside the cervix.
- Microscopic appearance
  - Mucinous adenocarcinoma: most common.
  - Malignant adenocarcinoma: Also known as micro-adenocarcinoma, a highly differentiated mucinous adenocarcinoma, endogenous, secreting a large amount of mucus, spreading early, with poor prognosis.
  - Adenosquamous carcinoma: Accounting for 3% ～ 5% of cervical cancers.
  - Others: Neuroendocrine carcinoma.

3.Metastatic spread

（1）Direct extension, most common.

（2）Lymphatic metastasis

- Class A: Lymph nodes adjacent to the uterus, and cervix, obturator lymph nodes, internal iliac lymph nodes, exlernal iliac lymph nodes, common iliac lymph nodes, and presacral lymph nodes.

- Class B: Including deep inguinal lymph nodes, superficial inguinal lymph nodes,

（3）血行转移，极少见。

4.临床分期

Ⅰ期 肿瘤局限于宫颈（扩展至宫体应被忽略）。

  ⅠA 镜下浸润癌（所有肉眼可见的病灶，包括表浅浸润，均为ⅠB期）。局限间质浸润，间质浸润深度＜5mm，宽度≤7mm。

  ⅠA1 间质浸润深度≤3mm，宽度≤7mm。

  ⅠA2 间质浸润深度＞3mm且＜5mm，宽度≤7mm。

  ⅠB 肉眼可见癌灶局限于子宫颈，或者镜下病灶＞ⅠA。

  ⅠB1 肉眼可见癌灶≤4cm。

  ⅠB2 肉眼可见癌灶＞4cm。

Ⅱ期 肿瘤超越子宫，但未达骨盆壁或未达阴道下1/3。

  ⅡA 肿瘤侵犯阴道上2/3，无明显宫旁浸润。

  ⅡA1 肉眼可见癌灶≤4cm。

  ⅡA2 肉眼可见癌灶＞4cm。

  ⅡB 有明显宫旁浸润，但未达到盆壁。

Ⅲ期 肿瘤已扩展到骨盆壁，在进行直肠指诊时，在肿瘤和盆壁之间无间隙。

and abdominal aortic lymph nodes.

（3）Hematogenous metastasis: Rare.

4.Clinical staging

Stage Ⅰ The carcinoma is strictly confined to the cervix（extension to the uterine corpus should be disregarded）

  ⅠA Invasive cancer identified only microscopically（All gross lesions even with superficial invasion are Stage ⅠB cancers）. Invasion is limited to measured stromal invasion with a maximum depth of 5 mm and ≤ 7 mm width.

  ⅠA1 Measured invasion of stroma ≤ 3 mm in depth and ≤ 7 mm width.

  ⅠA2 Measured invasion of stroma ＞ 3 mm and ＜ 5 mm in depth and ≤ 7 mm width.

  ⅠB Clinically visible lesion confined to the cervix, or preclinical lesions greater than stage ⅠA.

  ⅠB1 Clinically visible lesion ≤ 4 cm in size.

  ⅠB2 Clinically visible lesion ＞ 4 cm in size.

Stage Ⅱ The carcinoma extends beyond the uterus, but has not extended onto the pelvic wall or to the lower third of vagina.

  ⅡA Involvement of up to the upper 2/3 of the vagina, no obvious parametrial involvement.

  ⅡA1 Clinically visible lesion ≤ 4 cm.

  ⅡA2 Clinically visible lesion ＞ 4 cm.

  ⅡB Obvious parametrial involvement but not onto the pelvic sidewall.

Stage Ⅲ The carcinoma has extended onto the pelvic sidewall, on rectal examination, there is no cancer

肿瘤累及阴道下1/3。由肿瘤引起的肾盂积水或肾无功能的所有病例，除非已知由其他原因所引起。

ⅢA 肿瘤累及阴道下1/3，没有扩展到骨盆壁。

ⅢB 肿瘤扩展到骨盆壁，或引起肾盂积水或肾无功能。

Ⅳ期 肿瘤超出了真骨盆范围，或侵犯膀胱和（或）直肠黏膜。

ⅣA 肿瘤侵犯邻近的盆腔器官。

ⅣB 远处转移。

5.临床表现

（1）阴道出血：接触性出血（同房出血是最常见症状）。

（2）阴道排液。

（3）晚期宫颈癌的症状：食欲缺乏、体重减轻、乏力、盆腔疼痛、大量阴道出血、骨折。

6.诊断

强调早期诊断，强调"三阶梯"诊断程序。

（1）宫颈细胞学检查

■ 液基薄层细胞学检查（TCT）。

■ 宫颈刮片（巴氏法）

Ⅰ级 正常。

Ⅱ级 炎症。

Ⅲ级 可疑癌前病变。

Ⅳ级 可见1～2个恶性细胞，可疑阳性。

free space between the tumor and pelvic sidewall. The tumor involves the lower third of the vagina. All cases of hydronephrosis or non-functioning kidney should be included unless they are known to be due to other cause.

ⅢA Involvement of the lower vagina but no extension onto pelvic sidewall.

ⅢB Extension onto the pelvic sidewall, or hydronephrosis/non-functioning kidney.

Stage Ⅳ The carcinoma has extended beyond the true pelvis or has clinically involved the mucosa of the bladder and /or rectum.

ⅣA Spread to adjacent pelvic organs.

ⅣB Spread to distant organs.

5.Clinical manifestations

（1）Vaginal bleeding: Contact bleeding（one most common form being bleeding after sexual intercourse）.

（2）Vaginal discharge.

（3）Symptoms of advanced cervical cancer: Loss of appetite, weight loss, fatigue, pelvic pain, heavy vaginal bleeding, and bone fractures.

6.Diagnosis

Early diagnosis, the "three ladders" diagnostic program.

（1）Cervical cytology

■ Thinprep cytologic test（TCT）.

■ Pap smear, Bethesda system classification

Ⅰ—Normal.

Ⅱ—Inflammatory.

Ⅲ—Suspected precancerous lesion.

Ⅳ—1～2 malignant cells, suspected to be positive.

Ⅴ级　较多恶性细胞，阳性。

（2）高危型HPV-DNA检测。

（3）阴道镜检查。

■ TCT异常或Bethesda系统分类＞Ⅲ级，HPV16阳性。

（4）宫颈活检及宫颈管搔刮术：确诊方法。

（5）宫颈冷刀锥切术。

7.鉴别诊断

（1）宫颈柱状上皮异位与息肉。

（2）宫颈乳头状瘤。

（3）子宫黏膜下肌瘤。

（4）宫颈结核。

（5）宫颈与阴道穹窿的子宫内膜异位症。

8.处理原则

（1）手术和放疗为主、化疗为辅的综合治疗。

（2）根据患者的个体化，年龄，生殖目标，功能状态和获得医疗保健资源进行治疗。

（3）根据宫颈癌FIGO分期选择治疗方式：

■ 手术治疗适合ⅠA～ⅡA

- ⅠA1期：年轻患者可行筋膜外全子宫切除术；绝经后女性可行全子宫切除，卵巢正常者可予保留；要求保留生育者可行宫颈锥切术。

- ⅠA2期：改良根治性子宫切除术＋盆腔淋巴结切除术，卵巢正常者可予以保留。

- ⅠB1、ⅡA1期：广泛性子宫切除术＋盆腔淋巴结切除术，必要时腹主动脉旁淋巴结取样。

- ⅠB2、ⅡA2期：广泛性

Ⅴ—Many malignant cells, positive.

（2）High risk HPV-DNA detection.

（3）Colposcopy.

■ TCT abnormal or Bethesda system classification ＞Ⅲ or HPV16（＋）.

（4）Biopsy of cervix and endocervical curettage（ECC）: Diagnostic method.

（5）Cold knife conization（CKC）.

7.Differential diagnosis

（1）Cervical ectropion and polyp.

（2）Cervical papilloma.

（3）Submucosal myoma of uterus.

（4）Cervical tuberculosis.

（5）Endometriosis on cervix or vaginal fornix.

8.Principles of treatment

（1）Surgery and radiotherapy with chemotherapy.

（2）Treatment is individualized to the patients, based on age, reproductive goals, functional status, and access to health care resources.

（3）Treatment according to the FIGO stages of cervical carcinoma:

■ Surgical treatment for ⅠA～ⅡA

- Stage ⅠA1: In young individuals, extrafascial hysterectomy; in post reproductive age total-hysterectomy, ovarian normal can be reserved; conization for younger women who want to preserve fertility.

- Stage ⅠA2: Modified radical hysterectomy ＋pelvic lymphadenectomy, ovarian normal can be reserved.

- Stage ⅠB1 and ⅡA1: Radical hysterectomy ＋pelvic lymphadenectomy ＋abdominal aortic lymph node sampling if necessary.

- Stage ⅠB2 and ⅡA2: Radical

子宫切除术＋盆腔淋巴结切除术＋腹主动脉淋巴结取样，同期放、化疗后行全子宫切除术。

■ 化疗或姑息疗法（也取决于以前使用的治疗方法），ⅡB～ⅣA期

  • 主要用于ⅣB晚期或复发转移患者。

配伍方案：

  ①TP（顺铂和紫杉醇）。

  ②BVP（博来霉素、长春新碱、顺铂）。

  ③BP（博来霉素、顺铂）。

■ 一般采用放疗（顺铂作为放射增敏剂）。由于存在明显的阳性边缘和阳性淋巴结的风险，这组女性不接受手术。

9.预后（表19-1）

（1）预后与临床期别Ⅰ＞Ⅱ＞Ⅲ＞Ⅳ。

（2）病理类型。

（3）有无淋巴结转移。

（4）治疗是否合理。

10.预防

（1）普及防癌知识，开展性卫生教育，提倡晚婚，少育。

（2）定期开展宫颈癌的普查普治工作。

（3）积极治疗宫颈上皮瘤变，

hysterectomy ＋ pelvic lymphadenectomy ＋ abdominal aortic lymph node sampling, total hysterectomy after concurrent radiotherapy and chemotherapy.

■ Chemotherapy or palliative therapy（also depending on previous treatments）. Stage ⅡB～ⅣA

  • Stage ⅣB and recurrent cancer.

Protocol:

  ①TP（cisplatin and pacilitaxel）.

  ②BVP（bleomycin, vincristine and cisplatin）.

  ③BP（bleomycin and cisplatin）.

■ Generally radiotherapy（cisplatin used as radiosensitizer）. Surgery is not recommended due to the significant risk of positive margins and positive nodes.

9.Prognosis（Table 19-1）

（1）Prognosis and clinical staging Ⅰ＞Ⅱ＞Ⅲ＞Ⅳ.

（2）Pathological type.

（3）With or without lymph node metastasis.

（4）Reasonable treatment or not.

10.Prevention

（1）Popularizing the knowledge of preventing cancer, and education of sex hygiene, encourage late marriage and fewer childbearing.

（2）Regular screening and general treatment of cervical cancer.

（3）Active treatment of CIN and the use of

表19-1　宫颈癌5年生存率

Table 19-1　Five-year survival rate of cervical cancer

	Ⅰ	Ⅱ	Ⅲ	Ⅳ
手术 Surgery	＞90%	80%	40%	10%
放疗 Radiotherapy	93%	82%	63%	26%

HPV疫苗的使用。

（4）重视高危因素及高危人群，有异常症状者及时就医。

11.随访

（1）宫颈癌治疗后复发50%在1年内，75%～80%在2年内。

（2）出院后1个月随访，以后，2年内3个月1次；3～5年6个月1次；再以后每年1次。

重点专业词汇

1.子宫颈癌

2.子宫颈上皮内瘤变（CIN）

3.子宫颈鳞状上皮内病变（SIL）

4.转化区（移行带）

5.阴道镜检查

6.接触性出血

7.阴道排液

8.液基薄层细胞学检查

9.疫苗

10.随访

11.筛查

12.子宫颈环形电切术（LEEP）

13.子宫颈锥切术

14.冷灼法

15.微小浸润癌

16.外生型

17.菜花样

18.内生型

19.溃疡型

20.宫颈管型

21.腺癌

22.转移

练习题

1.普查宫颈癌时最有实用价值的检查方法是：（A）

HPV vaccine.

（4）Paying attention to high-risk factors and high-risk groups. Timely medical treatments for patients with abnormal symptoms.

11.Follow-up

（1）50% of cervical cancer recurrences within one year after surgery, and 75% ～ 80% within 2 years.

（2）Follow-up one month after discharge and once every 3 months within 2 years; once every 6 months in 3 ～ 5 years; once a year thereafter.

Key words

1.Cervical cancer

2.Cervical intraepithelial neoplasia（CIN）

3.Cervical squamous intraepithelial lesion（SIL）

4.Transformation zone

5.Colposcopy

6.Contact bleeding

7.Vaginal discharge

8.TCT

9.Vaccinum

10.Follow-up

11.Screening test

12.Loop electrosurgical excision procedure（LEEP）

13.Cervical conization

14.Cryocautery

15.Microinvasive carcinoma

16.Exophytic type

17.Cauliflower type

18.Entophytic type

19.Ulcerative type

20.Endocervical type

21.Adenocarcinoma

22.Metastasis

Exercises

1.The most valuable approach to screen cervical cancer is:（A）

A.宫颈细胞学检查

B.宫颈碘试验

C.妇科三合诊检查

D.阴道镜检查

E.宫颈活组织检查

2.女，45岁。性交后出血6个月。妇科检查：宫颈Ⅰ度糜烂状。宫颈细胞学检查结果为低度鳞状上皮内病变（LSIL）。为明确诊断，下一步首选的处理是：（C）

A.宫颈冷刀锥切（CKC）

B.宫颈环形电切除术（LEEP）

C.阴道镜下活检

D.宫颈管搔刮

E.HPV-DNA检测

3.女，38岁，接触性出血1个月余，白带有恶臭，妇科检查：宫颈Ⅱ度糜烂，前唇有5cm×3cm的质地脆赘生物，易出血。子宫正常大，三合诊（－）。确诊后，其临床期别为：（C）

A.ⅠA期

B.ⅠB1期

C.ⅠB2期

D.ⅡA期

E.ⅡB期

4.女，53岁。接触性出血1个月。妇科检查：宫颈后唇有一菜花样新生物，接触性出血阳性，宫体大小正常，双侧附件未触及异常。该患者最可能的诊断是：（D）

A.子宫内膜癌

B.急性宫颈癌

C.宫颈肌瘤

D.宫颈癌

E.慢性宫颈炎

A.Cervical cytology

B.Cervical iodine test

C.Trimanual gynecologic examination

D.Colposcopy

E.Biopsy of cervix

2.A 45-year-old female has bleeding after sexual intercourse for half a year. Gynecological examination: Cervix erosion degree Ⅰ, TCT: LSIL. For clear diagnosis, the next preferred treatment is: （C）

A.Cold knife conization （CKC）

B.Loop electrosurgical excision procedure （LEEP）

C.Biopsy under colposcope

D.Endocervical curettage

E.HPV-DNA detection

3.A 38-year-old female has contact bleeding for over a month with foul smelling leukorrhea. Gynecological examination: Cervix erosion degree Ⅱ, a 5cm×3cm fragile neoplasm in anterior lip, prone to bleeding. The size of uterus normal, trimanual gynecologic examination （－）. After diagnosed, the clinical stage is: （C）

A.Stage Ⅰ A

B.Stage Ⅰ B1

C.Stage Ⅰ B2

D.Stage Ⅱ A

E.Stage Ⅱ B

4.A 53-year-old female has contact bleeding for over a month. Gynecological examination: A cauliflower-like neoplasm in posterior lip of cervix, contact bleeding （＋）, the size of uterus normal, both sides of the annex area cannot be touched. The most likely diagnosis for the patient is: （D）

A.Endometrial carcinoma

B.Acute cervical cancer

C.Cervical myoma

D.Cervical cancer

E.Chronic cervicitis

5.宫颈癌普查最常用的方法是：（B）

A.宫颈针吸细胞学

B.宫颈细胞学涂片

C.宫颈组织学检查

D.宫颈碘试验

E.测阴道分泌物 pH

6.哪种方法诊断子宫颈癌最合适？（C）

A.分段诊断性刮宫

B.诊断性刮宫

C.宫颈活检

D.宫颈细胞学检查

E.超声

7.宫颈癌的好发部位：（A）

A.宫颈外口柱状上皮与鳞状上皮交界处

B.宫体内膜与宫颈黏膜交界处

C.宫颈外口与阴道鳞状上皮交界处

D.宫颈管内的柱状上皮

E.宫颈外口的鳞状上皮

（王学慧）

5.Which is the most common method used for cervical cancer screening?（B）

A.Cervical needle aspiration cytology

B.Cervical cytology smear

C.Cervical histology

D.Cervical iodine test

E.pH of vaginal discharge

6.Which method is the most appropriate for the diagnosis of cervical cancer?（C）

A.Fractional curettage

B.Diagnostic curettage

C.Cervical biopsy

D.Cervical smear cytology

E.Ultrasound

7.The most common site of cervical cancer is:（A）

A.The junction of columnar epithelium and squamous epithelium at the external cervical orifice

B.The junction of the endometrium and cervical mucosa

C.The junction of the external cervix and the squamous epithelium of the vagina

D.The columnar epithelium of the cervix

E.The squamous epithelium of the external cervix

第20章 子宫内膜异位症和子宫腺肌病

CHAPTER 20　Endometriosis and adenomyosis

第一节　子宫内膜异位症

1.概述

- 子宫内膜组织（腺体和间质）出现在子宫体以外的其他部位，称为子宫内膜异位症。异位内膜可侵犯全身任何部位，但绝大多数位于盆腔脏器和壁腹膜，以卵巢、宫骶韧带最常见；其次为子宫及其他脏腹膜、阴道直肠隔等部位。
- 子宫内膜异位症是激素依赖性疾病。在形态学上呈良性表现，但在临床行为学上具有类似恶性肿瘤的特点，如种植、侵袭及远处转移等。

发病率：在25～45岁女性中为76%。

2.病因

- 种植学说
  - 经血逆流。
  - 淋巴及静脉播散。
  - 医源性种植
    - 体腔上皮化生学说。

    - 诱导学说。
    - 遗传因素。
    - 免疫与炎症因素。
    - 其他因素。

3.病理

基本病理变化为异位子宫内膜

Section 1　Endometriosis

1.Introduction

- Endometrial tissue（gland and stroma）that appears outside the uterus which is called endometriosis. Ectopic endometrium can invade any part of the body but most of them are located in pelvic organs and wall peritoneum, with ovary and uterosacral ligaments being the most common, followed by uterus and other visceral peritoneum, vagina rectum diaphragm, etc.
- Endometriosis is the hormone-dependent disease. It is benign in morphology but similar to malignant tumors in clinical behavior such as implantation, invasion and distant metastasis.

Incidence: 76% in women aged 25～45.

2.Etiology

- Implantation theory
  - Retrograde menstruation.
  - Lymphatic and venous dissemination.
  - Iatrogenic planting
    - Metaplasia theory of coelomic epithelium.
    - Induction theory.
    - Genetic factors.
    - Immune and inflammatory factors.
    - Other factors.

3.Pathology

The basic pathological changes are that

随卵巢激素变化而发生周期性出血，导致周围纤维组织增生和囊肿、粘连形成，在病变区出现紫褐色斑点或小泡，最终发展成大小不等的紫褐色实质性结节或包块。

（1）大体病理

■ 卵巢子宫内膜异位症：约80%病变累及一侧，累及双侧占50%。

· 微小病变型：病灶只有数毫米大小。

· 典型病变型：又称囊肿型，直径多在5cm左右。

■ 腹膜子宫内膜异位症

· 色素沉着型：典型的蓝紫色或褐色腹膜异位结节。

· 无色素沉着型。

■ 深部浸润型异位症：指病灶浸润深度≥5cm。

■ 其他部位的内异症。

（2）镜下检查

■ 子宫内膜上皮、腺体、内膜间质、纤维素和红细胞/含铁血黄素。

4.临床表现

（1）症状：与月经周期密切相关，25%患者无任何症状。

■ 下腹痛和痛经：疼痛是内异症的主要症状，典型症状为继发性痛经，进行性加重。

■ 不孕：不孕率高达40%。

■ 性交不适：月经来潮前性交痛最明显。

■ 月经异常：15%～30%的患者有经量增多、经期延长或

the ectopic endometrium undergoes periodic hemorrhage with ovarian hormone changes, leading to the proliferation of surrounding fibrous tissue and the formation of cysts and adhesions. Purple-brown spots or vesicles appear in the lesion area and eventually develop into a purple-brown substantial nodules or masses of varying sizes.

（1）Gross pathology

■ Ovarian endometriosis: About 80% of the lesions involve one side and 50% involve both sides.

· Minimal lesion type: The lesion is only a few millimeters in size.

· Typical lesion type: Also known as cyst type, with diameter of about 5cm.

■ Peritoneal endometriosis

· Pigmentation: Typical blue-purple or brown ectopic peritoneal nodules.

· Non-pigmentation.

■ Deep invasive endometriosis: The depth of invasion of lesion ≥ 5 cm.

■ Others.

（2）Microscopic examination

■ Endometrial epithelium, glands, endometrial stroma, cellulose and erythrocytes/hemosiderin.

4.Clinical manifestations

（1）Symptoms: Closely related to menstrual cycle, with 25% of patients no symptoms.

■ Lower abdominal pain and dysmenorrhea: Pain is the main symptom of endometriosis. The typical symptom is secondary dysmenorrhea with progressive aggravation.

■ Infertility: Up to 40%.

■ Discomfort of sexual intercourse: Sexual intercourse pain is most obvious before menstruation.

■ Menstrual abnormalities: 15% ～ 30% of patients have increased menstrual volume,

月经淋漓不尽。

■ 其他。

除上述症状外，卵巢子宫内膜异位囊肿破裂时，可发生急腹痛。

（2）体征

■ 肿块、腹膜刺激征、触痛性结节。

■ 卵巢异位囊肿较大时，妇科检查可扪及与子宫粘连的肿块。囊肿破裂时腹膜刺激征阳性。典型盆腔内异症妇科检查可发现子宫后倾固定，触痛性结节，一侧或双侧囊实性包块，活动度差。

5.诊断

育龄期女性有继发性痛经，进行性加重，不孕或慢性盆腔痛、性交痛等，盆腔检查盆腔内有触痛性结节或子宫旁有不活动的囊性肿块，应高度怀疑。确诊首选腹腔镜检查。

（1）病史、妇科检查。

（2）影像学检查：超声检查可确定异位囊肿的位置、大小和形状，其诊断敏感度和特异度均在96%以上。

（3）腹腔镜检查：目前国际公认的内异症诊断的最佳方法。下列情况应首选腹腔镜检查：异位内异症的不孕患者、妇科检查及超声检查无阳性发现的慢性腹痛及痛经进行性加重者、有症状特别是血清CA125水平升高者。只有在腹腔镜检查或剖腹探查直视下才能确定内异症临床分期。

prolonged menstruation or endless menstrual dripping.

■ Others.

Acute abdominal pain may occur if the ovarian endometriotic cyst ruptures.

（2）Signs

■ Lump, peritoneal irritation, and tender nodules.

■ The gynecological examination may palpate the mass adhering to the uterus when the ovarian ectopic cyst is large. The peritoneal irritation sign is positive when the cyst is ruptured. Typical gynecological examination of pelvic endometriosis may reveal posterior uterine fixation, tender nodules, cystic and solid masses on one or both sides with poor mobility.

5.Diagnosis

If women at childbearing age have secondary dysmenorrhea, progressive aggravation, infertility or chronic pelvic pain, sexual pain, etc, and pelvic examination reveals tender nodules in the pelvic cavity or inactive cystic masses near the uterus, endometriosis should be highly suspected. Laparoscopy is the first choice for diagnosis.

（1）Medical history, pelvic examination.

（2）Imaging examination: Ultrasonic examination can determine the location, size and shape of ectopic cyst , with diagnostic sensitivity and specificity both more than 96%.

（3）Laparoscopy: The internationally recognized best method for diagnosis of endometriosis. Laparoscopy should be preferred in the following cases: Infertility with ectopic endometriosis, chronic abdominal pain and progressive dysmenorrhea without positive findings in gynecological and ultrasound examinations and with symptoms, especially with elevated serum CA125 level. The clinical stages of endometriosis can only be determined by laparoscopy

（4）CA125、HE4：CA125水平可能升高，重症患者更明显。HE4在内异症多在正常水平，可用于与卵巢癌的鉴别诊断。

6.鉴别诊断

（1）卵巢恶性肿瘤：早期无症状。有症状时多呈持续性腹痛、腹胀，病情发展快，一般情况差。超声图像显示包块为混合性或实性。血清CA125和HE4的表达水平多显著升高。腹腔镜检查或剖腹探查可鉴别。

（2）盆腔炎性包块：多有急性或反复发作的盆腔感染史，疼痛无周期性，平时亦有下腹部隐痛，可伴发热和白细胞增高等，抗生素治疗有效。

（3）子宫腺肌病：痛经症状与内异症相似，但多位于下腹正中且更剧烈，子宫多呈均匀性增大，质硬，经期检查时，子宫触痛明显。此病常与内异症并存。

（4）输卵管妊娠破裂。

7.临床分期

目前我国多采用美国生育学会（AFS）提出的"修正子宫内膜异位症分期法"（表20-1）。该分期法于1985年最初提出，1997年再次修正。内异症分期需在腹腔镜下或剖腹探查手术时进行，要求详细观察并对异位内膜的部位、数目、大小、粘连程度等进行记录，最后进行评分。该分期法有利于评估疾病严重程度、正确选择治疗方案、准确比较和评

or laparotomy.

（4）The levels of CA125 and HE4: CA125 may increase, especially in severe patients. HE4 is mostly at normal level in endometriosis and can be used for differential diagnosis with ovarian cancer.

6.Differential diagnosis

（1）Ovarian malignant tumor: Early asymptomatic. Symptoms are usually persistent abdominal pain, abdominal distension, rapid disease progression, with generally poor condition. Ultrasound images show that the mass is mixed or solid. The levels of serum CA125 and HE4 increase significantly. Laparoscopy or laparotomy can be used for differentiation.

（2）Pelvic inflammatory mass: Most of them have a history of acute or recurrent pelvic infections with non-periodic pain. Usually they also have dull pain in the lower abdomen, which can be accompanied by fever and leukocytosis. Antibiotic treatment is effective.

（3）Adenomyosis: The symptoms of dysmenorrhea similar to those of endometriosis, but most of them are located in the middle of the lower abdomen and more severe. The uterus is more uniform and hard. Uterine tenderness is obvious during menstrual examination. This disease often coexists with endometriosis.

（4）Rupture of tubal pregnancy.

7.Clinical stages

Fertility "Amended Endometriosis Staging Method" of the American Fertility Society（AFS）has been used in China（Table 20-1）. This method first proposed in 1985 and revised again in 1997. Endometriosis staging should be carried out under laparoscopy or laparotomy. Location, number, size and adhesion degree of ectopic endometrium should be observed in detail and recorded. The score should be evaluated finally. This staging method is helpful to evaluate the

表 20-1　ASRM 修正子宫内膜异位症分期法（1997 年）

Table 20-1　ASRM Amended Endometriosis Staging Method（1997）

异位病灶 Ectopic focus		病灶大小 Lesion size				粘连范围 Adhesion range		
		＜1cm	1～3cm	＞3cm		＜1/3 包裹 Enclosure	1/3～2/3 包裹 Enclosure	＞2/3 包裹 Enclosure
腹膜 Peritoneum	浅 Superficial	1	2	4				
	深 Deep	2	4	6				
卵巢 Ovary	右浅 Right superficial	1	2	4	薄膜 Filmy	1	2	4
	右深 Right deep	4	16	20	致密 Dense	4	8	16
	左浅 Left superficial	1	2	4	薄膜 Filmy	1	2	4
	左深 Left deep	4	16	20	致密 Dense	4	8	16
输卵管 Fallopian tube	右 Right				薄膜 Filmy	1	2	4
					致密 Dense	4	8	16
	左 Left				薄膜 Filmy	1	2	4
					致密 Dense	4	8	16
直肠子宫凹陷 Douglas' pouch	部分消失 Imcomplete disappearance	4			完全消失 Complete disappearance	40		

　注：1.若输卵管全部包入应改为 16 分

　2．Ⅰ期（微型）：1～5 分；Ⅱ期（轻型）：6～15 分；Ⅲ期（中型）：16～40 分；Ⅳ期（重型）：＞40 分

Note: 1. If the fimbriated end of the fallopian tube is completely enclosed, change the point assignment to 16.

　2. Stage Ⅰ（micro）：1～5 points; stage Ⅱ（mild）：6～15 points; stage Ⅲ（moderate）：16～40 points; stage Ⅳ（severe）：＞40 points

价各种治疗方法的疗效，并有助于判断患者的预后。

severity of the disease, select the correct treatment plan, accurately compare and evaluate the curative effects of various treatment methods and help judge the prognosis of patients.

8.治疗

根本目的：缩减和去除病灶、减轻和控制疼痛、治疗和促进生育，预防和减少复发。

（1）治疗方法

- 期待治疗：仅适用于轻症患者。

- 药物治疗：治疗的目的是抑制卵巢功能，阻止内异症的发生。
  - 口服避孕药、孕激素、米非司酮、孕三烯酮、达那唑、GnRH-a。

- 手术治疗：治疗的目的是切除病灶，恢复解剖。适用于药物治疗后症状不缓解、局部病变加剧或生育功能未恢复者，较大的卵巢内膜异位囊肿者。
  - 保留生育功能手术：切净或破坏所有可见的异位内膜病灶、分离粘连、恢复正常的解剖结构，但保留子宫、一侧或双侧卵巢，至少保留部分卵巢组织。适用于药物治疗无效、年轻和有生育要求的患者。术后复发率约40%，因此术后宜尽早妊娠或使用药物以减少复发。
  - 保留卵巢功能手术：切除盆腔内病灶及子宫，保留至少一侧或部分卵巢。适用于Ⅲ、Ⅳ期患者、症状明显且无生育要求的45岁以下患者。术后复发率约5%。
  - 根治性手术：将子宫、双附件及盆腔内所有异位内

8.Treatment

Fundamental purpose: Reduce and remove lesions, reduce and control pain; treat and promote fertility, and prevent and reduce recurrence.

（1）Therapeutic method

- Expected treatment: Only for mild cases.

- Medical treatement: With the purpose of inhibiting ovarian function and preventing the occurrence of endometriosis.
  - Oral contraceptives, progesterone, mifepristone, gestrione, danazol, and GnRH-a.

- Surgical treatment: To remove the focus and restore the anatomy, suitable for those who do not alleviate symptoms, have aggravated local lesions or have no recovery of fertility function after drug treatment, and those with large endometriosis cyst of ovary.
  - Fertility preservation surgery: Cutting or destroying all visible ectopic endometrial lesions, separating adhesions, restoring normal anatomical structure, but retaining uterus, one or both ovaries, and at least part of the ovarian tissue. Suitable for patients with ineffective drug treatment, young age and fertility requirements. Postoperative recurrence rate is about 40%, so early pregnancy or medication should be used to reduce recurrence.
  - Function preservation ovarian surgery: Excision of pelvic lesions and uterus, with preservation of at least one or part of the ovary, suitable for patients in stage Ⅲ and Ⅳ, under 45 years old, with obvious symptoms and no fertility requirement. Postoperative recurrence rate is about 5%.
  - Radical surgery: Excise and remove all ectopic endometrial lesions in uterus,

膜病灶予以切除和清除。适用于45岁以上重症患者。术后不用雌激素补充治疗者，几乎不复发。

■ 手术与药物联合治疗。

（2）内异症不同情况的处理

■ 内异症相关疼痛
  ● 未合并不孕及无附件包块者，首选药物治疗。一线药物包括：非甾体抗炎药、口服避孕药及高效孕激素。二线药物包括GnRH-a、左炔诺孕酮宫内缓释系统（LNG-IUS）。一线药物治疗无效改二线药物，若依然无效，应考虑手术治疗。所有的药物治疗都存在停药后疼痛的高复发率。

  ● 合并不孕或附件包块者，首选手术治疗。手术指征：①卵巢子宫内膜异位囊肿直径≥4cm；②合并不孕；③痛经药物治疗无效。手术以腹腔镜为首选。
■ 内异症相关不孕：排除其他不孕因素。腹腔镜是首选的手术治疗方式。
■ 内异症恶变：主要恶变部位在卵巢，其他部位少见。临床有以下情况应警惕内异症恶变。

  ● 绝经后内异症患者，疼痛节律改变。

bilateral adnexa and pelvis. Suitable for severe patients over 45 years old. No recurrence in patients who do not use estrogen supplement therapy after surgery.

■ Surgery combined with medication.

（2）Treatment of different endometriosis conditions

■ Endometriosis-related pain
  ● For patients without infertility or adnexal mass, drug treatment is preferred. First-line drugs include: Non-steroidal anti-inflammatory drugs, oral contraceptives and high-efficiency progestin. Second-line drugs include: GnRH-a and levonorgestrel intrauterine sustained-release system（LNG-IUS）. Surgical treatment should be considered if the first-line drug treatment is ineffective and the second-line is still ineffective. All drug treatments have a high recurrence rate of pain after drug withdrawal.

  ● For patients with infertility or adnexal mass, surgical treatment is preferred. Surgical indications:①The diameter of ovarian endometriosis cyst ≥ 4cm;②Infertility;③With dysmenorrhea medication ineffective. Laparoscopic surgery is the first choice.
■ Endometriosis-related infertility: Exclude other infertility factors. Laparoscopy is the preferred surgical treatment.
■ Malignant transformation of endometriosis: The main site of malignant transformation is ovary, other sites rare. Be alert to the malignant change of endometriosis in the following clinical conditions.
  ● Changes of pain rhythm in postmeno-pausal patients with endometriosis.

- 卵巢囊肿直径＞10cm。
- 影像学检查有恶性征象。
- 血清CA125水平＞200U/ml。

9.预防

（1）防止经血逆流。

（2）药物避孕。

（3）防止医源性异位内膜种植。

第二节 子宫腺肌病

1.概述

- 子宫内膜腺体和间质存在于子宫肌层中。病因不清，多发于30～50岁经产妇。

2.病因

- 多次妊娠、人工流产、慢性子宫内膜炎等造成子宫内膜基底层损伤。
- 高水平雌激素刺激。

3.病理

（1）巨检

- 子宫多呈均匀增大，呈球形，一般不超过12周妊娠子宫大小。
- 弥漫型和局限型。
- 子宫腺肌瘤。

（2）镜检

- 子宫肌层内呈岛状分布的子宫内膜腺体与间质是本病的镜下特征。

4.临床表现

（1）症状＋体征。

（2）主要症状：经量增多和经期延长（40%～50%）及逐渐加重的进行性痛经（15%～30%）。

5.诊断

- 进行性痛经、月经过多、妇科检查、影像学检查。

- Ovarian cyst diameter ＞ 10cm.
- Malignant signs in imaging examination.
- Serum CA125 ＞ 200U/ml.

9.Prevention

（1）Prevention of retrograde menstruation.

（2）Drug contraception.

（3）Prevention of iatrogenic endometriosis.

Section 2   Adenomyosis

1.Introduction

- Endometrial glands and stroma exist in the uterine myometrium. The cause is unknown, with 30 ～ 50 year old multipara mostly occurring.

2.Etiology

- Multiple pregnancy, induced abortion, chronic endometritis and so on cause damage to endometrial basal layer.
- High-level estrogen stimulation.

3.Pathology

（1）Gross appearance

- The uterus is usually uniformly enlarged and spherical, and less than 12 weeks pregnant uterus size generally.
- Diffuse and localized type.
- Adenomyoma.

（2）Microscopic appearance

- Endometrial glands and stroma in the uterine myometrium are island-shaped under microscopy.

4.Clinical manifestations

（1）Symptoms ＋ signs.

（2）The main symptoms: Increased menstrual volume, prolonged menstruation（40% ～ 50%）and progressive dysmenorrhea（15% ～ 30%）.

5.Diagnosis

- Progressive dysmenorrhea, menorrhagia, pelvic examination, and imaging examination.

6. 治疗

（1）期待疗法。

（2）药物治疗：曼月乐、GnRHa。

（3）手术治疗。

重点专业词汇

1. 子宫内膜异位症

2. 子宫腺肌症

3. 腺体和间质

4. 种植学说

5. 诱导学说

6. 周期性出血

7. 卵巢子宫内膜异位症

8. 腹膜子宫内膜异位症

9. 深部浸润型异位症

10. 红细胞/含铁血黄素

11. 痛经

12. 不孕

13. 月经紊乱

14. 触痛性结节

15. 腹腔镜检查

16. 卵巢肿瘤

17. 盆腔炎性包块

18. 输卵管妊娠破裂

练习题

1. 子宫内膜异位症较少累及的部位是：（A）

A. 输卵管

B. 直肠子宫陷凹

C. 宫骶韧带

D. 子宫后壁下段

E. 卵巢

2. 子宫内膜异位症的临床分期依据是：（D）

A. 彩色多普勒超声

B. 典型病史及妇科检查

C. 宫腔镜检查

D. 腹腔镜检查

E. 血清 CA125 测定

3. 子宫内膜异位症根治手术适

6. Treatment

（1）Expected treatment.

（2）Medical treatment: Mirena, GnRHa.

（3）Surgical treatment.

Key words

1. Endometriosis

2. Adenomyosis

3. Gland and stroma

4. Implantation theory

5. Induction theory

6. Periodic hemorrhage

7. Ovarian endometriosis

8. Peritoneal endometriosis

9. Deep invasive endometriosis

10. Erythrocytes/hemosiderin

11. Dysmenorrhea

12. Infertility

13. Menstrual disorder

14. Tender nodules

15. Laparoscopy

16. Ovarian tumor

17. Pelvic inflammatory mass

18. Rupture of tubal pregnancy

Exercises

1. The less involved part of endometriosis is: （A）

A. Fallopian tube

B. Rectouterine pouch

C. Uterosacral ligament

D. Inferior segment of posterior wall of uterus

E. Ovaries

2. The clinical stage of endometriosis is based on: （D）

A. Color Doppler ultrasound

B. Typical history and pelvic examination

C. Hysteroscopy

D. Laparoscopy

E. Determination of serum CA125

3. Radical surgery for endometriosis is suitable

用于:(A)

A.45岁以上重度患者

B.45岁以下轻度患者

C.45岁以上轻度患者

D.45岁以下重度患者

E.45岁以下中度患者

4.子宫腺肌病的典型症状是:(D)

A.月经周期逐渐延长

B.月经期延长伴月经量增多

C.阴道不规则出血

D.继发性痛经进行性加重

E.阴道分泌物增多

(贾琳钰)

for:(A)

A.Severe patients over 45 years old

B.Mild patients under 45 years old

C.Mild patients over 45 years old

D.Severe patients under 45 years old

E.Moderate patients under 45 years old

4.The typical symptom of adenomyosis is:(D)

A.Menstrual cycle gradually extended

B.Prolonged menstrual period with increased menstrual flow

C.Irregular vaginal bleeding

D.Progressive exacerbation of secondary dysmenorrhea

E.Increased vaginal secretions

第21章 盆底功能障碍

CHAPTER 21 Pelvic floor dysfunction

女性盆底支持组织因退化、创伤等因素导致其支持薄弱，从而发生盆底功能障碍。盆底功能障碍性疾病的治疗与否取决于是否影响患者的生活质量，治疗有非手术和手术治疗两种办法。

Female pelvic floor supporting tissues become weakened due to degeneration, trauma and other factors, which leads to pelvic floor dysfunction. The treatment of pelvic floor dysfunction depends on whether it affects the patients' quality of life. There are two ways to treat pelvic floor dysfunction: Non-surgical and surgical treatment.

第一节 盆腔器官脱垂

1.概述

- 盆腔器官脱垂（POP）指盆腔器官脱出于阴道内或阴道外。2001年美国国立卫生研究所提出：POP指任何阴道节段的前缘达到或超过处女膜缘外1cm以上。

- 阴道前壁脱垂也即阴道前壁膨出，阴道内2/3膀胱区域脱出称之膀胱膨出。若支持尿道的膀胱宫颈筋膜受损严重，尿道紧连的阴道前壁下1/3以尿道口为支点向下膨出，称尿道膨出。阴道后壁膨出又称为直肠膨出，常伴随子宫直肠陷凹疝。子宫从正常位置沿阴道下降，宫颈外口达到坐骨棘水平以下，甚至子宫全部脱出阴道口以外，称子宫脱垂。子宫切除术后若阴道顶端支持结构受损，则发生阴道穹窿脱垂。

Section 1 Pelvic organ prolapse

1.Introduction

- Pelvic organ prolapse（POP）refers to pelvic organ prolapse out of the vagina or outside the vagina. In 2001, the National Institutes of Health（NIH）proposed that POP means that the leading edge of any vaginal segment reaches or exceeds 1 cm beyond the edge of the hymen.

- Vaginal anterior wall prolapse is also known as anterior vaginal wall bulging. Prolapse of 2/3 of the bladder area in the vagina is called cystocele. If the vesicocervical fascia supporting the urethra is severely damaged, the lower 1/3 of the anterior vaginal wall tightly connected to the urethra, bulges downward with the urethral orifice as the fulcrum, which is called urethrocele.Vaginal posterior wall bulge also known as rectocele, is often accompanied by hernia of Douglas' pouch. The uterus descends from the normal position along the vagina, and the external orifice of the cervix reaches below the level of the sciatic spine, and even the uterus is completely out of the vaginal orifice, which is called uterine prolapse. Vault prolapse occurs after hysterectomy if the top supporting structure of the vagina is damaged.

2.病因

（1）妊娠、分娩、产后过早参加体力劳动。

（2）衰老。

（3）慢性咳嗽、腹腔积液、腹型肥胖、持续负重或便秘而造成腹腔内压力增加，可致腹压增加导致脱垂。

（4）医源性原因。

3.临床表现

（1）症状

■ 轻者无症状。

■ 重度脱垂韧带筋膜有牵拉，盆腔充血，患者有不同程度的腰骶部酸痛或下坠感，久站或劳累后症状明显，卧床休息则症状减轻。阴道前壁膨出常伴有尿频、排尿困难、残余尿增加，部分患者可发生压力性尿失禁，尿路感染。阴道后壁膨出常表现为便秘，甚至需要手助压迫阴道后壁帮助排便。暴露在外的宫颈和阴道黏膜长期与衣裤摩擦，可导致溃疡发生。子宫脱垂程度一般不影响月经，轻度子宫脱垂也不影响受孕、妊娠及分娩。

（2）体征

■ 脱垂的阴道前后壁、宫颈黏膜常有增厚角化，可有溃疡和出血。阴道前壁呈球状膨

2.Etiology

（1）Pregnancy, childbirth, physical labor too early after delivery.

（2）Aging.

（3）Chronic cough, peritoneal effusion, abdominal obesity, persistent weight-bearing or constipation can increase intra-abdominal pressure which leads to prolapse.

（4）Iatrogenic causes.

3.Clinical manifestations

（1）Symptoms

■ Mild cases have no symptoms.

■ Severe prolapsed ligament fascia has traction, and pelvic congestion. Patients have varying degrees of lumbosacral pain or sense of falling, with symptoms obvious after long standing or fatigue, and alleviated after bed rest. Vaginal anterior wall bulge is often accompanied by frequent urination, dysuria and increased residual urine. Some patients may suffer from stress urinary incontinence and urinary tract infection. Vaginal posterior wall bulge is often manifested as constipation, and even hand-assisted compression of the posterior wall of the vagina is needed to help defecate. Exposure of cervical and vaginal mucosa may cause ulcers due to long-term friction with clothing. Uterine prolapse generally does not affect menstruation, and mild uterine prolapse does not affect conception, pregnancy and childbirth generally.

（2）Signs

■ Prolapsed vaginal anterior and posterior walls and cervical mucosa often have hyperkeratosis, ulcers and bleeding. The anterior vaginal

出。阴道后壁膨出肛门检查手指向前方可触及向阴道凸出的直肠。不能回纳的子宫脱垂常伴宫颈肥大并延长。

wall is spherically bulging. Prolapse of the posterior vaginal wall: In an anus examination, fingers can touch the rectum protruding to the vagina. Unacceptable uterine prolapse is often accompanied by cervical hypertrophy and elongation.

4.临床分期

- 国际上应用最多的是POP-Q分期（表21-1、表21-2）。中国沿用传统分度，将盆腔脏器脱垂分为3度（表21-3、表21-4、表21-5）。程度评

4.Clinical staging

- The POP-Q staging is widely used in the world（Table 21-1, Table 21-2）. According to Chinese traditional grading, pelvic organ prolapse is divided into 3 degrees（Table 21-3, Table 21-4, Table 21-5）. Degree

表21-1　盆腔器官脱垂评估指示点（POP-Q分期）

Table 21-1　Indicators for pelvic organ prolapse assessment（POP-Q staging）

指示点 Indicator	内容描述 Description	范围 Range
Aa	阴道前壁中线距处女膜3cm处，相当于尿道膀胱沟内 The midline of the anterior vaginal wall is 3 cm away from the hymen, which is equivalent to the urethral bladder groove	$-3 \sim +3cm$
Ba	阴道顶端或前穹窿到Aa点之间阴道前壁上段中的最远点 The farthest point in the upper segment of the anterior vaginal wall between the top of the vagina or the anterior fornix and point Aa	在无阴道脱垂时，此点位于-3cm，在子宫切除术后阴道完全外翻时，此点将为+TVL In the absence of vaginal prolapse, this point is -3cm, which will be + TVL when the vagina is completely valgus after hysterectomy
C	宫颈或子宫切除后阴道顶端所处的最远端 The farthest end of the vagina after cervicectomy or hysterectomy	$-TVL \sim +TVL$
D	有宫颈时的后穹窿的位置，它提示了子宫骶骨韧带附着到近端宫颈后壁的水平 The position of the posterior fornix in the presence of the cervix indicates the level at which the uterosacral ligament attaches to the posterior wall of the proximal cervix	$-TVL \sim +TVL$ 或空缺（子宫切除后） $-TVL \sim +TVL$ or vacancy（after hysterectomy）
Ap	阴道后壁中线距处女膜3cm处，Ap与Aa点相对应 The midline of the posterior vaginal wall is 3 cm away from the hymen, and Ap corresponds to point Aa	$-3 \sim +3cm$
Bp	阴道顶端或后穹窿到Ap点之间阴道后壁上段中的最远点，Bp与Ba点相对应 The farthest point in the upper segment of the posterior vaginal wall between the top of the vagina or the posterior fornix and point Ap，the Bp corresponds to point Ba	在无阴道脱垂时，此点位于-3cm，在子宫切除术后阴道完全外翻时，此点将为+TVL In the absence of vaginal prolapse, this point is -3cm, which will be + TVL when the vagina is completely valgus after hysterectomy

阴道总长度（TVL）

Total vaginal length（TVL）

表21-2 盆腔器官脱垂分期（POP-Q分期法）

Table 21-2 Pelvic organ prolapse staging（POP-Q staging）

分期 Staging	内容 Contents
0	无脱垂，Aa、Ap、Ba、Bp均在-3cm处，C、D两点在阴道总长度和阴道总长度-2cm之间，即C或D点量化值<（TVL-2）cm No prolapse. Aa, Ap, Ba and Bp are all at −3 cm, while C and D are between the total vaginal length −2 cm and the total length of vagina, i.e. the quantized value of point C or D <（TVL-2）cm
I	脱垂最远端在处女膜平面上>1cm，即量化值<-1cm The farthest part of prolapse > 1 cm on the hymen plane, i.e.the quantized value < −1 cm
II	脱垂最远端在处女膜平面上<1cm，即量化值>-1cm，但<+1cm The farthest part of prolapse < 1 cm on the hymen plane, i.e. the quantized value > −1 cm, but <+ 1 cm
III	脱垂最远端超过处女膜平面>1cm，但<阴道总长度-2cm，即量化值>+1cm，但<（TVL-2）cm The farthest part of prolapse beyond the hymen plane > 1 cm, but < the total length of vagina−2 cm, i.e. quantized value >+ 1 cm, but <（TVL-2）cm
IV	下生殖道呈全长外翻，脱垂最远端及宫颈或阴道残端脱垂超过阴道总长度-2cm，即量化值>（TVL-2）cm The lower genital tract shows full-length valgus. Prolapse of the most distal part and the cervical or vaginal stump exceeds the total length of the vagina −2 cm, i.e. the quantized value >（TVL-2）cm.

表21-3 子宫脱垂中国传统分度

Table 21-3 Chinese traditional grading of uterine prolapse

I 度
I degree

轻型 / Mild type
宫颈外口距处女膜缘<4cm，未达处女膜缘
The outer cervical orifice away from the hymen margin < 4cm, but not reaching the hymen margin

重型 / Severe type
宫颈已达处女膜缘，阴道口可见宫颈
The cervix has reached the hymen margin, with the cervix visible at the vaginal orifice

II 度
II degree

轻型 / Mild type
宫颈脱出阴道口，宫体仍在阴道内
The cervix falls out of the vaginal orifice, and the uterus body is still in the vagina

重型 / Severe type
宫颈及部分宫体脱出阴道口
The cervix and part of the uterine body prolapse from the vaginal orifice.

III 度 / III degree
宫颈和宫体全部脱出阴道口外
The cervix and the uterine body are all out of the vagina

表21-4　阴道前壁膨出中国传统分度

Table 21-4　Chinese traditional grading of anterior vaginal wall bulge

Ⅰ度	阴道前壁形成球状物，向下突出，达处女膜缘，但仍在阴道内
Ⅰ degree	The anterior wall of the vagina forms globular mass, protruding downward, reaching the hymen margin but still in the vagina
Ⅱ度	阴道壁展平或消失，部分阴道前壁突出于阴道外
Ⅱ degree	The vaginal wall flattens or disappears, and part of the vaginal anterior wall protrudes outside the vagina
Ⅲ度	阴道前壁全部突出于阴道外
Ⅲ degree	The anterior vaginal wall all protrudes outside the vagina

表21-5　阴道后壁膨出中国传统分度

Table 21-5　Chinese traditional grading of posterior vaginal wall bulge

Ⅰ度	阴道后壁达处女膜缘，但仍在阴道内
Ⅰ degree	The posterior wall of the vagina reaches the hymen margin but is still in the vagina
Ⅱ度	阴道壁后壁部分脱出阴道外
Ⅱ degree	The posterior wall of the vagina partially protrudes outside the vagina
Ⅲ度	阴道后壁全部脱出于阴道外
Ⅲ degree	The posterior wall of the vagina all protrudes outside the vagina

价均以患者平卧最大用力向下屏气时程度为准。

evaluation is based on the degree of breath holding with maximum effort in supine position.

5.诊断

（1）病史。

（2）妇科检查。

6.鉴别诊断

（1）阴道壁肿物。

（2）宫颈延长。

（3）子宫黏膜下肌瘤。

（4）慢性子宫内翻。

7.治疗

（1）非手术疗法

■ 为盆腔器官脱垂的一线治疗方法。通常用于POP-QⅠ～Ⅱ度有症状的患者，也适用于希望保留生育功能、不能耐受手术治疗或者不愿意手术治疗的重度（POP-QⅢ～

5.Diagnosis

（1）Medical history.

（2）Gynecological examination.

6.Differential diagnosis

（1）Vaginal wall mass.

（2）Cervical elongation.

（3）Submucosal myoma of uterus.

（4）Chronic inversion of uterus.

7.Treatment

（1）Non-surgical treatment

■ First-line treatment of pelvic organ prolapse, usually used for patients with symptoms of POP-QⅠ～Ⅱ degree, and for patients with severe prolapse（POP-QⅢ～Ⅳ degree or traditional grading mild or below Ⅱ degree）, who want to retain fertility

Ⅳ度，或传统Ⅱ度轻型及以下）脱垂患者。非手术的目标为缓解症状，增加盆底肌肉的强度、耐力和支持力，预防脱垂加重，避免或延缓手术干预。目前的非手术治疗方法包括应用子宫托、盆底康复治疗和行为指导。

- 盆底肌肉锻炼和物理疗法：增加盆底肌肉群的张力。
- 放置子宫托：子宫托是一种支持子宫和阴道壁并使其维持在阴道内而不脱出的工具。
- 支撑型和填充型
  · 适用情况：患者全身状况不适宜做手术；妊娠期和产后；膨出面溃疡：手术前促进溃疡面愈合。
- 中药和针灸

（2）手术治疗

■ 目的：缓解症状，恢复正常的解剖位置和脏器功能，有满意的性功能并能够维持效果。
- 合并压力性尿失禁患者应同时行膀胱颈悬吊手术或悬带手术。

■ 术式
- 阴道封闭术：全封闭和半封闭术。
- 盆底重建手术
  · 曼氏手术：适用于年龄较轻，宫颈延长患者。
  · 经阴道子宫全切除及阴道前后壁修补术：适用

function or can not be treated by surgery, or are unwilling to undergo surgery. The goals of non-surgical treatment are to alleviate symptoms, increase the strength, endurance and support of pelvic floor muscles, prevent aggravating of prolapse and avoid or delay surgical intervention. Current non-surgical treatments include the use of pessaries, pelvic floor rehabilitation and behavior guidance.

- Pelvic floor muscle training and physical therapy: To strengthen the tension of pelvic floor muscles.
- Pessary: A device that supports the uterus and vaginal wall to keep them in the vagina without prolapse.

- Supporting type and filling type
  · Indications: The patient's general condition is not suitable for surgery; during pregnancy and postpartum; promoting ulcer healing before surgery.
- Chinese medicine and acupuncture.

（2）Surgical treatment

■ Purpose: To alleviate symptoms, and restore normal anatomical position and organ function, with satisfactory sexual function and maintaining the effect.
- Patients with stress urinary incontinence should undergo bladder neck suspension or suspensory surgery at the same time.

■ Surgical method
- Colpocleisis: Total and partial surgery.

- Pelvic floor reconstructive surgery
  · Manchester operation: Suitable for younger patients with cervical elongation.
  · Transvaginal hysterectomy and anterior and posterior vaginal wall repair:

于年龄较大，无生育要求的患者。

8.预防

■ 预防和治疗增加腹压的疾病。

第二节　压力性尿失禁

压力性尿失禁（SUI）：腹压突然增加导致尿液不自主流出，而不是由逼尿肌收缩压或膀胱壁对尿液的张力压引起。

特点：正常状态下无遗尿，而腹压突然增高时尿液自动流出。

1.病因

（1）解剖型（＞90%）：盆底组织松弛引起，如妊娠、分娩损伤。

（2）尿道内括约肌障碍型（＜10%）：先天发育异常所致。

2.临床表现

■ 几乎所有的下尿路症状及许多阴道症状；腹压增加下不自主溢尿；膀胱膨出（80%）。

3.分度

（1）主观分度

■ Ⅰ级：尿失禁只有发生在剧烈压力下，如咳嗽、打喷嚏、慢跑。

■ Ⅱ级：尿失禁发生在中度压力下，如快速运动、上下楼梯。

■ Ⅲ级：尿失禁发生在轻度压力下，如站立时。患者在仰卧位时可控制尿液。

（2）客观分度：基于尿垫试验。

For older patients without fertility requirements.

8.Prevention

■ Prevention and treatment of diseases that increase abdominal pressure.

Section 2　Stress urinary incontinence

Stress urinary incontinence（SUI）: A sudden increase in abdominal pressure causes an involuntary outflow of urine, but not caused by detrusor systolic pressure or bladder wall tension pressure on the urine.

Characteristics: No enuresis in normal condition, urine automatically flows out when abdominal pressure suddenly increases.

1.Etiology

（1）Anatomic type（＞90%）: Pelvic floor tissue loosening, for example pregnancy and birth injury

（2）Internal urethral sphincter disorder（＜10%）: Congenital dysplasia.

2.Clinical manifestations

■ Almost all lower urinary tract symptoms and many vaginal symptoms; involuntary overflow with increased abdominal pressure; cystocele（80%）.

3.Staging

（1）Subjective staging:

■ Stage Ⅰ: Urinary incontinence only occurs under severe pressure, such as cough, sneezing and jogging.

■ Stage Ⅱ: Urinary incontinence occurs under moderate pressure, such as rapid movement, up and down stairs.

■ Stage Ⅲ: Urinary incontinence occurs under mild stress, while standing. Patients can control urine in supine position.

（2）Objective staging: Based on urine pad test.

4.诊断

（1）症状。

（2）妇科检查。

（3）相关神经系统检查。

（4）压力试验。

（5）指压试验。

（6）棉签试验。

（7）尿动力学检查。

（8）尿道膀胱镜检查。

5.鉴别诊断

■ 急迫性尿失禁。

6.治疗

（1）非手术治疗

■ 适用于轻度、中度患者。生活方式干预、盆底康复锻炼、膀胱训练、局部雌激素治疗。

（2）手术治疗

■ 耻骨后膀胱尿道悬吊术：Burch手术。

■ 阴道无张力尿道中段悬吊带术。

7.预防

■ 预防和治疗增加腹压的疾病。

重点专业词汇

1.盆底功能障碍（PFD）

2.膀胱膨出

3.耻骨宫颈韧带

4.膀胱宫颈筋膜

5.泌尿生殖膈

6.分娩

7.处女膜

8.直肠膨出

9.会阴裂伤

10.子宫脱垂

11.压力性尿失禁（SUI）

12.压力试验

4.Diagnosis

（1）Symptoms.

（2）Pelvic examinations.

（3）Related neurological examinations.

（4）Stress test.

（5）Bonney test.

（6）Q-tip test.

（7）Urodynamics.

（8）Cystoscopy.

5.Differential diagnosis

■ Urgent urinary incontinence.

6.Treatment

（1）Non-surgical treatment

■ Suitable for mild and moderate patients. Lifestyle intervention, pelvic floor muscle exercises, bladder training, and topical estrogen therapy.

（2）Surgical treatment

■ Posterior pubic vesicourethral suspension: Burch operation.

■ Tension-free vaginal tape suspension.

7.Prevention

■ Prevention and treatment of diseases that increase abdominal pressure.

Key words

1.Pelvic floor dysfunction（PFD）

2.Cystocele

3.Pubocervical ligament

4.Vesicocervical fascia

5.Urogenital diaphragm

6.Labor

7.Hymen

8.Rectocele

9.Perineal lacerations

10.Uterine prolapse

11.Stress urinary incontinence（SUI）

12.Stress test

练习题

1.子宫脱垂最常见的病因是：
（D）

A.慢性咳嗽

B.肥胖体型

C.习惯性便秘

D.分娩损伤

E.长期重体力劳动

2.女，58岁，绝经8年，发现阴道脱出肿物3个月，休息后可消失。妇科检查：平卧位屏气向下用力时，宫颈脱出阴道口外，宫体仍在阴道内。该患者子宫脱垂的临床分期是：（D）

A. Ⅲ度型

B. Ⅱ度重型

C. Ⅰ度轻型

D. Ⅱ度轻型

E. Ⅰ度重型

（贾琳钰）

Exercises

1.The most common cause of uterine prolapse is:（D）

A.Chronic cough

B.Obese figure

C.Habitual constipation

D.Labor injury

E.Long-term heavy manual labor

2.A 58-year-old female has menopause for 8 years. Prolapse mass was found outside the vagina for 3 months, and disappeared after rest. Pelvic examination: When in supine position with breath-holding and force downward, the cervix prolapsed outside the vagina, with the uterine body still in the vagina. The clinical stage of uterine prolapse in this patient is:（D）

A. Ⅲ degree

B. Ⅱ degree severe

C. Ⅰ degree mild

D. Ⅱ degree mild

E. Ⅰ degree severe

第22章 妊娠滋养细胞疾病

CHAPTER 22 Gestational trophoblastic diseases

第一节 葡 萄 胎

葡萄胎因妊娠后胎盘绒毛滋养细胞增生、间质水肿，而形成大小不一的水泡，水泡间借蒂相连成串，形如葡萄而名之。

1.病因

（1）完全性葡萄胎：种族、营养状况、社会经济。

- 染色体核型为二倍体，均来自父系。

（2）部分性葡萄胎：染色体核型为三倍体。

2.病理（表22-1）

（1）完全性葡萄胎：大体检查水泡状物形如成串葡萄，大小直径不等。

（2）部分性葡萄胎：仅部分绒毛为水泡状，合并胚胎或胎儿组织，胎儿多已死亡，常伴发育迟缓或多发性畸形。

3.临床表现

（1）完全性葡萄胎

- 停经后阴道出血：停经8～12周。
- 子宫异常增大、变软。

- 妊娠呕吐。
- 子痫前期征象。
- 甲状腺功能亢进。

Section 1　Hydatidiform mole

Proliferation of trophoblasts and interstitial edema of placenta villi after pregnancy results in the formation of vesicles of different sizes with grape-like shape, which is termed as hydatidiform mole.

1.Etiology

（1）Complete hydatidiform mole: Race, nutrition, and social economy.

- The karyotype in diploid, all from the paternal line.

（2）Partial hydatidiform mole: The karyotype in triploid.

2.Pathology（Table 22-1）

（1）Complete hydatidiform mole: Gross examination reveals that the shape of vesicles is like clusters of grapes, with varying sizes and diameters.

（2）Partial hydatidiform mole: Only part of the villi vesicular, with embryo or fetal tissue. Most fetuses have died, often accompanied by growth retardation or multiple malformations.

3.Clinical manifestations

（1）Complete hydatidiform mole

- Vaginal bleeding after menopause: 8～12 weeks after menopause.
- Abnormal enlargement and softening of the uterus.
- Vomiting during pregnancy.
- Signs of preeclampsia.
- Hyperthyroidism.

表22-1　完全性和部分性葡萄胎核型和病理特征比较

Table 22-1　Comparison of karyotypes and pathological characteristics of
complete and partial hydatidiform moles

特征 Characteristic	完全性葡萄胎 Complete hydatidiform mole	部分性葡萄胎 Partial hydatidiform mole
核型 Karyotype	46，XX（90%）和46，XY 46, XX（90%）and 46, XY	常见为69，XXX和69，XXY Common 69, XXX and 69, XXY
病理特征 Pathological characteristics		
胎儿组织 Fetal tissue	缺乏 Absent	存在 Present
胎膜、胎儿红细胞 Fetal membranes and fetal erythrocyte	缺乏 Absent	存在 Present
绒毛水肿 Villus edema	弥漫 Diffuse	局限，大小和程度不一 Limited, different in size and degree
滋养细胞包涵体 Trophoblast inclusion body	缺乏 Absent	存在 Present
扇贝样轮廓绒毛 Scallop-like villi	缺乏 Absent	存在 Present
滋养细胞增生 Trophoblastic proliferation	弥漫，轻-重度 Diffuse, mild to severe	局限，轻-中度 Localized, mild to moderate
滋养细胞异型性 Trophoblast atypia	弥漫，明显 Diffuse, obvious	局限，轻度 Localized and mild

■ 腹痛：常发生于阴道出血前。

■ 卵巢黄素化囊肿。

（2）部分性葡萄胎：可有完全性葡萄胎的大多数症状，但程度较轻。

4. 自然转归

■ 正常情况下，葡萄胎排空后hCG稳定下降，首次降至正常的平均时间大约为9周，一般最长不超过14周。若葡萄胎排空后hCG持续异常考虑妊娠滋养细胞肿瘤。

■ 高危葡萄胎：hCG > 100 000U/L；子宫明显大于相应孕周；

■ Abdominal pain: Usually before vaginal bleeding.

■ Theca lutein ovarian cyst.

（2）Partial hydatidiform mole: Most symptoms of complete hydatidiform mole may exist, but to mild degree.

4.Natural course

■ Normally, hCG decreases steadily after hydatidiform mole emptying, and the average time for the first time to fall to normal is about 9 weeks, with the maximum no longer than 14 weeks. If hCG continues to be abnormal after hydatidiform mole emptying, gestational trophoblastic tumor should be considered.

■ High-risk hydatidiform mole: hCG > 100,000U/L; uterus significantly larger

卵巢黄素化囊肿直径＞6cm；年龄＞40岁和重复葡萄胎。

5.诊断

（1）上述症状＋体征。

（2）超声检查：落雪状、蜂窝状。

（3）hCG测定。

（4）DNA倍体分析。

（5）母源表达印迹基因检测。

（6）其他。

6.鉴别诊断

（1）流产。

（2）双胎妊娠。

7.治疗

（1）清宫：一经诊断，及时清宫。清宫前先对症处理，稳定病情。一般选用吸刮术，具有手术时间短、出血少、不易发生子宫穿孔等优点。清宫应在手术室进行。一般推荐缩宫素在充分扩张宫颈管和开始吸宫后使用。子宫＜12孕周可一次刮净，＞12孕周或术中感到一次刮净有困难时，可一周后行第二次刮宫。

（2）卵巢黄素化囊肿的处理：因囊肿在葡萄胎清宫后会自行消退，一般不需处理。若发生急性扭转，可在超声或腹腔镜下做穿刺抽液，囊肿多能自然复位。若扭转时间较长发生坏死，需做患侧附件切除。

（3）预防性化疗：不常规推荐。

（4）子宫切除术。

than the corresponding gestational weeks; theca lutein ovarian cyst diameter ＞ 6 cm; age ＞ 40 years old and with a history of hydatidiform mole.

5.Diagnosis

（1）The above symptoms ＋ signs.

（2）Ultrasound examination: Snow-like and honeycomb-like.

（3）Determination of hCG.

（4）DNA ploidy analysis.

（5）Maternal expressed imprinted genes detection.

（6）Others.

6.Differential diagnosis

（1）Abortion.

（2）Twin pregnancy.

7.Treatment

（1）Curettage: Timely curettage once diagnosed. Symptomatic treatment is needed to stabilize the condition before the curettage. Generally suction and curettage is used, which has the advantages of short operation time, less bleeding, less prone to uterine perforation and so on. Curettage should be carried out in operation room. Oxytocin is generally recommended to be used after the full dilation of the cervical canal and the start of uterine aspiration. If uterine ＜ 12 gestational weeks, curettage, ＞ 12 gestational weeks or one curettage is not enough, a second curettage can be performed a week later.

（2）Treatment of theca lutein ovarian cyst: After uterine curettage, the cyst in hydatidiform mole will resolve by itself, and generally no treatment is needed. Puncture and aspiration can be performed under ultrasound or laparoscopy in case of acute torsion and if necrosis occurs, the side appendages should be removed.

（3）Preventive chemotherapy: Not recommended.

（4）Hysterectomy.

8.随访

（1）hCG测定：葡萄胎清宫后每周1次，连续3次阴性后，每个月1次共6个月，再每2个月1次共6个月。

（2）月经、阴道出血、咳嗽、咯血、转移病灶等。

（3）妇科检查、超声、胸片等。

（4）葡萄胎随访期间可靠避孕1年。避孕方法可选避孕套或口服避孕药。

第二节 妊娠滋养细胞肿瘤

妊娠滋养细胞肿瘤60%继发于葡萄胎妊娠，30%继发于流产，10%继发于足月妊娠或异位妊娠。侵蚀性葡萄胎全部继发于葡萄胎妊娠，绒癌可继发于葡萄胎妊娠，也可继发于非葡萄胎妊娠。

1.病理

- 侵蚀性葡萄胎大体检查：子宫肌壁内有大小不等、深浅不一的水泡状组织。镜下可见绒毛结构及滋养细胞增生和异型性。绒毛膜癌镜下可见细胞滋养细胞和合体滋养细胞，而没有水泡状结构或绒毛。

2.临床表现

（1）无转移滋养细胞肿瘤：大多数继发于葡萄胎妊娠。

- 阴道出血、子宫复旧不全或不均匀性增大、卵巢黄素化

8.Follow-up

（1）hCG determination: After hydatidiform mole removal, once a week, after 3 consecutive negatives, once a month for 6 months, and then once every 2 months for 6 months.

（2）Menstruation, vaginal bleeding, cough, hemoptysis, metastasis, etc.

（3）Gynecological examination, ultrasound, chest X-ray, etc.

（4）Reliable contraception during follow-up for 1 year. Contraceptive methods include condoms or oral contraceptives.

Section 2　Gestational trophoblastic neoplasia

60% of gestational trophoblastic tumors secondary to hydatidiform mole pregnancy, 30% secondary to abortion, and 10% secondary to full-term pregnancy or ectopic pregnancy. Invasive moles are all secondary to hydatidiform mole pregnancy. Choriocarcinoma can be secondary to hydatidiform mole pregnancy or non-hydatidiform mole pregnancy.

1.Pathology

- Gross examination of invasive mole: Vesicular tissues of varying size and depths in the wall of uterus. The villus structure and trophoblast proliferation and atypia can be observed under microscope. Microscopically, cytotrophoblasts and syncytiotrophoblasts can be seen in choriocarcinoma without vesicular structure or villi.

2.Clinical manifestations

（1）Non-metastatic trophoblastic tumors: Most secondary to hydatidiform mole pregnancy.

- Vaginal bleeding, incomplete or uneven uterine involution, luteinized ovarian cysts,

囊肿、腹痛、假孕症状。

（2）转移滋养细胞肿瘤：除肺转移外，大多数继发于非葡萄胎妊娠或绒癌。

■ 主要经血行转移。肺转移（80%）、阴道转移（30%）、肝转移（20%）、脑转移（20%）、其他转移。

3.诊断

（1）临床诊断

■ 葡萄胎排空后或流产、足月分娩、异位妊娠后出现阴道出血和（或）转移灶及其相应症状和体征，考虑妊娠滋养细胞肿瘤。

■ hCG测定：hCG是葡萄胎妊娠后滋养细胞肿瘤的主要诊断依据。凡符合下列标准中任何一项且排除妊娠物残留或妊娠即可诊断妊娠滋养细胞肿瘤：①hCG测定4次高水平呈平台状态（±10%）并持续3周或更长时间，即1、7、14、21日；②hCG测定3次升高（>10%），并至少持续2周或更长时间，即1、7、14日。

■ 非葡萄胎妊娠后滋养细胞肿瘤诊断标准：足月产、流产、异位妊娠后hCG多在4周左右转为阴性，若超过4周hCG仍持续高水平，或一度下降后又上升，在除外妊娠物残留或妊娠可诊断妊娠滋养细胞肿瘤。

■ 超声检查、X线胸片、CT和

abdominal pain, and pseudopregnancy symptoms.

（2）Metastatic trophoblastic tumors: Most secondary to non-hydatidiform mole pregnancy or choriocarcinoma with the exception of lung metastasis.

■ Mainly hematogenous metastasis. Lung metastases（80%）, vaginal metastases（30%）, liver metastases（20%）, brain metastases（20%）and other metastases.

3.Diagnosis

（1）Clinical diagnosis

■ The gestational trophoblastic tumors should be considered, if vaginal bleeding and/or metastases and their symptoms and signs occur after hydatidiform emptying, abortion, full-term delivery and ectopic pregnancy.

■ Determination of hCG: The main diagnostic basis. Gestational trophoblastic tumors can be diagnosed if any of the following criteria is met and pregnancy residues or pregnancies are excluded: ①4 high levels of hCG in a plateau state（＋10%）for 3 weeks or longer, i.e. 1, 7, 14, 21 days; ②3 hCG increase（＞10%）for at least 2 weeks or longer, i.e. 1, 7, 14 days.

■ Diagnostic criteria for trophoblastic tumors in non-hydatidiform mole pregnancy: After full-term delivery, abortion, and ectopic pregnancy hCG usually turns negative in about 4 weeks. If the level of hCG remains high for more than 4 weeks or increases again after a decline, gestational trophoblastic tumors can be diagnosed excluding pregnancy residues or pregnancy.

■ Ultrasound, X-ray, CT and MRI.

磁共振检查。

（2）组织学诊断

- 绒毛或退化的绒毛阴影：侵蚀性葡萄胎。
- 成片滋养细胞浸润及坏死出血，未见绒毛结构者：绒癌。

4.临床分期（表22-2）

5.治疗

原则：化疗为主，手术和放疗为辅的综合治疗。

（1）化疗：单一药物化疗、联合化疗（EMA-CO为首选）

- 甲氨蝶呤（MTX）、放线菌素D（Act-D）、氟尿嘧啶（5-FU）、环磷酰胺（CTX）、长春新碱（VCR）、依托泊苷（VP-16）等。

- 疗效评估：每疗程结束后，每周测1次hCG。每疗程化疗结束至18日内，血hCG下降至少1个对数称为有效。

- 化疗药毒副作用：主要毒副作用为骨髓抑制，其次为消化道反应。

- 停药指征：hCG连续3次阴

（2）Histological diagnosis

- Shadow of villi or vestigial villi: Invasive mole.
- Trophoblast cells infiltrated, necrotic and bleeding, and no villi structure: Choriocarcinoma.

4.Clinical stage （Table 22-2）

5.Treatment

Principle: Chemotherapy as the main treatment, and surgery and radiotherapy as the complementary.

（1）Chemotherapy: Single drug chemotherapy, and combined chemotherapy（with EMA-CO the first choice）

- Methotrexate(MTX), dactinomycin(Act-D), fluorouracil（5-FU）, cyclophosphamide（CTX）, vincristine（VCR）, etoposide（VP-16）and so on.

- Efficacy evaluation: hCG is measured once a week after each course. Within 18 days of the end of each course of chemotherapy, decrease in the blood hCG by at least 1 logarithm is considered effective.

- Toxicity and side effects: Myelosuppression is the main toxicity and side effects, followed by digestive tract reactions.

- Drug withdrawal indications: After 3

表22-2　滋养细胞肿瘤解剖学分期（FIGO，2000年）

Table 22-2　Anatomical stages of trophoblastic neoplasm（FIGO, 2000）

Ⅰ期 Stage I	病变局限于子宫 Lesion confined to the uterus
Ⅱ期 Stage II	病变扩散，但仍局限于生殖器官（附件、阴道、阔韧带） Lesions spread but still limited to reproductive organs（adnexa, vagina, broad ligament）
Ⅲ期 Stage III	病变转移至肺，有或无生殖系统病变 Metastasis to the lung with or without reproductive system lesions
Ⅳ期 Stage IV	所有其他转移 All other metastasis

性后，低危患者至少给予一个化疗周期，而对化疗过程中hCG下降缓慢和病变广泛者可给予2～3个疗程的化疗；高危患者必须化疗3个疗程，且第一疗程必须是联合化疗。

（2）手术：子宫切除，肺切除术，开颅手术。

（3）放射治疗。

（4）耐药复发病例治疗。

6.随访

■ 严密随访。第1次在出院后3个月，然后每6个月1次至3年，此后每年1次至5年，以后可每2年1次。随访内容同葡萄胎。随访期间可靠避孕，一般于化疗停止≥12个月才可妊娠。

重点专业词汇

1.葡萄胎

2.完全性葡萄胎

3.部分性葡萄胎

4.胚胎

5.核型

6.绒毛水肿

7.绒毛滋养细胞

8.子痫前期

9.卵巢黄素化囊肿

10.流产

11.双胎妊娠

12.缩宫素

13.妊娠滋养细胞肿瘤（GTN）

14.异位妊娠

15.侵蚀性葡萄胎

16.绒癌

consecutive hCG negatives, low-risk patients are given at least one cycle of chemotherapy while those with slow hCG decline and extensive lesions during chemotherapy can be given 2 ～ 3 courses of chemotherapy; high-risk patients must be given 3 courses of chemotherapy, with the first course combined chemotherapy.

（2）Surgery: Hysterectomy, pneumonectomy and craniotomy.

（3）Radiotherapy.

（4）Treatment of drug-resistant recurrence cases.

6.Follow-up

■ Close follow-up. The first time is 3 months after discharge, then once every 6 months for 3 years, then once a year till 5 years, after that, once every 2 years. Follow-up is the same as that of hydatidiform mole. Reliable contraception should be used during follow-up and pregnancy is allowed after chemotherapy has ceased for ≥ 12 months.

Key words

1.Hydatidiform mole

2.Complete hydatidiform mole

3.Partial hydatidiform mole

4.Embryo

5.Karyotype

6.Villus edema

7.Villous trophoblast

8.Preeclampsia

9.Theca lutein ovarian cyst

10.Abortion

11.Twin pregnancy

12.Oxytocin

13.Gestational trophoblastic neoplasia（GTN）

14.Ectopic pregnancy

15.Invasive mole

16.Choriocarcinoma

练习题

1.下列关于葡萄胎的处理措施，哪项正确？（A）

A.先备血，再吸宫

B.先静脉滴注缩宫素，再吸宫

C.先化疗，再吸宫

D.先吸氧，再吸宫

E.先行子宫动脉栓塞，再吸宫

2.葡萄胎患者清宫后最理想的避孕方法是：（D）

A.长效口服避孕药

B.短效口服避孕药

C.放置宫内节育器

D.避孕套

E.避孕针

3.关于妊娠滋养细胞肿瘤的发生，下列哪项正确？（D）

A.侵蚀性葡萄胎可继发于流产后

B.侵蚀性葡萄胎不会发生子宫外转移

C.绝经后女性不会发生绒毛膜癌

D.绒毛膜癌可继发于足月妊娠或异位妊娠后

E.侵蚀性葡萄胎多继发于葡萄胎清宫后1年以上

4.绒毛膜癌最常见的转移部位依次是：（B）

A.肺、盆腔、肝、脑、阴道

B.肺、阴道、盆腔、肝、脑

C.肺、脑、盆腔、肝、阴道

D.阴道、肺、盆腔、肝、脑

E.肺、肝、阴道、盆腔、脑

（贾琳钰）

Exercises

1.Which of the following treatments of hydatidiform mole is correct?（A）

A.Blood preparation first, then uterine aspiration

B.Intravenous drip of oxytocin, and then uterine aspiration

C.Chemotherapy first, then uterine aspiration

D.First oxygen inhalation, and then uterine aspiration

E.Uterine artery embolization before uterine aspiration

2.The best contraceptive method for hydatidiform mole patients after curettage is:（D）

A.Long-acting oral contraceptives

B.Short-acting oral contraceptives

C.Placement of intrauterine device

D.Condom

E.Contraceptive injection

3.Which of the following is true about the occurrence of gestational trophoblastic tumor?（D）

A.Invasive hydatidiform mole can be secondary to abortion

B.Invasive hydatidiform mole does not cause extrauterine metastasis

C.Postmenopausal women do not have choriocarcinoma

D.Choriocarcinoma can be secondary to full-term pregnancy or ectopic pregnancy

E.Invasive hydatidiform mole usually occurs more than 1 year after curettage

4.The most common metastatic sites of choriocarcinoma are:（B）

A.Lung, pelvis, liver, brain, vagina

B.Lung, vagina, pelvis, liver and brain

C.Lung, brain, pelvis, liver and vagina

D.Vagina, lung, pelvis, liver and brain

E.Lung, liver, vagina, pelvis and brain

第23章　生殖内分泌疾病

CHAPTER 23　Reproductive endocrine diseases

<table>
<tr><td>

第一节　异常子宫出血

无排卵性异常子宫出血

1.病因及分类（图23-1）

■ 下丘脑-垂体-卵巢轴的功能失调，靶细胞效应异常，月经失调。占所有异常子宫

</td><td>

Section 1　Abnormal uterine bleeding

Anovulatory abnormal uterine bleeding

1.Etiology and classification (Table 23-1)

■ Hypothalamic-pituitary-ovarian axis dysfunction, abnormal target cell effects, menstrual disorders, accounting for 85% of

</td></tr>
</table>

异常子宫出血（AUB）
· 月经过多（AUB/HMB）
· 月经周期间出血（AUB/IMB）
Abnormal uterine bleeding（AUB）
· Heavy menstrual bleeding（AUB/HMB）
· Intermenstrual bleeding（AUB/IMB）

PALM：器质性病变 PALM：Structural causes	COEIN：非器质性病变 COEIN：Nonstructural causes
子宫内膜息肉（AUB-P） Polyp（AUB-P） 子宫腺肌病（AUB-A） Adenomyosis（AUB-A） 子宫肌瘤（AUB-L） Leiomyoma（AUB-L） 　黏膜下肌瘤（AUB-LSM） 　Submucosal myoma（AUB-LSM） 　其他部位肌瘤（AUB-LO） 　Other myoma（AUB-LO） 子宫内膜恶变和不典型增生（AUB-M） Malignancy and hyperplasia（AUB-M）	凝血功能障碍（AUB-C） Coagulopathy（AUB-C） 排卵功能障碍（AUB-O） Ovulatory dysfunction（AUB-O） 子宫内膜异常（AUB-E） Endometrial（AUB-E） 医源性因素（AUB-I） Iatrogenic（AUB-I） 未分类（AUB-N） Not yet classified（AUB-N）

图23-1　病因及分类

Table 23-1　Etiology and classification

出血（AUB）的85%。

- 青春期：下丘脑-垂体-卵巢轴激素间的反馈调节尚未成熟，大脑中枢对雌激素的正反馈作用反应低下，无LH高峰而不能排卵。
- 绝经过渡期：卵巢对垂体促性腺激素反应低下，卵泡发育受阻而不能排卵。
- 生育年龄女性：应激等因素如压力、紧张等也可以发生无排卵。

2.病理生理

（1）出血类型
- 撤退性出血：雌激素水平急剧下降引起的出血。
- 突破性出血：低水平雌激素内膜修复慢引起少量间断性出血，高水平雌激素引起闭经后的内膜不牢固引起的大量出血。

（2）出血的机制
- 缺乏孕激素导致月经的自限性机制缺陷
  - 子宫内膜组织脆弱，缺乏基质支持。
  - 子宫内膜脱落不完全，缺乏足够刺激，上皮再生修复困难。
  - 血管结构与功能异常，小血管多处断裂缺乏螺旋化。
  - 凝血与纤溶异常。
  - 血管舒张因子异常。

3.子宫内膜病理改变

（1）子宫内膜增生症
- 简单型增生：1%发展为子宫内膜癌。

all abnormal uterine bleeding（AUB）.

- Adolescence: Immaturity of the hypothalamic-pituitary-ovarian axis. Low response of hypothalamus and pituitary gland to positive feedback from estrogen, no LH peak and no ovulation.
- Menopause transition period: Low response of gonadotropins, follicle dysplasia without ovulation.
- Women of childbearing age: Anovulation can occurs also due to stress, tension, etc.

2.Pathophysiology

（1）Patterns of bleeding
- Withdrawal bleeding: Bleeding caused by a sharp drop in estrogen levels.
- Breakthrough bleeding: Low-level estrogen, and slow endometrial repair causing a small amount of intermittent bleeding; high-level estrogen causing massive hemorrhage due to unstable endometrium after amenorrhea.

（2）Mechanism of bleeding
- Lack of progesterone causes defects in the self-limiting mechanism of menstruation
  - Friability of endometrial tissue and lack of stromal support.
  - Incomplete shedding of endometrium, and no enough stimulation for epithelial regeneration.
  - Abnormal structure and function of blood vessels; lack of spiralization of the arteries.
  - Abnormal coagulation and fibrinolysis defects.
  - Abnormal vasodilator factors.

3.Endometrial pathological changes

（1）Endometrial hyperplasia
- Simple hyperplasia: 1% developing endometrial carcinoma.

- 复杂型增生：3%发展为子宫内膜癌。
- 不典型增生：23%发展为子宫内膜癌。

（2）增生期子宫内膜。

（3）萎缩型子宫内膜。

4.临床表现

（1）无排卵性功血患者可有各种不同的临床表现。

（2）最常见的症状是子宫不规则出血。

（3）特点是月经周期紊乱，经期长短不一，经量不定，甚至大量出血可导致贫血。

5.诊断

详细询问病史、体格检查、辅助检查方法。

（1）询问病史：异常子宫出血类型（月经过多、月经过频、子宫不规则出血过多、子宫不规则出血）、避孕措施、相关疾病及用药等。

（2）体格检查：包括全身检查、妇科检查等，以除外全身性疾病及生殖道器质性病变。

（3）辅助检查方法

- 诊断性刮宫：为明确子宫内膜病理和达到止血目的，必须进行全面刮宫。
- 超声检查：可了解子宫大小、形状，宫腔内有无赘生物，子宫内膜厚度等。
- 宫腔镜检查：直视下选择病变区域进行活检。
- 基础体温测定：基础体温呈单相型，提示无排卵。
- 激素测定：经前测定血清孕

- Complex hyperplasia: 3% developing endometrial carcinoma.
- Atypical hyperplasia: 23% developing endometrial carcinoma.

(2) Proliferative phase endometrium.

(3) Atrophic endometrium.

4.Clinical manifestations

(1) Anovulatory AUB patients may have a variety of clinical manifestations.

(2) The most common symptom is irregular uterine bleeding.

(3) Characterized by menstrual cycle disorder, menstrual periods of varying length, irregular menstrual flow, and even anemia caused by massive bleeding.

5.Diagnosis

Detailed inquiry of medical history, physical examination, auxiliary examination methods.

(1) Medical history: AUB types (menorrhagia, polymenorrhea, menometrorrhagia, metrorrhagia); contraception; related diseases; drug used, etc.

(2) Physical examination: Including systemic examination and pelvic examination, to exclude systemic diseases and reproductive tract organic diseases.

(3) Auxiliary examination methods

- Diagnostic curettage: Complete curettage is necessary to clarify endometrial pathology and achieve hemostasis.
- Ultrasound: The size and shape of the uterus, intrauterine cavity without neoplasm, endometrial thickness and so on.
- Hysteroscopy: The lesion area selected for biopsy under direct vision.
- Basal body temperature: Monophasic, indicating anovulation.
- Hormone determination: Premenstrual

酮值，若为卵泡期水平为无排卵。

- 妊娠试验：以排除妊娠及妊娠相关疾病。
- 血红细胞计数及血细胞比容：了解贫血情况。
- 血凝功能测定：排除凝血功能障碍疾病。

6.鉴别诊断

（1）全身性疾病：如血液病、肝损害、甲状腺功能亢进或低下等。

（2）异常妊娠或妊娠并发症：如流产、宫外孕、滋养细胞疾病、子宫复旧不良、胎盘残留、胎盘息肉等。

（3）生殖器官感染：如急性或慢性子宫内膜炎、子宫肌炎等。

（4）生殖器官肿瘤：如子宫内膜癌、子宫肌瘤、卵巢肿瘤等。

（5）其他：性激素类药物使用不当及宫内节育器或异物引起的子宫不规则出血。

7.治疗

（1）一般治疗：改善全身情况。

（2）药物治疗：治疗原则（止血，调经，促排卵）。

- 青春期及生育年龄：止血、调整周期、促排卵为主。
- 绝经过渡期：止血、调整周期、减少经量，防止子宫内膜病变为原则。
- 止血：对少量出血患者，使用最低有效量激素，减少药物不良作用。大量出血患者，要求在性激素治疗8小

serum progesterone value, if the level of follicular phase, indicating anovulation.

- Pregnancy test: Excluding pregnancy and pregnancy-related diseases.
- Red blood cell count and hematocrit: Anemia or not.
- Blood coagulation test: Excluding coagulation dysfunction.

6.Differential diagnosis

（1）Systemic diseases: Such as hematopathy, liver damage, hyperthyroidism or hypothyroidism, etc.

（2）Abnormal pregnancy or pregnancy complications: Such as abortion, ectopic pregnancy, trophoblastic diseases, uterus subinvolution, placental residue, placental polyp, etc.

（3）Genital infection: Such as acute or chronic endometritis, myometritis, etc.

（4）Genital tumors: Such as endometrial cancer, uterine myoma, ovarian tumors, etc.

（5）Others: Improper use of sex hormones and irregular bleeding caused by intrauterine devices or foreign bodies.

7.Treatment

（1）General treatment: Improving overall condition.

（2）Medical treatment: Principles of treatment （hemostasis, cycle adjustment and ovulation induction）

- Adolescence and childbearing age: Hemostasis, cycle adjustment and ovulation induction mainly.
- Menopause transition period: Hemostasis, cycle adjustment, reducing bleeding, preventing endometrial lesions.
- Hemostasis: For patients with a small amount of bleeding, use the lowest effective dose of hormone to reduce drug side effects. For patients with massive

时内明显见效，24～48小时血止，若96小时以上仍不止血，应考虑更改AUB诊断。

①性激素联合用药：性激素联合用药的止血效果优于单一用药。口服避孕药。

②单一激素：雌激素治疗（内膜修复法），适用于大量出血患者。孕激素治疗（内膜脱落法或称药物刮宫），适用于体内有一定水平雌激素患者。

③刮宫：可以快速止血，了解子宫内膜病理情况，除外恶性病变。

④辅助治疗：一般止血药、雄激素、凝血药、纠正贫血、抗感染。

● 调整月经周期：使用性激素止血后必须调整月经周期。

①雌孕激素序贯法、雌孕激素联合用药。

②后半周期疗法：适用于青春期或绝经过渡期AUB。

③宫内孕激素释放系统（曼月乐）。

● 促排卵：青春期不提倡用促排卵药物，生育期有生育要求的可采用。

hemorrhage, it is required to have obvious effect within 8 hours of hormone treatment, and stop bleeding within 24～48 hours. If bleeding does not stop for more than 96 hours, change of AUB diagnosis should be considered.

①Sex hormone combination: Sex hormone combination of hemostatic effect superior to the single drug use. Oral contraceptive pill.

②Single hormone: Estrogen therapy (endometrial repair method): Suitable for patients with massive hemorrhage. Progesterone therapy (endometrial shedding method also known as drug curettage): Suitable for patients with a certain level of estrogen.

③Curettage: Rapid hemostasis, understanding the endometrium pathology, and excluding malignant lesions.

④Adjuvant therapy: General hemostatic, androgen, coagulation drug, anemia correction, and anti-infection.

● Adjustment of menstrual cycle: After hemostasis with sex hormones, menstrual cycle must be adjusted.

①Estrogen-progestogen sequential method, and estrogen-progesterone combination.

②Half cycle therapy: Suitable for patients in puberty or menopause transition.

③Intrauterine progestogen release system (Mirena).

● Ovulation induction: Ovulation induction drugs are not recommended in puberty, but can be used for women in childbearing age with fertility needs.

（3）手术治疗：药物治疗疗效不佳、不宜用药、无生育要求、不宜随访的年龄较大者（子宫内膜切除术、子宫切除术）。

排卵性异常子宫出血

1.类型

（1）月经过多。

（2）月经周期间出血。

■ 黄体功能异常：黄体功能不足，子宫内膜不规则脱落。

■ 围排卵期出血。

2.月经过多

（1）育龄期19%发生率。

（2）子宫内膜纤溶酶活性高或ER、PR增高。

（3）月经规律，经期正常，经量增多，排除器质性疾病。

（4）止血药、避孕药、曼月乐治疗。

3.月经周期间出血

（1）黄体功能不足（LPD）

■ 病因及临床特点

• 卵泡期FSH缺乏，使卵泡发育缓慢，雌激素分泌减少，从而对垂体及下丘脑正反馈不足，LH脉冲峰值不高及排卵峰后LH低脉冲缺陷。

• 卵巢本身发育不良，卵泡期颗粒细胞LH受体缺陷，也可使排卵后颗粒细胞黄素化不良，孕激素分泌减少，致子宫内膜分泌的反应不足。

（3）Surgical treatment: Older patients with poor curative effects of medication, unsuitable for drug use and follow-up, and with no fertility requirements（endometrial resection, and hysterectomy）.

Ovulatory AUB

1.Classification

（1）Menorrhagia.

（2）Hemorrhage between menstrual cycles

■ Corpus luteum dysfunction: Luteum phase defect（LPD）, irregular shedding of endometrium.

■ Periovulation bleeding.

2.Menorrhagia

（1）Incidence of 19% in childbearing age.

（2）High endometrial fibrinolytic enzyme activity or increased ER and PR.

（3）Normal menstrual cycle, normal duration of bleeding, increased volume, excluding organic diseases.

（4）Hemostatic, contraceptive pills, Mirena therapy.

3.Hemorrhage between menstrual cycles

（1）Luteal phase defect（LPD）

■ Etiology and clinical features

• FSH deficiency in follicular stage and slow follicular development cause decreased estrogen secretion, resulting in insufficient positive feedback to pituitary and hypothalamus, low LH pulse peak and low LH pulse defect after ovulation peak.

• Ovarian dysplasia, and granulosa cell LH receptor defect in follicular phase, can also cause poor luteinization of granular cells after ovulation, and reduce progesterone secretion, thus resulting in insufficient response to endometrial

- 孕激素分泌减少，导致黄体期缩短（＜11日）。
- 分泌期内膜腺体呈分泌不良，内膜活检显示分泌反应落后2日。

- 月经周期短，尤其黄体期短，易发生不孕或流产，双相体温，但高相期小于11日。
- 治疗
  - 促进卵泡发育。
  - 促进月经周期中LH峰形成。
  - 黄体功能刺激疗法。
  - 黄体功能替代疗法。
  - 黄体功能不足合并高催乳激素血症的治疗。
  - 避孕药。

（2）子宫内膜不规则脱落

- 由于下丘脑-垂体-卵巢轴调节功能紊乱或溶黄体机制异常引起黄体萎缩不全，子宫内膜持续受孕激素影响，以致不能如期完整脱落。

- 于月经期第5～6日仍能见呈分泌反应的内膜，子宫内膜表现为混合型。
- 经期延长，长达9～10日，且出血量多。
- 基础体温双相，但下降缓慢。

- 孕激素、绒促性素、避孕药治疗。

（3）围排卵期出血

- 即排卵期出血。
- 排卵期雌激素水平短暂下降。
- 出血量少、出血期少于7日、

secretion.

- Low production of progesterone leading to shortened luteal phase（＜11 days）.
- During the period of secretion, the membrane glands show poor secretion, and endometrial biopsy shows a 2-day delay in secretory response.
- Short menstrual cycle, especially short luteal phase, is prone to infertility or abortion, with biphasic body temperature, but the high phase less than 11 days.
- Treatment
  - Stimulating follicular development.
  - Enhancing the LH peak.
  - Luteal stimulation therapy.
  - Luteal replacement therapy.
  - Treatment of luteal dysfunction with hyperprolactinemia.
  - Contraceptive pills.

（2）Irregular shedding of endometrium

- Due to the dysfunction of hypothalamic-pituitary-ovary axis regulation or abnormal luteolysis mechanism causing luteal atrophy, the endometrium continues to be affected by progesterone, so that it cannot be completely exfoliated as scheduled.
- On the 5th ～ 6th day of menstruation, the secretory endometrium is still visible, and the endometrium is mixed.
- The period is prolonged, for 9 ～ 10 days, and the amount of bleeding is large.
- Basal body temperature is biphasic but drops slowly.
- Progesterone, gonadotropin, and contraceptive treatment.

（3）Periovulation bleeding

- Ovulation bleeding.
- A brief estrogen level drop during ovulation.
- Less bleeding, less than 7 days of bleeding,

时有时无。

■ 避孕药治疗。

重点专业词汇

1. 异常子宫出血（AUB）

2. 无排卵性异常子宫出血

3. 排卵性异常子宫出血

4. 单纯型增生

5. 复杂型增生

6. 不典型增生

7. 月经过多

8. 雌孕激素序贯疗法（人工周期）

练习题

1. 最常见的两类排卵性异常子宫出血是（   ）和（   ）。

2. BBT 单相型提示：（D）

A. 流产

B. 分娩发作

C. 有排卵

D. 无排卵

E. 异位妊娠

3. 如果月经周期为32日，排卵发生在月经周期第几日？（D）

A.9日

B.14日

C.16日

D.18日

E.20日

（温　菁）

第二节　闭　　经

1.定义

■ 闭经：无月经或月经停止。

■ 原发性闭经：年龄超过14岁，第二性征未发育；或年龄超过16岁，第二性征已发育，月经还未来潮。

with no bleeding sometimes.

■ Contraceptive treatment.

Key words

1. Abnormal uterine bleeding（AUB）

2. Anovulatory abnormal uterine bleeding

3. Ovulatory abnormal uterine bleeding

4. Simple hyperplasia

5. Complex hyperplasia

6. Atypical hyperplasia

7. Menorrhagia

8. Sequential therapy with E and P（artificial cycle）

Exercises

1. The two most common types of ovulatory abnormal uterine bleeding are（   ）and（   ）.

2. BBT monophasic type indicates:（D）

A. Abortion

B. Onset of labor

C. Ovulation

D. Anovulation

E. Ectopic pregnancy

3. If menstrual period is 32 days, ovulation occurs on which day of the menstrual cycle?（D）

A. Ninth

B. Fourteenth

C. Sixteenth

D. Eighteenth

E. Twentieth

Section 2　Amenorrhea

1.Definition

■ Amenorrhea: Absence or cessation of menstruation.

■ Primary amenorrhea: A young woman has never menstruated by age 14 years without secondary sexual development or by age 16 years with secondary sexual development.

■ 继发性闭经：正常月经建立后月经停止6个月，或按自身原有月经周期计算停止3个周期以上。

2.病因

（1）原发性闭经

■ 第二性征存在的原发性闭经

- 米勒管发育不全综合征（MRKH）。

- 雄激素不敏感综合征。
- 对抗卵巢综合征。
- 生殖道闭锁。
- 真两性畸形。

■ 第二性征缺乏的原发性闭经

- 低促性腺激素性腺功能减退
  ·最常见体质性青春发育延迟，其次为嗅觉缺失综合征。
- 高促性腺激素性腺功能减退，为性腺衰竭所致。
  ①特纳综合征。
  ②46，XX单纯性腺发育不全。
  ③46，XY单纯性腺发育不全，又称Swyer综合征。

（2）继发性闭经

■ 下丘脑性闭经
- 最常见，以功能性原因为主。下丘脑合成和分泌GnRH缺陷或下降导致垂体卵泡刺激素（FSH）和黄体生成素（LH）的分泌功能低下。
  ①精神应激。
  ②体重下降和神经性厌食。

■ Secondary amenorrhea: A menstruating woman has not menstruated for 6 months or for the duration of three typical menstrual cycles.

2.Etiology

（1）Primary amenorrhea

■ Primary amenorrhea with secondary sexual characteristics
- Müllerian agenesis syndrome or Mayer-Rokitansky-Kuster-Hauser syndrome（MRKH）.
- Androgen insensitivity syndrome.
- Savage syndrome.
- Atresia of genital tract.
- True hermaphroditism.

■ Primary amenorrhea without secondary sexual characteristics
- Hypogonadotropic hypogonadism

  · Constitutional delayed adolescence is common, and then Kallmann's syndrome.
- Hypergonadotropic hypogonadism, caused by gonadal failure.
  ①Turner's syndrome.
  ②46, XX gonadal dysgenesis.

  ③46, XY gonadal dysgenesis（Swyer syndrome）.

（2）Secondary amenorrhea

■ Hypothalamic amenorrhea
- Most common, mainly for functional reasons. Deficiency or decline in hypothalamic synthesis and secretion of GnRH results in hyposecretion of pituitary follicle stimulating hormone（FSH）and luteinizing hormone（LH）.
  ①Psychogenic stress.
  ②Weight loss and anorexia nervosa.

③运动性闭经。

④药物性闭经。

⑤颅咽管瘤。

- 垂体性闭经
  - 腺垂体器质性病变或功能失调，均可影响促性腺激素分泌，继而影响卵巢功能引起闭经。

    ①垂体梗死：希恩综合征（Sheehan syndrome），由于产后大出血休克，导致垂体尤其是腺垂体促性腺激素分泌细胞缺血坏死，引起腺垂体功能低下。

    ②垂体肿瘤：催乳素腺瘤，引起闭经溢乳综合征。

    ③空蝶鞍综合征。

- 卵巢性闭经
  - 卵巢分泌的性激素水平低下，子宫内膜不发生周期性变化而导致闭经，促性腺激素升高。

    ①卵巢早衰：40岁前卵巢功能衰竭，称为卵巢早衰。高促性腺激素水平，FSH＞40U/L，伴雌激素水平下降。

    ②卵巢功能性肿瘤。

    ③多囊卵巢综合征。

- 子宫性闭经
  - 感染、创伤导致宫腔粘连引起的闭经。月经调节功能正常，第二性征发育也正常。

    ①Asherman综合征：为子宫性闭经最常见原因，多因刮宫过度损伤子宫内膜，导致宫腔粘

③Exercise induced amenorrhea.

④Drug induced amenorrhea.

⑤Craniopharyngioma.

- Pituitary amenorrhea
  - Organic disease or dysfunction of anterior pituitary gland can affect gonadotropin secretion and ovarian function, leading to amenorrhea.

    ①Pituitary infarction: Sheehan syndrome, due to postpartum hemorrhagic shock, leads to hypophysis, especially adenohypophysis gonadotropin secreting cells ischemia necrosis, resulting in hypopituitarism.

    ②Pituitary tumor: Prolactin（PRL）adenoma causes amenorrhea galactorrhea syndrome.

    ③Empty sella syndrome.

- Ovarian amenorrhea
  - The level of sex hormones secreted by ovaries is low, and the endometrium does not change periodically, which leads to amenorrhea and gonadotropin elevation.

    ①Premature ovarian failure: Ovarian failure before the age of 40 is known as premature ovarian failure. High gonadotropin level, FSH＞40U/L, decreased estrogen level.

    ②Functional ovarian tumor.

    ③Polycystic ovary syndrome.

- Uterine amenorrhea
  - Infection and trauma lead to amenorrhea caused by intrauterine adhesions. Menstrual regulation is normal and secondary sexual development is normal.

    ①Asherman syndrome: The most common cause of uterine amenorrhea, mostly due to excessive curettage of endometrium, resulting in intrauterine

连而闭经。

②手术切除子宫或放疗。

■ 甲状腺、肾上腺、胰腺等功能紊乱也可引起闭经。

3.诊断

（1）病史：详细询问月经史、生育史、其他疾病及家族史。

（2）体格检查：包括全身检查及妇科检查，注意第二性征发育情况。

（3）辅助检查：生育年龄女性闭经首先应排除妊娠。

■ 功能试验
  ● 药物撤退试验：用于评估体内雌激素水平，以确定闭经程度。
    ①孕激素试验：停药后出现撤药性出血（阳性反应），提示子宫内膜已受一定水平雌激素影响。停药后无撤药性出血（阴性反应），应进一步行雌孕激素序贯试验。
    ②雌孕激素序贯试验：撤药无出血，提示子宫性闭经。
  ● 垂体兴奋试验：又称GnRH刺激试验。
■ 血清激素测定
  ● 血甾体激素测定。
  ● 催乳素及垂体促性腺激素测定。
  ● 雄激素测定、口服葡萄糖耐量试验、胰岛素释放试验等。

adhesion and amenorrhea.

②Hysterectomy or radiotherapy.

■ Dysfunction of thyroid, adrenal gland and pancreas can also cause amenorrhea.

3.Diagnosis

（1）Medical history: Detailed inquiry of menstrual history, reproductive history, other diseases and family history.

（2）Physical examination: Including general examination and pelvic examination, paying attention to the development of secondary sexual characteristics.

（3）Auxiliary examination: For amenorrhea in women of childbearing age, pregnancy should be excluded at first.

■ Function test
  ● Drug withdrawal test: Used to assess the level of estrogen in the body to determine amenorrhea.
    ①Progestational challenge: Drug withdrawal bleeding（positive reaction）indicating that endometrium has been affected by a certain level of estrogen. No bleeding after withdrawal（negative reaction）, a further sequential test of estrogen and progestogen should be carried out.
    ②Sequential test of estrogen and progestogen: No bleeding after withdrawal, indicating uterine amenorrhea.
  ● Pituitary stimulation test: Also known as GnRH stimulation test.
■ Serum hormone determination
  ● Serum steroid hormone determination.
  ● Prolactin and pituitary gonadotropin determination.
  ● Serum androgen assay, OGTT, IRT.

- 影像学检查
  - 盆腔超声检查。
  - 子宫输卵管造影。
  - 计算机断层扫描（CT）或磁共振显像（MRI）。
  - 静脉肾盂造影。
- 宫腔镜检查
- 腹腔镜检查
- 染色体检查
- 基础体温测定、子宫内膜取样、内膜培养等

4.治疗

（1）全身治疗
- 积极治疗全身性疾病，提高机体体质。

（2）激素治疗
- 性激素补充治疗
  - 目的：
    ①维持女性全身健康及生殖健康。
    ②促进和维持第二性征和月经。
  - 雌激素补充治疗。
  - 雌、孕激素人工周期疗法。
  - 孕激素疗法。
- 促排卵：适用于有生育要求的患者。卵巢功能衰竭，不建议采用促排卵药物治疗。
  - 氯米芬。
  - 促性腺激素：并发症为多胎妊娠和卵巢过度刺激综合征。
  - 促性腺激素释放激素。
- 溴隐亭。
- 其他激素治疗
  - 肾上腺皮质激素：适用于

- Imaging examination
  - Pelvic ultrasound examination.
  - Hysterosalpingography.
  - Compute tomography（CT）or magnetic resonance imaging（MRI）.
  - Intravenous pyelography.
- Hysteroscopy
- Laparoscopy
- Chromosome examination
- Basal body temperature measurement, endometrial sampling, endometrial culture, etc.

4.Treatment

（1）General treatment
- Active treatment of systemic diseases, to improve body constitution.

（2）Hormone therapy
- Sex hormone replacement therapy
  - Purpose:
    ①To keep overall and reproductive health for women.
    ②To promote and maintain secondary sexual characteristics and menstruation.
  - Estrogen replacement therapy.
  - Artificial cycle therapy of estrogen and progestogen.
  - Progestogen therapy.
- Ovulation induction: Suitable for patients with fertility requirements. Ovulation induction drugs are not recommended to patients with ovarian failure.
  - Clomiphene.
  - Gonadotropin: Complications are multiple pregnancy and ovarian hyperstimulation syndrome.
  - Gonadotropin releasing hormone(GnRH).
- Bromocriptine.
- Other hormone therapies
  - Adrenal cortex hormone: Suitable for

先天性肾上腺皮质增生所致的闭经。

- 甲状腺素：适用于甲状腺功能减退引起的闭经。

（3）辅助生殖技术

（4）手术治疗

- 生殖器畸形。
- Asherman综合征。
- 肿瘤。

重点专业词汇

1.闭经

2.原发性闭经

3.继发性闭经

4.特纳综合征

5.希恩综合征

6.卵巢早衰

7.月经稀发

8.经量过少

9.下丘脑-垂体-卵巢轴（H-P-O轴）

练习题

1.关于闭经的分类，正确的有：（ABCD）

A.子宫性闭经

B.卵巢性闭经

C.垂体性闭经

D.下丘脑性闭经

E.输卵管性闭经

2.关于闭经的诊断，下列哪项是错误的？（C）

A.孕激素试验（＋）——卵巢能分泌雌激素

B.雌激素试验（–）——原因在子宫

C.刮取内膜检查可确定闭经类型

D.女性第二性征发育良好——原因在子宫

E.基础体温双相——原因在

amenorrhea due to congenital adrenal hyperplasia.

- Thyroxine: Suitable for amenorrhea due to hypothyroidism.

（3）Assisted reproductive technology

（4）Surgical treatment

- Genital malformation.
- Asherman syndrome.
- Tumor.

Key words

1.Amenorrhea

2.Primary amenorrhea

3.Secondary amenorrhea

4.Turner's syndrome

5.Sheehan syndrome

6.Premature ovarian failure

7.Oligomenorrhea

8.Hypomenorrhea

9.Hypothalamic-pituitary-ovarian axis

Exercises

1.Which is right about the types of amenorrhea? （ABCD）

A.Uterine amenorrhea

B.Ovarian amenorrhea

C.Pituitary amenorrhea

D.Hypothalamic amenorrhea

E.Tubal amenorrhea

2.Which one is wrong about the diagnosis of amenorrhea?（C）

A.Progesterone challenge test（＋）—Ovaries produce estrogen

B.Estrogen challenge test（–）—The cause is in uterus

C.The type of amenorrhea can be determined by curettage examination

D.Good female secondary sexual development—The cause is in uterus

E.Basal body temperature is biphasic—The

子宫

3.未婚女性，28岁，闭经2年，肛诊：子宫正常大小，孕激素试验阴性，下一步最佳方法是：（E）

A.垂体兴奋试验

B.基础体温测定（BBT）

C.染色体检查

D.激素水平测定

E.雌激素试验

（魏　巍）

第三节　多囊卵巢综合征

多囊卵巢综合征（PCOS）是常见的妇科内分泌疾病，以雄激素过高的临床或生化表现、持续无排卵、卵巢多囊样改变为特征，常伴有胰岛素抵抗和肥胖。

1.内分泌特征与病理生理

（1）内分泌特征

■ 雄激素过多。

■ 雌酮过多。

■ 黄体生成激素/卵泡刺激素比值增大。

■ 胰岛素过多。

（2）产生这些内分泌变化的机制可能有：

■ 下丘脑–垂体–卵巢轴调节功能异常。

■ 胰岛素抵抗和高胰岛素血症。

■ 肾上腺内分泌功能异常。

2.病理

（1）卵巢变化：双侧卵巢均匀

cause is in uterus

3.An-unmarried female of 28 years old, has been amenorrhea for 2 years. The size of uterus is normal by anal examination, and progesterone challenge test is negative. The next best examination is：（E）

A.Pituitary stimulation test

B.Basal body temperature（BBT）

C.Chromosome examination

D.Hormone determination

E.Estrogen challenge test

Section 3　Polycystic ovarian syndrome

Polycystic ovarian syndrome（PCOS）is a common gynecological endocrine disorder, characterized by clinical or biochemical manifestations of excessive androgen, persistent anovulation, polycystic ovarian changes, and often accompanied by insulin resistance and obesity.

1.Endocrine characteristics and pathophysiology

（1）Endocrine characteristics

■ Androgen excess.

■ Estrone excess.

■ Ratio increase in luteinizing hormone（LH）/follicle-stimulating hormone（FSH）.

■ Hyperinsulinemia.

（2）The mechanisms responsible for these endocrine changes may include:

■ Abnormal regulation of hypothalamic-pituitary-ovarian axis.

■ Insulin resistance and hyperinsulinemia.

■ Abnormal adrenal endocrine.

2.Pathology

（1）Ovarian changes: Bilateral ovarian

性增大，白膜增厚，≥12个囊性卵泡及闭锁卵泡，无成熟卵泡及排卵迹象。

（2）子宫内膜变化：因无排卵子宫内膜呈现不同程度增殖性改变，长期持续无排卵，增加子宫内膜癌的发生概率。

3.临床表现

（1）PCOS多起病于青春期，主要临床表现包括月经失调、雄激素过量和肥胖。

（2）月经失调：月经稀发或闭经，也可表现为不规则子宫出血。

（3）不孕：生育期女性排卵障碍性不孕。

（4）多毛、痤疮：高雄激素血症最常见表现。

（5）肥胖：50%以上患者肥胖且常呈腹部肥胖型。

（6）黑棘皮症。

- 附：多囊卵巢综合征并发症

- 近期并发症
  - 肥胖。
  - 不孕。
  - 抑郁。
  - 睡眠呼吸暂停。
  - 月经紊乱。
  - 血脂异常。
  - 非酒精性脂肪肝。
  - 多毛/痤疮/雄激素性脱发。
  - 胰岛素抵抗/黑棘皮症。
- 远期并发症
  - 糖尿病。
  - 子宫内膜癌。
  - 心血管疾病。

4.辅助检查

（1）基础体温测定：呈单相型基础体温曲线。

uniform enlargement, white membrane thickened, ≥12 cystic follicles and atresia follicles, no mature follicles and signs of ovulation.

（2）Endometrial changes: Endometrium shows different proliferative changes due to anovulation. Long-term persistent anovulation increases the risk of endometrial cancer.

3.Clinical manifestations

（1）PCOS often occurs in adolescence. The main clinical manifestations include menstrual disorders, androgen excess and obesity.

（2）Menstrual disorders: Oligomenorrhea or amenorrhea and irregular uterine bleeding.

（3）Infertility: Anovulatory infertility in reproductive women.

（4）Hirsute and acne: The most common manifestation of androgen excess.

（5）Obesity: More than 50% patients are obese and are often of abdominal obesity type.

（6）Acanthosis nigricans.

- Appendix: Complications of polycystic ovarian syndrome
- Short-term complications
  - Obesity.
  - Infertility.
  - Depression.
  - Sleep apnea.
  - Menstrual disorder.
  - Abnormal lipid levels.
  - Non-alcoholic fatty liver disease.
  - Hirsutism/acne/androgenic alopecia.
  - Insulin resistance/acanthosis nigricans.
- Long-term complications
  - Diabetes mellitus.
  - Endometrial cancer.
  - Cardiovascular disease.

4.Auxiliary examination

（1）Basal body temperature measurement: A monophasic basal body temperature curve.

（2）超声检查：见卵巢增大，一侧或两侧卵巢各有12个以上直径为2～9mm无回声区，围绕卵巢边缘，呈车轮状排列，称为"项链征"。连续监测未见主导卵泡发育及排卵迹象。

（3）诊断性刮宫：子宫内膜呈不同程度增殖改变，无分泌期变化。

（4）腹腔镜检查。

（5）内分泌测定

■ 血清雄激素：睾酮、雄烯二酮升高，脱氢表雄酮、硫酸脱氢表雄酮正常或轻度升高。

■ 血清FSH、LH：血清FSH正常或偏低，LH升高，但无排卵前LH峰值出现。LH/FSH比值增加。

■ 血清雌激素：雌酮（E1）升高，雌二醇（E2）正常或轻度升高，E1/E2＞1。

■ 尿17-酮类固醇：正常或轻度升高，升高时提示肾上腺功能亢进。

■ 血清催乳素：可轻度增高。

■ 肥胖患者，应检测空腹血糖（FBG）及口服葡萄糖耐量试验（OGTT），胰岛素释放试验（IRT）及血脂。

5.诊断

■ PCOS是排除性诊断，欧洲生殖和胚胎医学会与美国生殖医学会提出PCOS的诊断标准应符合下列3项中的2项：

（2）Ultrasound examination: Ovarian enlargement, with more than 12 follicles in diameter of 2 ～ 9mm on one or both ovaries, arranged in wheel shape around the ovarian margin, known as "necklace sign". Continuous monitoring shows no sign of dominant follicular development and ovulation.

（3）Diagnostic curettage: Endometrium shows different degrees of proliferation and no changes in secretory phase.

（4）Laparoscopy examination.

（5）Endocrine determination

■ Serum androgen: Testosterone and andros-tenedione increased, dehydroepiandroste-rone and dehydroepiandrosterone sulfate normal or slightly elevated.

■ Serum FSH and LH: Serum FSH normal or low, LH increased, but without the LH peak before ovulation. LH: FSH ratios elevated.

■ Serum estrogen: Estrone（E1）increased, estradiol（E2）normal or slightly elevated, E1/E2＞1.

■ Urinary 17-ketosteroids: Normal or slightly elevated. Adrenal hyperfunction indicated when elevated.

■ Serum prolactin: Slightly increased.

■ For obese patients, fasting blood glucose（FBG）, oral glucose tolerance test（OGTT）, insulin release test（IRT）, and blood lipids should be tested.

5.Diagnosis

■ PCOS is an exclusion diagnosis. The joint ESHRE/ASRM（European Society of Human Reproduction and Embryology/ American Society for Reproductive Medicine）consensus defined PCOS as requiring the presence of two out of the following three criteria:

- 稀发排卵或无排卵。
- 高雄激素的临床表现和（或）高雄激素血症。
- 卵巢多囊样改变。

■ 并排除其他高雄激素病因，如先天性肾上腺皮质增生（CAH）、库欣综合征、分泌雄激素的肿瘤。

6.鉴别诊断
（1）卵泡膜细胞增殖症。
（2）肾上腺皮质增生或肿瘤。

（3）分泌雄激素的卵巢肿瘤。
（4）垂体催乳素腺瘤。

7.治疗
（1）调整生活方式：应控制饮食和增加运动以降低体重和缩小腰围，可增加胰岛素敏感性，降低胰岛素、睾酮水平，从而恢复排卵及生育功能。
（2）药物治疗
■ 调节月经周期
- 口服避孕药：为雌孕激素联合周期疗法，疗程一般为3～6个月，可重复使用。能有效抑制毛发生长和治疗痤疮。
- 孕激素后半周期疗法：调节月经并保护子宫内膜。

■ 降低血雄激素水平
- 糖皮质类固醇：适用于雄激素过多为肾上腺来源或肾上腺和卵巢混合来源者。
- 环丙孕酮。
- 螺内酯。

■ 改善胰岛素抵抗：对肥胖或有胰岛素抵抗患者常用胰岛

- Oligo-ovulation or anovulation.
- Clinical manifestations of hyperandrogens and hyperandrogenism.
- Polycystic ovaries assessed by ultrasound.

■ Excluding other hyperandrogenic causes, such as congenital adrenal hyperplasia （CAH）, cushing syndrome and androgen-secreting tumors.

6.Differential diagnosis
（1）Ovarian hyperthecosis.
（2）Congenital adrenal hyperplasia or adrenal tumors.
（3）Androgen-secreting ovarian tumors.
（4）Pituitary prolactinoma.

7.Treatment
（1）Lifestyle modification: Diet and exercise should be controlled to reduce weight and waist circumference, which increases insulin sensitivity, reduce insulin and testosterone levels and restore ovulation and fertility function.
（2）Medical treatment
■ Regulating menstrual cycle
- Oral contraceptives: Estrogen-progestin combination cycle therapy, with treatment course usually 3 ～ 6 months and reuse. It can treat hirsutism and acne effectively.
- Progesterone second half cycle therapy: Menstruation regulation and endometrium protection.

■ Decrease in serum androgen level
- Glucocorticoid: Suitable for those with androgen excess from adrenal gland or mixed source of adrenal and ovary.
- Cyproterone.
- Spironolactone.

■ Insulin resistance improvement: Insulin sensitizers used for obese or insulin-

素增敏剂。

■ 诱发排卵：有生育要求者在生活方式调整、抗雄激素和改善胰岛素抵抗等基础治疗后，进行促排卵治疗。

（3）手术治疗

■ 腹腔镜下卵巢打孔术。

■ 卵巢楔形切除术。

重点专业词汇

1. 多囊卵巢综合征（PCOS）

2. 胰岛素抵抗

3. 胰岛素受体

4. 多毛症

5. 痤疮

6. 口服避孕药

练习题

1. 多囊卵巢综合征多起病于：（B）

A. 儿童期

B. 青春期

C. 妊娠期

D. 围绝经期

E. 哺乳期

2. 多囊卵巢综合征患者月经失调多表现为：（D）

A. 月经频发

B. 月经量多

C. 痛经

D. 月经稀发或闭经

E. 不规则出血

3. 多囊卵巢综合征患者行诊断性刮宫时机应选择在：（C）

A. 月经第 4 日

B. 月经干净后 3 ～ 5 日

C. 在月经前数日或月经来潮 6 小时内

resistant patients.

■ Ovulation induction: After basic treatment such as lifestyle modification, anti-androgen therapy and insulin resistance improvement, those with fertility requirements are given ovulation induction therapy.

（3）Surgical treatment

■ Laparoscopic ovarian drilling.

■ Ovarian wedge resection.

Key words

1. Polycystic ovarian syndrome（PCOS）

2. Insulin resistance

3. Insulin receptor

4. Hirsutism

5. Acne

6. Oral contraceptives

Exercises

1. Polycystic ovarian syndrome usually occurs in:（B）

A. Childhood

B. Adolescence

C. Pregnancy

D. Perimenopause

E. Lactation

2. Irregular menstruation in patients with polycystic ovarian syndrome is mostly manifested as:（D）

A. Polymeorrhea

B. Menorrhagia

C. Dysmenorrhea

D. Oligomenorrhea or amenorrhea

E. Irregular bleeding

3. The time of diagnostic curettage for patients with polycystic ovary syndrome should be chosen on:（C）

A. The 4th day of menstruation

B. 3 ～ 5 days after menstruation

C. Several days before menstrual period or within 6 hours of menstrual onset

D.月经第2日

E.无特殊要求

（魏　巍）

第四节　绝经综合征

月经永久性停止，称为绝经。

绝经综合征（menopause syndrome）指妇女绝经前后出现性激素波动或减少所致的一系列躯体及精神心理症状。

1.内分泌变化

（1）雌激素：绝经过渡早期雌激素水平波动很大，甚至可高于正常卵泡期水平；在卵泡完全停止生长发育后，雌激素水平才迅速下降。绝经后卵巢极少分泌雌激素。

（2）孕激素：分泌减少。

（3）雄激素：绝经后总体雄激素水平下降。雄烯二酮下降，而睾酮水平增高。

（4）促性腺激素：绝经过渡期FSH水平升高，呈波动型，LH仍在正常范围内，FSH/LH仍＜1。绝经后FSH和LH增加。其中FSH升高较LH更显著，FSH/LH＞1（表23-1）。

（5）促性腺激素释放激素：增加。

（6）抑制素：下降。

2.临床表现

（1）近期症状

■ 月经紊乱：月经紊乱是绝经过渡期的常见症状，由于稀发排卵或无排卵，表现为月经周期不规则、经期持续时间长及经量增多或减少。

D.The 2nd day of menstruation

E.No special requirement

Section 4　Menopause syndrome

Menopause is the permanent cessation of menses.

Menopause syndrome: A series of physical and psychological symptoms caused by fluctuation and reduction of sex hormones before and after menopause.

1.Endocrine changes

（1）Estrogen: The level of estrogen fluctuates greatly in the early stage of menopausal transition, even higher than that in normal follicular phase. The level of estrogen decreases rapidly after follicles stop growing completely. The ovaries rarely produce estrogen after menopause.

（2）Progesterone: Decreased.

（3）Androgen: The overall androgen level decreases after menopause. Androstenedione decreases while testosterone increases.

（4）Gonadotropin: The level of FSH increases and fluctuates in menopausal transition period, and LH is still within the normal range, FSH/LH＜1. Both FSH and LH increase after menopause, and the increase of FSH is more significant than that of LH, and FSH/LH＞1（Table 23-1）.

（5）Gonadotropin-releasing hormone（GnRH）: Increased.

（6）Inhibin: Decreased.

2.Clinical manifestations

（1）Short-term symptoms

■ Menstrual disorders: Common symptoms in menopausal transition period, caused by oligo-ovulation or anovulation, with irregular menstrual cycle, long duration of menstrual period and increased or

表23-1　不同生命阶段中FSH值的相关变化

Table 23-1　Relative changes in FSH of life stages

生命阶段 Life stages	FSH（mU/ml）
儿童期 Childhood	＜4
育龄期 Childbearing age	6 ～ 10
围绝经期 Perimenopause	14 ～ 24
绝经期 Menopause	＞30

■ 血管舒缩症状：潮热，是雌激素降低的特征性症状。

■ 自主神经失调症状：如心悸、眩晕、头痛、失眠、耳鸣等自主神经失调症状。

■ 精神神经症状：围绝经期女性常表现为注意力不易集中，并且情绪波动大，如激动易怒、焦虑不安或情绪低落、抑郁、不能自我控制等情绪症状。记忆力减退也较常见。

（2）远期症状

■ 泌尿生殖道症状：由于雌激素水平下降，出现泌尿生殖道萎缩症状，如阴道干燥、性交困难及反复阴道感染。泌尿道萎缩可能出现排尿困难、尿痛、尿急等症状。

■ 骨质疏松：与绝经后女性雌激素缺乏有关，一般发生在绝经后5 ～ 10年。50岁以上女性50%以上会发生绝经后

decreased menstrual volume.

■ Vasomotor symptoms: Hot flush is a characteristic symptom of decreased estrogen.

■ Autonomic nervous disorder symptoms: Such as palpitation, dizziness, headache, insomnia, tinnitus, etc.

■ Psychoneurological symptoms: Women in the perimenopausal period often poorly show concentration and mood changes, such as irritability, anxiety, depression, feeling out of control, etc. Memory loss is also common.

（2）Long-term symptoms

■ Urogenital symptoms: With decreasing estrogen production, urogenital tissues become atrophic resulting in various symptoms, vaginal dryness, dyspareunia and recurrent vaginal infection. Because of atrophy of the lining of the urinary tract, there may be symptoms of dysuria, urinary frequency and urgency.

■ Osteoporosis: Osteoporosis is associated with decreased estrogen production in the first 5 ～ 10 years following menopause. More than 50% of women over age of 50

骨质疏松。

- 阿尔茨海默病：可能与绝经后内源性雌激素水平降低有关。
- 心血管病变：绝经后女性糖脂代谢异常增加，动脉硬化、冠心病的发病风险较绝经前明显增加，可能与雌激素低下有关。

3.诊断

根据病史及临床表现不难诊断，实验室检查有助于诊断。

（1）血清FSH值及E2值测定：绝经过渡期血清 FSH＞10U/L，提示卵巢储备功能下降。闭经，FSH＞40U/L且E2＜10～20pg/ml，提示卵巢功能衰竭。

（2）氯米芬兴奋试验：月经第5日起口服氯米芬，每日50mg，共5日，停药第1日测血清FSH＞12 U/L，提示卵巢储备功能降低。

4.治疗

（1）一般治疗：心理疏导，锻炼身体，健康饮食，预防骨质疏松。

（2）激素替代治疗（HRT）
- 适应证
  - 绝经相关症状：如潮热、睡眠障碍、疲倦、易激动、焦虑、情绪低落等。
  - 泌尿生殖道萎缩相关的问题。
  - 骨质疏松症。
- 禁忌证：已知或可疑妊娠、原因不明的阴道出血、已知或可疑患有乳腺癌、已知或可疑患有性激素依赖性恶性

experience postmenopausal osteoporosis.

- Alzheimer's disease: Alzheimer's disease may be associated with low endogenous estrogen level after menopause.
- Cardiovascular disease: Under menopause, changes occur in the cardiovascular lipid profile. The risk of arteriosclerosis and coronary heart disease is significantly higher than that before menopause, which may be associated with low estrogen.

3.Diagnosis

Diagnosis is not difficult to make based on the medical history and clinical manifestations. Laboratory examination is helpful for diagnosis.

（1）Serum FSH, E_2 determination: Menopausal serum FSH > 10U/L, indicating a decline in ovarian reserve. Amenorrhea, FSH > 40 U/L and E_2 < 10 ～ 20pg/ml, indicating ovarian failure.

（2）Clomiphene challenge test: Clomiphene, 50mg, po, 5 days, from the 5th day of the menstrual period. If the first day after drug withdrawal FSH > 12 U/L, indicating reduced ovarian reserve.

4.Treatment

（1）General treatment: Psychological counseling, physical exercise, healthy diet, and prevention of osteoporosis.

（2）Hormone replacement therapy（HRT）
- Indications
  - Menopausal symptoms: Hot flushes, insomnia, tiredness, irritability, anxiety, and depression.
  - Symptoms associated with urogenital atrophy.
  - Osteoporosis.
- Contraindications: Pregnancy or suspected pregnancy, unexplained vaginal bleeding, breast cancer or suspected breast cancer, known or suspected hormone-dependent

肿瘤、最近6个月内患有活动性静脉或动脉血栓栓塞性疾病、严重肝及肾功能障碍、血卟啉症、耳硬化症、脑膜瘤等。

- 慎用情况：慎用情况并非禁忌证，但在HRT应用前和应用过程中，应该咨询相关专业的医师，共同确定应用HRT的时机和方式，并采取更为严密的措施，监测病情的进展。慎用情况包括：子宫肌瘤、子宫内膜异位症、子宫内膜增生史、尚未控制的糖尿病及严重高血压、有血栓形成倾向、高催乳素血症、系统性红斑狼疮、乳腺良性疾病、乳腺癌家族史，及已完全缓解的部分妇科恶性肿瘤等。

- 制剂选择
  - 雌激素制剂：戊酸雌二醇、结合雌激素、尼尔雌醇。
  - 组织选择性雌激素活性调节剂：替勃龙。
  - 孕激素制剂：醋酸甲羟孕酮，地屈孕酮。

- 用药途径
  - 口服。
  - 胃肠道外途径：经阴道给药，经皮肤给药。

- 用药剂量与时间：在卵巢功能开始衰退并出现相关症状时即可使用。停止雌激素治疗时，应缓慢减量或间歇用药，逐步停药。

- 不良反应
  - 子宫出血。

malignancy, active venous or arterial thromboembolic disease within the last 6 months, severe liver and kidney dysfunction, hematoporphyria, otosclerosis, meningioma, etc.

- The cautions: Cautions are not contraindications, but before and during HRT, doctors with relevant expertise should be consulted to jointly determine the timing and method of HRT, and take more rigorous monitor the progress of the disease. Cautions include: Uterine myoma, endometriosis, history of endometrial hyperplasia, uncontrolled diabetes and severe hypertension, tendency to thrombosis, hyperprolactinemia, systemic lupus erythematosus, benign breast diseases, family history of breast cancer, and some gynecological malignancies that have been completely relieved.

- Preparation:
  - Estrogen preparations: Estradiol valerate, conjugated estrogen and nilestriol.
  - Selective tissue estrogenic activity regulator: Tibolone.
  - Progesterone preparations: Medroxyprogesterone acetate（MPA）, dydrogesterone.

- Route of administration
  - Take orally.
  - Parenteral administration: Intravaginal preparation, and transdermal preparations.

- Dosage and time: Drugs are used when ovarian failure begins and relevant symptoms occur. When estrogen treatmentends, drugs should be reduced slowly or intermittently, with gradual withdrawal.

- Side effects
  - Uterus bleeding.

- 性激素不良反应
  ①雌激素：剂量过大可引起乳房胀、头痛、水肿等。
  ②孕激素：不良反应包括抑郁、易怒、乳房痛和水肿等。
  ③雄激素：有发生高血脂、动脉粥样硬化、血栓栓塞性疾病危险，大量应用出现体重增加、多毛及痤疮。
- 子宫内膜癌：长期单用雌激素，可使子宫内膜癌危险性增加，而联合应用雌孕激素，不增加子宫内膜癌发病风险。

- 卵巢癌：长期应用HRT，卵巢癌的风险可能增加。
- 乳腺癌：应用天然雌孕激素可使增加乳腺癌的发病风险减小，但乳腺癌患者仍是HRT的禁忌证。

- 心血管疾病及血栓性疾病：HRT对降低心血管疾病发生有益，但一般不主张HRT作为心血管疾病的二级预防。没有证据证明天然雌孕激素会增加血栓风险，但对于有血栓疾病患者尽量选择经皮给药。

- 糖尿病：HRT能通过改善胰岛素抵抗而明显降低糖尿病风险。

- The side effects of hormone
  ① Estrogen: Excessive dose can cause breast distension, headache, edema, etc.
  ② Progesterone: Side effects include depression, irritability, breast pain, edema, etc.
  ③ Androgen: Risk of hyperlipidemia, atherosclerosis, thromboembolic disease. Excessive dose can cause weight gain, hirsutism and acne.

- Endometrial carcinoma: Long-term use of estrogen alone can increase the risk of endometrial carcinoma, while combined estrogen and progestin therapy does not increase the risk of endometrial carcinoma.
- Ovarian cancer: Long-term use of HRT may increase the risk of ovarian cancer.
- Breast cancer: The use of natural estrogen and progesterone can reduce the risk of breast cancer, but patients with breast cancer are still contraindication to HRT.
- Cardiovascular disease and thromboembolic disease: HRT is beneficial to reduce the occurrence of cardiovascular disease, but it is generally not recommended as secondary prevention of cardiovascular disease. No evidence indicates natural estrogens and progesterones can increase the risk of thromboembolism. However, for patients with thromboembolic disease, transdermal administration should be the best choice.
- Diabetes: HRT can significantly reduce the risk of diabetes by improving insulin resistance.

（3）非激素类药物

■ 选择性5-羟色胺再摄取抑制剂。

■ 钙剂。

■ 维生素D。

重点专业词汇

1.绝经综合征

2.绝经过渡期

3.雌激素

4.孕激素类（孕激素，孕酮）

5.雄激素

6.促性腺激素

7.月经紊乱

8.绝经后骨质疏松

9.激素补充治疗（HRT）

练习题

1.哪一项与绝经期患者雌激素下降无关？（C）

A.潮热

B.易怒

C.子宫内膜增生

D.性交困难

E.骨质疏松

2.属于HRT适应证的是:（E）

A.严重高血压

B.血栓性静脉炎

C.重症肝炎

D.患乳腺癌的绝经后期患者

E.骨质疏松

3.下列哪项不属于HRT禁忌证？（E）

A.妊娠

B.血栓性静脉炎

C.肝炎

D.乳腺癌病史

E.骨质疏松

4.HRT治疗主要的药物是:（B）

A.孕激素

B.雌激素

（3）Non-hormonal drugs

■ Selective serotonin reuptake inhibitors（SSRIs）.

■ Calcium preparations.

■ Vitamin D.

Key words

1.Menopause syndrome

2.Menopausal transition period

3.Estrogen

4.Progestogen（progesterone, progestin）

5.Androgen

6.Gonadotropin

7.Menstrual disorder

8.Postmenopausal osteoporosis

9.Hormone replacement therapy（HRT）

Exercises

1.Which one has nothing to do with decreased estrogen in menopausal patients?（C）

A.Hot flush

B.Irritability

C.Endometrial hyperplasia

D.Dyspareunia

E.Osteoporosis

2.Indication of HRT is:（E）

A.Severe hypertension

B.Thrombophlebitis

C.Severe hepatitis

D.Postmenopausal patients with breast cancer

E.Osteoporosis

3.Which one is not the contraindication of HRT?（E）

A.Pregnancy

B.Thrombophlebitis

C.Hepatitis

D.History of breast cancer

E.Osteoporosis

4.What is the main drug for HRT ?（B）

A.Progesterone

B.Estrogen

C.雄激素

D.FSH

E.GnRH

（陈艺华）

第五节　经前期综合征

经前期综合征（PMS）是指反复在黄体期出现周期性以情感、行为和躯体障碍为特征的综合征。多见于25～45岁女性，月经来潮后，症状自然消失。

1.病因

（1）精神社会因素。

（2）卵巢激素失调。

（3）神经递质异常。

2.临床表现

（1）躯体症状：头痛、乳房胀痛、腹部胀满、肢体水肿、运动协调功能减退。

（2）精神症状：易怒、焦虑、紧张、抑郁、情绪不稳定、疲乏及饮食、睡眠、性欲改变。

（3）行为改变：注意力不集中、工作效率低、记忆力减退、神经质、易激动等。

3.诊断与鉴别诊断

（1）根据经前期出现周期性典型症状，诊断多不困难。

（2）鉴别诊断：需与轻度精神障碍及心、肝、肾等疾病引起的水肿相鉴别。

4.治疗

（1）心理治疗有助于减轻症状。

（2）调整生活状态：可以有效改善症状，包括营养饮食及适当的

C.Androgen

D.FSH

E.GnRH

Section 5　Premenstrual syndrome

Premenstrual syndrome（PMS）is a group of mood-related, behavioral and physical changes that occur in a regular, cyclic relationship to the luteal phase of the menstrual cycle. These symptoms often occur in 25～45 years old women, resolving with onset of menses usually.

1.Etiology

（1）Psychosocial factors.

（2）Ovarian hormone disorder.

（3）Neurotransmitter dysregulation.

2.Clinical manifestations

（1）Somatic symptoms: Headache, breast tenderness, abdominal bloating, swelling of extremities and hypokinesia.

（2）Psychological symptoms: Irritability, anxiety, tension, depression, emotional lability, fatigue, and changes in diet, sleep and libido.

（3）Behavioral changes: Lack of concentration, low work efficiency, hypomnesis, nervousness, temperament.

3.Diagnosis and differential diagnosis

（1）Diagnosis is not difficult to make according to the typical and cyclic occurrence of the symptoms prior to the onset of menses.

（2）Differential diagnosis: Differentiation from mild mental disorders, and edema caused by heart, liver or kidney diseases.

4.Treatment

（1）Psychotherapy has been shown to provide symptomatic relief.

（2）Lifestyle interventions that have demonstrated significant improvement in symptoms

身体锻炼，限制糖和脂肪的摄入。降低食盐的摄入有助于消除水肿，限制咖啡因及酒精的摄入可以减轻紧张及焦虑的症状。

（3）药物治疗

■ 抗焦虑药：阿普唑仑（alprazolam）经前用药，0.25mg，每日2～3次口服，逐渐增量，最大剂量为每日4mg，用至月经来潮第2～3日。

■ 抗抑郁症药：氟西汀能选择性抑制中枢神经系统5-羟色胺的再摄取。黄体期用药，20mg，每日1次口服，能明显缓解精神症状及行为改变，但对躯体症状疗效不佳。

■ 醛固酮受体的竞争性抑制剂：螺内酯20～40mg，每日2～3次口服，减轻水肿症状，对改善精神症状也有效。

■ 维生素B$_6$：10～20mg，每日3次口服，可改善症状。

■ 口服避孕药通过抑制排卵缓解症状。也可用促性腺激素释放激素激动剂（GnRH-a）抑制排卵。

重点专业词汇

1.经前期综合征

2.黄体期

3.口服避孕药

4.抑制排卵

5.促性腺激素释放激素（GnRH）

练习题

1.治疗经前期综合征不可选用哪一种？（E）

including nutritional diet, proper physical exercise, and minimizing the intake of refined sugars and fats. Minimizing salt intake may help with bloating, and eliminating caffeine and alcohol from the diet can reduce nervousness and anxiety.

（3）Medical treatment

■ Antianxietic: Alprazolam 0.25mg, bid or tid po gradually. The maximum dose 4mg per day taken during the luteal phase until 2～3 days after the onset of menses.

■ Antidepressant drugs: Elevating serotonin levels in the central nervous system readily be achieved by the use of fluoxetine. Fluoxetine 20mg daily usually is effective to improve psychological symptoms and behavior changes rather than somatic symptoms.

■ Competitive inhibitors of aldosterone receptors: Antisterone 20～40mg, bid or tid po, can relieve swelling and improve psychological symptoms.

■ Vitamin B$_6$: 10～20mg tid po, improve symptoms.

■ Suppressing ovulation is beneficial for some patients with premenstrual syndrome and can be accomplished by using oral contraceptives, or gonadotropin-releasing hormone（GnRH）agonists.

Key words

1.Premenstrual syndrome

2.Luteal phase

3.Oral contraceptives

4.Inhibition of ovulation

5.Gonadotropin-releasing hormone（GnRH）

Exercises

1.Which of the following can not be chosen to treat the premenstrual syndrome?（E）

A.氟西汀

B.螺内酯

C.GnRH-a

D.阿普唑仑

E.维生素 C

2.经前期综合征特征错误的是哪一种？（A）

A.月经前1～2日出现症状

B.月经来潮后症状迅速消失

C.周期性发生

D.生活负性事件

E.躯体症状明显

3.PMS治疗原则是:（A）

A.心理疏导为主

B.适当镇静

C.对症治疗

D.人工绝经疗法

E.子宫切除

4.经前期综合征出现在:（B）

A.卵泡期

B.黄体期

C.月经早期

D.月经中期

E.月经后期

（陈艺华）

第六节　不　孕　症

夫妻正常性生活、未避孕12个月后未受孕，称为不孕症。分为原发性和继发性两大类。

1.不孕的原因

有女性因素、男性因素及不明原因。

（1）女性因素

■ 盆腔因素（35%）

A.Fluoxetine

B.Antisterone

C.GnRH-a

D.Alprazolam

E.Vitamin C

2.Which one is not the characteristic of premenstrual syndrome?（A）

A.Symptoms appearing 1 ～ 2 days prior to the onset of menses

B.Symptoms disappearing rapidly with onset of menses

C.Periodic occurrence

D.Negative life events

E.Obvious somatic symptoms

3.The principle of PMS treatment is:（A）

A.Psychological counseling

B.Proper sedative treatment

C.Symptomatic treatment

D.Artificial menopause

E.Hysterectomy

4.Premenstrual syndrome occurs in:（B）

A.Follicular phase

B.Luteal phase

C.The early phase of menstruation

D.The middle phase of menstruation

E.The late phase of menstruation

Section 6　Infertility

Infertility is the failure for a couple to conceive after 12 months of frequent, unprotected intercourse, which is classified as primary infertility and secondary infertility.

1.Causes of infertility

Including female factors, male factors and unexplained infertility.

（1）Female factors

■ Pelvic factors（35%）

- 输卵管阻塞或积水。
- 盆腔和输卵管功能和结构的破坏。
- 子宫内膜异位症。
- 子宫内膜病变。
- 子宫肌瘤。
- 生殖器官肿瘤。
- 生殖道发育畸形。
■ 排卵障碍（25% ～ 35%）
  - 持续性无排卵。
  - 多囊卵巢综合征（PCOS）。
  - 卵巢早衰（POF）和卵巢功能减退。
  - 先天性性腺发育不良。
  - 低促性腺激素性性腺功能不良（HH）。
  - 高催乳素血症。
  - 黄素化卵泡不破裂综合征（LUFS）。

（2）男性因素：精液异常、男性性功能障碍及免疫因素（表23-2）。

（3）不明原因不孕（UI, 10% ～ 20%）。

对夫妻双方进行综合评估，未

- Fallopian tube obstruction or hydrosalpinx.
- Destruction of pelvic and fallopian tube function and structure.
- Endometriosis.
- Lesion of endometrium.
- Myoma.
- Tumor of genital organ.
- Malformation of genital tract.
■ Ovulation dysfunction（25% ～ 35%）
  - Chronic anovulation.
  - Polycystic ovarian syndrome（PCOS）.
  - Premature ovarian failure（POF）and hypoovarianism.
  - Congenital gonadal dysplasia.
  - Hypogonadotropic hypogonadism(HH).
  - Hyperprolactinemia.
  - Luteinized unruptured follicle syndrome（LUFS）.

（2）Male factors: Abnormal semen, male sexual dysfunction and immune factors（Table 23-2）.

（3）Unexplained infertility（UI,10% ～ 20%）.

A comprehensive assessment for couples

表23-2　精液分析

Table 23-2　Semen analysis

内容 Element	参考值 Reference value
射出的精液体积（ml） Ejaculate volume	＞1.5
精子密度（10^6/ml） Sperm concentration	15
总活力（%） Motility	＞40%
快速前向运动（%） Rapid progressive motility	＞32%
正常精子形态（%） Normal morphology	＞4%

能得到不孕症的确切病因，可考虑为不明原因性不孕。尤其是检查提示精液分析结果正常、有排卵证据、宫腔形态正常、双侧通畅的输卵管。

2.检查与诊断

（1）男方

■ 病史。

■ 体格检查。

■ 精液常规。

（2）女方

■ 病史。

■ 体格检查。

■ 女性不孕特殊检查
  ● 基础体温测定。
  ● 超声监测优势卵泡发育。

  ● 基础激素水平测定。
  ● 评估输卵管通畅度的诊断性试验。
  ● 宫腔镜检查。
  ● 腹腔镜检查。

3.治疗

（1）治疗生殖道器质性病变

■ 输卵管因素不孕的治疗
  ● 一般疗法。
  ● 输卵管成形术。

■ 卵巢肿瘤。

■ 子宫病变。

■ 子宫内膜异位症。

■ 生殖系统结核。

（2）诱发排卵（OI）

■ 氯米芬。

■ 绒促性素（hCG）。

■ 绝经后促性腺激素，又称尿促性素（hMG）。

（3）不明原因不孕治疗：经过3～6个月的人工授精诊断性治疗

fails to find out the exact cause of infertility, which can be considered as unexplained infertility. In particular, the examination shows a normal semen analysis result, evidence of ovulation, a normal uterine cavity, and patent fallopian tubes.

2.Examination and diagnosis

（1）Male

■ Medical history.

■ Physical examination.

■ Seminal routine examination.

（2）Female

■ Medical history.

■ Physical examination.

■ Special examination for female infertility.
  ● Basal body temperature.
  ● Monitoring the development of a dominant follicle by ultrasound.
  ● Basal hormone level.
  ● Diagnostic test to assess tubal patency.

  ● Hysteroscopy.
  ● Laparoscopy.

3.Treatment

（1）Treatment of genital tract organic diseases

■ Treatment of tubal infertility.
  ● General treatment.
  ● Salpingoplasty.

■ Ovarian tumor.

■ Uterus lesion.

■ Endometriosis.

■ Genital tuberculosis.

（2）Ovulation induction（OI）

■ Clomifene.

■ Human chorionic gonadotrophin（hCG）.

■ Human menopausal gonadotrophin（hMG）.

（3）Treatment of unexplained infertility: After 3～6 months, diagnostic treatment of artificial

后仍未成功，可采用体外受精-胚胎移植（IVF-ET）或单精子卵母细胞浆内注射（ICSI）。

（4）辅助生殖技术（ARTs）：包括人工授精、体外受精胚胎移植及其衍生技术。

重点专业词汇

1.不孕症

2.子宫内膜异位症

3.排卵障碍

4.持续性无排卵

5.卵巢早衰（POF）

6.低促性腺激素性性腺功能不良（HH）

7.黄素化卵泡不破裂综合征（LUFS）

8.基础体温（BBT）

9.诱导排卵（OI）

练习题

1.男性不育因素包括：（ABC）

A.生精障碍

B.输精障碍

C.免疫因素

D.阑尾炎

2.女性不孕因素包括：（ABCD）

A.子宫内膜异位症

B.多囊卵巢综合征（PCOS）

C.卵巢早衰（POF）

D.黄素化卵泡不破裂综合征（LUFS）

（佟春艳）

第七节　辅助生殖技术

辅助生殖技术（ARTs）是为了

insemination（AI）with husband's sperm is still unsuccessful, in vitro fertilization-embryo transfer（IVF-ET）or intracytoplasmic sperm injection（ICSI）can be performed.

（4）Assisted reproductive techniques（ARTs）: Including artificial insemination, in vitro fertilization-embryo transfer and derivative technology.

Key words

1.Infertility

2.Endometriosis

3.Ovulation dysfunction

4.Chronic anovulation

5.Premature ovarian failure（POF）

6.Hypogonadotropic hypogonadism（HH）

7.Luteinized unruptured follicle syndrome（LUFS）

8.Basal body temperature（BBT）

9.Ovulation induction（OI）

Exercises

1.Causes of male sterility include:（ABC）

A.Dyszoospermia

B.Semen deposition dysfunction

C.Immune factors

D.Appendicitis

2.Causes of female infertility include:（ABCD）

A.Endometriosis

B.Polycystic ovarian syndrome（PCOS）

C.Premature ovarian failure（POF）

D.Luteinized unruptured follicle syndrome（LUFS）

Section 7　Assisted reproductive techniques

All fertility procedures that involve

获得妊娠而对配子、合子或胚胎进行显微操作的全部生殖步骤。包括人工授精、体外受精胚胎移植及其衍生技术等。

1.人工授精

（1）人工授精包括各种操作，均包含将处理后的精子置入到女性生殖道，这可以在没有性交的情况下使精子和卵子发生反应。目前，常见的人工授精形式包括从男性伴侣或捐赠者获得的处理后的精子。

（2）宫腔内人工授精（IUI）适用于轻度少弱精，男性性功能障碍，宫颈因素，不明原因性不孕等。

2.体外受精与胚胎移植（图23-2）

（1）体外受精（IVF）的过程包括产生多个卵泡的促排卵、取卵，实验室内的卵子受精、胚胎孵化，以及通过女性宫颈将胚胎移植到子宫内。

（2）IVF适用于双侧输卵管缺如或阻塞，输卵管绝育术，复通失败，严重的盆腔粘连，严重的子宫内膜异位症，卵巢低反应，排卵过少，严重的男性不育，不明原因性不孕及非手术治疗失败。

并发症：
- 卵巢过度刺激综合征（OHSS）。
- 多胎妊娠。

3.卵细胞质内单精子注射（ICSI）

（1）将获得单精子直接注入到

manipulation of gametes, zygotes, or embryos to achieve conception comprise the assisted reproductive techniques（ARTs）. It includes artificial insemination, in vitro fertilization-embryo transfer and derivative technology.

1.Artificial insemination（AI）

（1）Artificial insemination encompasses a variety of procedures. All involve the placement of processed sperm into the female reproductive tract, which permits sperm-ovum interaction in the absence of intercourse. Currently, all of the common forms of artificial insemination involve processed sperm obtained from the male partner or a donor.

（2）Indications for intrauterine insemination（IUI）: Mild oligospermia and asthenospermia, male sexual dysfunction, cervical factors, unexplained infertility, etc.

2.In vitro fertilization and embryo transfer（IVF-ET）（Figure 23-2）

（1）The process of in-vitro fertilization（IVF）involves ovarian stimulation to produce multiple follicles, retrieval of the oocytes from the ovaries, oocyte fertilization in vitro in the laboratory, embryo incubation in the laboratory, and transfer embryos into a woman's uterus through the cervix.

（2）Indications of IVF include absent or blocked fallopian tubes, tubal sterilization, failed surgery to achieve tubal patency, severe pelvic adhesions, severe endometriosis, poor ovarian response to stimulation, oligo-ovulation, severe male infertility, unexplained infertility, and failed treatment with less aggressive therapies.

Complications:
- Ovarian hyperstimulation syndrome（OHSS）.
- Multiple pregnancy.

3.Intracytoplasmic sperm injection（ICSI）

（1）This micromanipulation technique is

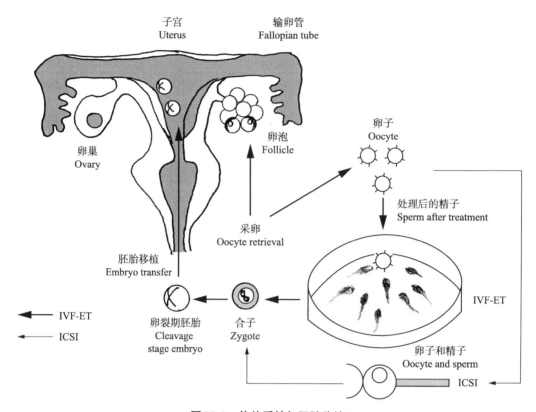

图23-2　体外受精与胚胎移植

Figure 23-2　In vitro fertilization and embryo transfer

卵子中，此项显微操作技术的目的是增加ATR过程中取卵的受精率。因此从理论上来讲，避免了精子活力、精子获能或顶体反应的缺陷以及精子结合透明带受限。

（2）操作步骤包括剥除围绕在卵子周围、构成卵丘的所有颗粒细胞，目的是使显微操作可以在卵子自身上进行。然后将有活力的精子注入到卵细胞浆（卵浆）。

（3）卵泡浆内单精子注射（ICSI）的绝对指征包括严重的少、弱、畸形精子症，精子缺失顶体，精子完全不活动，以及外科手术取出的附睾或睾丸中的精子。ICSI的其他绝对指征是非男方因素不孕，应用传

performed to increase the fertilization rate of oocytes retrieved during ART by direct injection of a live sperm into the oocyte, thereby theoretically bypassing limitations imposed by sperm motility, defective capacitation or acrosome reaction, and sperm binding the zona pellucida.

（2）The procedure includes stripping all granulosa cells surrounding ovum and forming cumulus, so that micromanipulation can be performed on the egg itself. Then aviable sperm is inserted into the cytoplasm of the egg（ooplasm）.

（3）Absolute indications for ICSI include severe oligospermia, asthenospermia, and teratozoospermia, the presence of spermatozoa lacking an acrosome or those that are completely immotile as well as the use of surgically recovered epididymal or testicular sperm. Other absolute

统IVF治疗受精失败和植入前基因诊断的卵子受精。

indications for ICSI are non-male factor-related and include a history of fertilization failure with conventional IVF and the fertilization of oocytes before preimplantation genetic diagnosis.

4.胚胎植入前遗传学诊断

（1）植入前基因诊断/筛查是一种临床诊断性操作，可以在胚胎植入子宫之前进行自身筛查，以明确是否存在特定的基因异常。最常用的是卵裂球/囊胚活检后对取得的细胞进行基因检测。

（2）植入前基因诊断的发展增加了某些特定遗传病高危家庭拥有健康儿的概率。

4.Preimplantation genetic diagnosis

（1）Preimplantation genetic diagnosis/screening（PGD/PGS）is a clinical diagnostic procedure that is performed on the embryo itself to determine whether a particular genetic abnormality is present before its transfer into the uterus.The most common method is gene detection of cells obtained after blastomere/blastocyst biopsy.

（2）Preimplantation genetic diagnosis developed in the effort to improve the chances of having healthy infants in families at high risk for a particular genetic disease.

重点专业词汇

1.辅助生殖技术（ARTs）

2.人工授精（AI）

3.丈夫精液人工授精（AIH）

4.供精者精液人工授精（AID）

5.体外受精与胚胎移植（IVF-ET）

6.卵巢过度刺激综合征（OHSS）

7.多胎妊娠

8.卵细胞质内单精子注射（ICSI）

9.胚胎植入前遗传学诊断/筛查（PGD/PGS）

Key words

1.Assisted reproductive techniques（ARTs）

2.Artificial insemination（AI）

3.Artificial insemination by husband sperm（AIH）

4.Artificial insemination by donor（AID）

5.In vitro fertilization and embryo transfer（IVF-ET）

6.Ovarian hyperstimulation syndrome（OHSS）

7.Multiple pregnancy

8.Intracytoplasmic sperm injection（ICSI）

9.Preimplantation genetic diagnosis/screening（PGD/PGS）

练习题

1.体外受精-胚胎移植术的并发症包括:（BD）

A.子宫内膜异位症

B.卵巢过度刺激综合征（OHSS）

C.子宫肌瘤

D.多胎妊娠

E.异位妊娠

Exercises

1.IVF-ET complications include:（BD）

A.Endometriosis

B.Ovarian hyperstimulation syndrome（OHSS）

C.Myoma of uterus

D.Multiple pregnancy

E.Ectopic pregnancy

2.属于辅助生殖技术的有:(AC)

A.丈夫精液人工授精(AIH)

B.多胎妊娠

C.体外受精与胚胎移植技术(IVF-ET)

D.卵巢过度刺激综合征(OHSS)

（佟春艳）

2.The technologies of ART include:（AC）

A.Artificial insemination by husband sperm（AIH）

B.Multiple pregnancy

C.In vitro fertilization and embryo transfer（IVF-ET）

D.Ovarian hyperstimulation syndrome（OHSS）

第24章 计划生育

CHAPTER 24 Family planning

第一节 避 孕

宫内节育器（IUD）

1.种类

（1）惰性IUD（第一代）由惰性材料金属、硅胶、塑料等制成，现已停止生产。

（2）活性IUD（第二代）内含有活性物质，如铜离子、激素、药物或磁性物质等。

- 含铜宫内节育器：T形、V形、母体乐、宫铜IUD、含铜无支架IUD。
- 含药宫内节育器：含孕激素IUD（曼月乐）、含吲哚美辛IUD。

2.作用机制

（1）对精子和胚胎的毒性作用：压迫局部产生炎症反应；铜离子使精子头尾分离。

（2）干扰着床。

（3）左炔诺孕酮IUD的避孕作用：可使一部分女性抑制排卵。

（4）含吲哚美辛IUD。

3.宫内节育器放置术

（1）适应证

- 育龄女性无禁忌证，要求放置IUD者。

（2）禁忌证

- 妊娠或可疑妊娠。

Section 1　Contraception

Intrauterine device（IUD）

1.Types

（1）Inert IUD（first generation）is made of inert materials such as metal, silica gel, plastic, etc. and has been discontinued.

（2）Active IUD（second generation）contains active substances such as copper ions, hormones, drugs or magnetic substances.

- Copper-containing IUD: T-shaped, V-shaped, MUTILE, uterine copper IUD, copper-containing stentless IUD.
- Drugs-containing IUD: IUD containing progesterone（Mirena）and indomethacin.

2.Mechanism of action

（1）Toxic effects on sperm and embryo: Local pressure produces inflammatory reaction; copper ions separate the head and tail of sperm.

（2）Interfere with implantation.

（3）The contraceptive effect of levonorgestrel IUD: For some women ovulation can be inhibited.

（4）Indomethacin-containing IUD.

3.Intrauterine device placement

（1）Indications

- No contraindications for women of childbearing age, and IUD required.

（2）Contraindications

- Pregnancy or suspected pregnancy.

- 生殖道急性炎症。
- 人工流产出血多，怀疑有妊娠组织物残留或感染可能；中期妊娠引产、分娩或剖宫产胎盘娩出后，子宫收缩不良有出血或潜在感染可能。
- 生殖器官肿瘤。
- 生殖器官畸形。
- 宫颈内口过松、重度陈旧性宫颈裂伤或子宫脱垂。
- 严重的全身性疾病。
- 宫腔＜5.5cm或＞9cm。
- 近3个月内有月经失调、阴道不规则出血。
- 铜过敏史。

（3）放置时间

- 月经干净3～7日无性交；人工流产后立即放置；产后42日恶露已净，会阴伤口愈合，子宫恢复正常；剖宫产后半年；含孕激素IUD在月经第3日放置；自然流产于转经后放置，药物流产2次正常月经后放置；哺乳期放置应先排除早孕；性交后5日内放置为紧急避孕方法之一。

4.宫内节育器取出术

（1）适应证

- 生理情况：计划再生育或已无性生活不再须避孕者；放置期已满须更换者；绝经过渡期停经1年内；拟改用其他避孕措施或绝育者。

- Acute inflammation of reproductive tract.
- Excessive bleeding from induced abortion, suspicion of residual pregnancy tissue or infection; bleeding or potential infection caused by uterine dyssystole after induced labor, delivery or cesarean section.
- Reproductive organ tumors.
- Reproductive organ malformation.
- Loose cervical, severe old cervical laceration or uterine prolapse.
- Severe systemic disease.
- Uterine cavity ＜ 5.5 cm or ＞ 9 cm.
- Menstrual disorders and irregular vaginal bleeding occurred in the past 3 months.
- A history of copper allergy.

（3）Placement time

- 3 ～ 7 days after menstruation without sexual intercourse; immediate placement after induced abortion; 42 days after delivery lochia being resolved, perineal wound healing, uterus returned to normal; six months after cesarean section; progesterone-releasing IUD placed on the 3rd day of menstruation; for spontaneous abortion placed after menstruation, while for drug abortion placed after 2 normal periods; early pregnancy should be excluded before placing IUD in lactation; placed within 5 days after sexual intercourse as one of the emergency contraception methods.

4.Intrauterine device removal

（1）Indications

- Physiological conditions: Women who plan to reproduce or no longer need contraception in their asexual life; who need to be replaced at the end of their placement period; who have menopause within one year; who plan to switch to other contraceptive measures or sterilization.

- 病理情况：有并发症及副作用，经治疗无效；带器妊娠，包括宫内或宫外妊娠。

（2）禁忌证
- 并发生殖道炎症时，先抗感染治疗，治愈后再取出IUD；全身情况不良或在疾病急性期，应待病情好转后再取出。

（3）取器时间
- 月经干净3～7日；带器早期妊娠行人工流产同时取器；带器异位妊娠术前行诊断性刮宫时，或在术后出院前取出IUD；子宫不规则出血者，随时可取，取IUD同时需行诊断性刮宫，刮出组织送病理。

5.宫内节育器的副作用
- 不规则阴道出血（最常见），白带增多，下腹痛。

6.并发症
（1）节育器异位。
（2）节育器嵌顿或断裂。

（3）节育器下移或脱落。

（4）带器妊娠。

激素避孕

1.作用机制
（1）抑制排卵。
（2）改变宫颈黏液性状。

- Pathological conditions: With complications and side effects, and ineffective after treatment; pregnancy with device, including intrauterine or extrauterine pregnancy.

（2）Contraindications
- When complicated with genital tract inflammation, anti-infection treatment should be given first and IUD should be removed after cure. If the condition of the body is not good or in the acute stage of disease, it should be taken out after the improvement of the condition.

（3）Time for removal
- 3～7 days after menstruation; simultaneous removal of device during early pregnancy with device; for ectopic pregnancy with device, removal of IUD during diagnostic curettage before operation or before discharge after operation; for irregular uterine bleeding at any time, it is desirable to remove IUD and make diagnostic curettage at the same time, scrape out the tissue and send it for pathological test.

5.Side effects of intrauterine device
- Irregular vaginal bleeding（most common）, increased leucorrhea, lower abdominal pain.

6.Complications
（1）Ectopic intrauterine device.
（2）Intrauterine device incarcerated or broken.

（3）The birth control device falling down or falling off.

（4）Pregnancy with IUD.

Hormonal contraception

1.Mechanism of action
（1）Inhibit ovulation.
（2）Change cervical mucus properties.

（3）改变子宫内膜形态与功能。

（4）改变输卵管功能。

2.种类

（1）口服避孕药

- 复方短效口服避孕药：雌、孕激素组成的复合制剂，如复方炔诺酮片、复方甲地孕酮片等。
- 单相片：整个周期中雌、孕激素含量是固定的。
- 三相片：每一相雌、孕激素含量，是根据女性生理周期而制定不同的剂量。
- 复方长效口服避孕药：市场上已少见。

（2）长效避孕针。

（3）探亲避孕药。

（4）缓释避孕药。

3.禁忌证

（1）严重心血管疾病、血栓性疾病不宜使用，如高血压、冠心病、静脉栓塞等。雌激素有促凝功能，增加心肌梗死及静脉栓塞的发生率。

（2）急、慢性肝炎或肾炎。

（3）恶性肿瘤、癌前病变。

（4）内分泌疾病：如糖尿病、甲状腺功能亢进症。

（5）哺乳期不宜使用复方口服避孕药，因雌激素可抑制乳汁分泌。

（6）年龄大于35岁的吸烟女性服用避孕药，增加心血管疾病的发病率，不宜长期服用。

（7）精神病患者。

（3）Change the morphology and function of endometrium.

（4）Change the function of fallopian tube.

2.Types

（1）Oral contraceptives

- Compound short-acting oral contraceptives: Estrogen and progestogen compound preparation, such as compound norethisterone tablets and compound megestrol tablets.
- Monophasic tablet: The ratio of estrogen and progestogen is fixed in the whole cycle.
- Triphasic tablets: The ratio of estrogen and progestogen in each phase is determined by the physiological cycle of women.
- Compound long-acting oral contraceptives: Rare in the market.

（2）Long-acting contraceptive injection.

（3）Vacation pill.

（4）Slow-release contraceptives.

3.Contraindications

（1）Severe cardiovascular diseases and thrombotic diseases should not be used, such as hypertension, coronary heart disease, venous embolism, etc. Estrogen promotes coagulation and increases the incidence of myocardial infarction and venous embolism.

（2）Acute or chronic hepatitis or nephritis.

（3）Malignant tumors and precancerous lesions.

（4）Endocrine diseases: Such as diabetes and hyperthyroidism.

（5）Compound oral contraceptives should not be used during lactation, as estrogen can inhibit milk secretion.

（6）Smoking women over 35 years old take contraceptives, which increases the incidence of cardiovascular diseases, and is not suitable for long-term use.

（7）Psychiatric patients.

（8）有严重偏头痛，反复发作者。

4.副作用及处理

（1）类早孕反应。

（2）不规则阴道出血。

（3）闭经。

（4）体重及皮肤变化。

（5）其他。

5.长期应用甾体激素避孕药对人体的影响

（1）对机体代谢的影响。

（2）对心血管系统的影响。

（3）对凝血功能的影响。

（4）对肿瘤的影响。

（5）对子代的影响。

其他避孕

- 包括紧急避孕、外用避孕与自然避孕法等。

第二节 输卵管绝育术

输卵管绝育术是一种安全、永久性节育措施，通过手术将输卵管结扎或用药物使输卵管腔粘连堵塞，阻断精子与卵子相遇而达到绝育。

1.经腹输卵管结扎术

（1）适应证

要求接受手术而无禁忌证者；患严重全身疾病不宜生育者。

（2）禁忌证

- 24小时内2次体温达37.5℃或以上。
- 全身状况不佳，如心力衰竭、血液病等，不能胜任手术。
- 患严重的神经官能症。

（8）Severe migraine with recurrent attacks.

4.Side effects and treatment

（1）Similar to morning sickness.

（2）Irregular vaginal bleeding.

（3）Amenorrhea.

（4）Changes in weight and skin.

（5）Others.

5.Effects of use of long-term steroid hormone contraceptives on the human body

（1）Effect on body metabolism.

（2）Effect on cardiovascular system.

（3）Effect on coagulation function.

（4）Effect on tumor.

（5）Effect on the offspring.

Other contraception

- It includes emergency contraception, external contraception and natural contraception.

Section 2　Tubal sterilization operation

It is a safe and permanent contraceptive measure, which achieves sterilization by ligating the fallopian tube surgically or blocking the oviduct cavity with drugs, preventing the sperm from meeting the ovum.

1.Abdominal tubal ligation

（1）Indications

Those who require surgery without contraindications; those suffering from serious systemic diseases that are not suitable for childbirth.

（2）Contraindications

- Temperature of 37.5 ℃ or above twice within 24 hours.
- Poor general condition with heart failure, hematological diseases, etc, not be operated on.
- Severe neurosis.

- 各种疾病急性期。
- 腹部皮肤有感染病灶或患有急、慢性盆腔炎。

（3）术前准备

- 手术时间选择。
- 解除患者思想顾虑，做好解释和咨询。
- 病史、检查、化验。

- 妇科腹部手术前常规准备。

- 麻醉：局部浸润麻醉或硬膜外麻醉。

（4）手术步骤

- 排空膀胱，取仰卧位，留置导尿管。
- 常规消毒铺巾。
- 切口：下腹正中耻骨联合上2横指（3～4cm）做2cm长纵切口。

- 寻找提取输卵管。
- 结扎输卵管：包埋抽芯法，输卵管银夹法，输卵管折叠结扎切除法。

（5）术后并发症

- 一般不发生。出血或血肿；感染；损伤；输卵管再通。

（6）术后处理。

2.经腹腔镜输卵管绝育术

（1）禁忌证：主要为腹腔粘连、心肺功能不全、膈疝等，余同经腹输卵管结扎术。

（2）术前准备：同经腹输卵管结扎术，受术者应取头低臀高仰卧位。

- Acute stage of various diseases.
- Infection lesions on abdominal skin, or acute and chronic pelvic inflammation.

（3）Preoperative preparation

- Operation time selection.
- Relieving patients' concerns, with full explanation and consultation.
- Medical history, examination and laboratory tests.

- Routine preparation before gynecologic abdominal surgery.

- Anesthesia: Local infiltration anesthesia or epidural anesthesia.

（4）Surgical procedures

- Empty the bladder, be in a supine position, and have indwelling catheter in place.
- Conventional disinfection towel.
- Incision: 2 cm longitudinal incision in the middle of the lower abdomen at the upper 2 transverse fingers（3～4cm）of the pubic symphysis.
- Searching for fallopian tubes.
- Ligation of fallopian tubes: Embedding core pulling method, oviduct silver clip method and tubal ligation and resection.

（5）Postoperative complications

- No complications occur generally. Hemorrhage or hematoma; infection; injury; fallopian tube recanalization.

（6）Postoperative management.

2.Laparoscopic sterilization of fallopian tubes

（1）Contraindications: Mainly abdominal adhesions, cardiopulmonary insufficiency, diaphragmatic hernia, etc, others the same as abdominal tubal ligation.

（2）Preoperative preparation: With abdominal tubal ligation, recipients should take Trendelenburg position.

（3）麻醉：局部麻醉、硬膜外麻醉或全身麻醉。

（4）手术步骤：同经腹输卵管结扎术。

（5）术后处理：静卧4～6小时后可下床活动；观察生命体征有无改变。

第三节　避孕失败的补救措施

人工流产指因意外妊娠、疾病等原因而采用人工方法终止妊娠，是避孕失败的补救方法。

手术流产：负压吸引术、钳刮术

1.负压吸引术

利用负压吸引原理，将妊娠物从宫腔吸出。

（1）适应证：妊娠10周内要求终止妊娠而无禁忌证，患有某种严重疾病不宜继续妊娠。

（2）禁忌证：生殖道炎症；各种疾病的急性期；全身情况不良，不能耐受手术；术前2次体温在37.5℃以上。

（3）术前准备：病史、体格检查、妇科检查；血或尿hCG测定，超声检查确诊；实验室检查包括阴道分泌物常规、血常规及凝血功能检查；术前测量体温、脉搏、血压；排空膀胱；解除思想顾虑。

（3）Anesthesia: Local anesthesia, epidural anesthesia or general anesthesia.

（4）Surgical procedures: The same as abdominal tubal ligation.

（5）Postoperative treatment: Lying down for 4 ～ 6 hours before getting out of bed and observing for changes in vital signs.

Section 3　Contraceptive failure remedies

Artificial abortion refers to termination of pregnancy by artificial methods due to unexpected pregnancy, disease and other reasons, which is a remedy for contraceptive failure.

Surgical abortion: Vacuum aspiration and forcep curettage

1.Vacuum aspiration

The principle of negative pressure suction, is utilized to suck the pregnant substance out of the uterine cavity.

（1）Indications: Termination of pregnancy is required without contraindications within 10 weeks of gestation, or not suitable to continue pregnancy with certain serious disease.

（2）Contraindications: Genital tract inflammation; acute stage of various diseases; poor general condition, unable to tolerate surgery; preoperative body temperature above 37.5 C twice.

（3）Preoperative preparation: Medical history, physical examination, pelvic examination; determination of hCG in blood or urine and diagnosis by ultrasonography; laboratory tests including routine vaginal secretions, blood routine and coagulation function tests; preoperative temperature, pulse and blood pressure measurement; emptying bladder; relieving mental concerns.

（4）手术步骤：

■ 患者取膀胱截石位。

■ 消毒外阴、阴道、铺无菌巾。

■ 双合诊检查子宫位置等。

■ 上阴道窥器、消毒阴道及宫颈管。

■ 宫颈钳夹持宫颈前唇。

■ 探针探宫腔深度、扩棒扩张宫颈。

■ 吸管连接负压吸引器（负压400～500mmHg）。

■ 顺时针吸宫腔1～2圈，感到宫壁粗糙，提示组织吸净。

■ 取出吸管，小号刮匙轻轻搔刮宫底及宫角。

■ 检查出血量，吸出组织有无绒毛。

（5）注意事项

■ 子宫大小及方位。

■ 扩宫颈管时用力均匀，以防宫颈内口撕裂。

■ 严格无菌操作。

■ 麻醉及监护。

■ 孕周≥10周应采用钳刮术。

2.人工流产术并发症及处理

（1）出血。

（2）子宫穿孔。

（3）人工流产综合反应。

（4）漏吸或空吸：施行人工流

（4）Surgical procedures:

■ Ask the patient to lie with the bladder lithotomy position.

■ Disinfect vulva, vagina and spread sterile towel.

■ Determine the position of uterus by bimanual examination.

■ Use vaginal speculum, and disinfect vagina and cervical canal.

■ Clamp the anterior lip of the cervix with cervical forceps.

■ Detect the uterine cavity depth with a probe and dilating the cervix with a rod.

■ Connect the suction pipe to the negative pressure aspirator（with negative pressure 400～500 mmHg）.

■ Suck the uterine cavity clockwise 1～2 times, and the rough uterine wall means that the tissue is sucked clean.

■ Withdraw the suction pipe and gently scrape the fundus uteri and cornua uteri with a small curette.

■ Check for blood loss and chorionic villi in the sucked tissue.

（5）Attentions

■ The size and orientation of the uterus.

■ The dilatation of the cervical canal should be taken with uniform force to prevent tearing of the cervical internal orifice.

■ Strict aseptic operation.

■ Anesthesia and monitoring.

■ Forceps curettage should be used for gestational weeks ≥ 10 weeks.

2.Complications and management of induced abortion

（1）Bleeding.

（2）Uterine perforation.

（3）Artificial abortion syndrome.

（4）Leakage or empty suction: Artificial abor-

产术未吸出胚胎或绒毛而导致继续妊娠或胚胎停止发育，称为漏吸。误诊为宫内妊娠行人工流产术，称为空吸。

（5）吸宫不全。

（6）感染。

（7）羊水栓塞。

（8）远期并发症：宫颈粘连、宫腔粘连、慢性盆腔炎、月经失调、继发性不孕等。

药物流产

（1）主要配伍药物

- 米非司酮：是一种类固醇类的抗孕激素制剂，具有抗孕激素及抗糖皮质激素的作用。
- 米索前列醇：是前列腺素类似物，具有子宫兴奋和宫颈软化作用。

（2）适应证

- 妊娠≤49日，本人自愿、年龄＜40岁的健康女性。
- 血或尿hCG阳性，超声检查确诊为宫内妊娠。
- 人工流产高危因素者，如瘢痕子宫、哺乳期、宫颈发育不良或严重骨盆畸形。
- 有多次人工流产史，对手术流产有恐惧和顾虑心理者。

（3）禁忌证

- 有使用米非司酮禁忌证，如肾上腺及其他内分泌疾病、妊娠期皮肤瘙痒史、血液病、血管栓塞等病史。
- 有使用前列腺素药物禁忌证，如心血管疾病、青光眼、哮喘、癫痫、结肠炎等。

tion does not suck out the embryo or villi leading to continued pregnancy or embryo development stop, which is called leakage. Artificial abortion is made for misdiagnosed intrauterine pregnancy which is called empty suction.

（5）Incomplete aspiration of uterus.

（6）Infection.

（7）Amniotic fluid embolism.

（8）Long-term complications: Cervical adhesions, intrauterine adhesions, chronic pelvic inflammation, menstrual disorders, secondary infertility, etc.

Medical abortion

（1）Main compatibility of drugs

- Mifepristone: A steroid antiprogesterone preparation which has the effects of anti-progesterone and anti-glucocorticoid.
- Misoprostol: A prostaglandin analogue with uterine excitation and cervical softening effects.

（2）Indications

- Pregnancy≤49 days, voluntary healthy women＜40 years old.
- Blood or urine hCG positive, ultrasound diagnosis of intrauterine pregnancy.
- High-risk factors of induced abortion, such as scarred uterus, lactation, cervical dysplasia or severe pelvic malformation.
- Multiple history of induced abortion, fear and worry about surgical abortion.

（3）Contraindications

- Contraindications for mifepristone, such as adrenal and other endocrine diseases, history of skin itching during pregnancy, blood diseases, and vascular embolism, etc.
- Contraindications for prostaglandins, such as cardiovascular diseases, glaucoma, asthma, epilepsy, colitis, etc.

■ 带器妊娠、宫外孕。

■ 其他：过敏体质，妊娠剧吐，长期服用抗结核、抗癫痫、抗抑郁、抗前列腺素药等。

（4）用药方法

■ 米非司酮：分顿服法和分服法。

第四节　避孕节育 措施的选择

（1）新婚期：选用复方短效口服避孕药、阴茎套。

（2）哺乳期：选用阴茎套，宫内节育器。

（3）生育后期：宫内节育器、皮下埋植剂、复方短效口服避孕药，阴茎套等均适用。

（4）绝经过渡期：选用阴茎套。

重点专业词汇

1.计划生育

2.避孕

3.宫内节育器（IUD）

4.激素避孕

5.口服避孕药

6.闭经

7.紧急避孕

8.输卵管绝育术

9.人工流产

10.负压吸引术

11.钳刮术

12.子宫穿孔

13.人工流产综合反应

14.漏吸或空吸

15.羊水栓塞

16.米非司酮

17.米索前列醇

■ Pregnancy with IUD, and ectopic pregnancy.

■ Others: Allergic constitution, hyperemesis gravidarum, long-term use of anti-tuberculosis, anti-epilepsy, anti-depression, anti-prostaglandin drugs, etc.

（4）Medication method

■ Mifepristone: One dose, one dose at a time.

Section 4　Choice of contraceptive measures

（1）Newlywed period: Combined oral contraceptives（COC）and condoms.

（2）Lactation period: Condoms and intrauterine devices（IUD）.

（3）Post-reproductive period: Intrauterine devices, subdermal implants, combined oral contraceptives and condoms.

（4）Menopausal transition period: Condoms.

Key words

1.Family planning

2.Contraception

3.Intrauterine device（IUD）

4.Hormonal contraception

5.Oral contraceptive

6.Amenorrhea

7.Emergency contraception

8.Tubal sterilization operation

9.Artificial abortion（induced abortion）

10.Vacuum aspiration

11.Forceps curettage

12.Uterine perforation

13.Artificial abortion syndrome

14.Leakage or empty suction

15.Amniotic fluid embolism

16.Mifepristone

17.Misoprostol

练习题

1.IUD取出的时间一般选择在：（D）

A.月经来潮6小时内

B.月经期第2～4日

C.月经前4～6日

D.月经干净3～7日

E.月经期第5～6日

2.IUD的避孕原理主要是：（A）

A.干扰受精卵着床

B.抑制卵巢排卵

C.影响精子获能

D.阻止精子和卵子相遇

E.改变宫颈黏液性状

3.短效口服避孕药含：（E）

A.雌激素

B.孕激素

C.雄激素＋雌激素

D.孕激素＋雄激素

E.孕激素＋雌激素

4.口服避孕药的副作用不包括：（C）

A.短期闭经

B.体重增加

C.卵巢肿瘤

D.类早孕反应

E.色素沉着

5.属于人工流产负压吸引术禁忌证的是：（E）

A.哺乳期

B.慢性宫颈炎

C.剖宫产术后1年

D.妊娠9周

E.间隔4小时再次体温超过37.5℃

6.剖宫产术后3个月哺乳期女性，最恰当的避孕方法应选择：（E）

Exercises

1.The time for IUD removal is usually selected at:（D）

A.Within 6 hours of menstrual onset

B.2～4 days of menstrual period

C.4～6 days before menstruation

D.3～7 days after menstruation clean

E.5～6 days of menstrual period

2.The main contraceptive principle of IUD is:（A）

A.Interfering with fertilized egg implantation

B.Inhibiting ovulation

C.Affecting sperm capacitation

D.Preventing sperm and eggs from meeting each other

E.Changing cervical mucus properties

3.Short-acting oral contraceptives contain:（E）

A.Estrogen

B.Progesterone

C.Androgen ＋ estrogen

D.Progesterone ＋ androgen

E.Progesterone ＋ estrogen

4.The side effects of oral contraceptives do not include:（C）

A.Short-term amenorrhea

B.Weight gaining

C.Ovarian tumor

D.Similar to morning sickness

E.Pigmentation

5.The contraindication of negative pressure suction for induced abortion is:（E）

A.Lactation period

B.Chronic cervicitis

C.1 year after cesarean section

D.9 weeks of gestation

E.Body temperature is above 37.5 ℃ again at intervals of 4 hours.

6.The most appropriate method of contraception for lactating women 3 months after

A.短效口服避孕药

B.安全期避孕法

C.IUD

D.皮下埋植法

E.阴茎套

（马晓秋）

cesarean section should be:（E）

A.Short-acting oral contraceptives

B.Safe period contraception

C.IUD

D.Subcutaneous implantation

E.Condom